Resource Manual for

Nursing Research

GENERATING AND ASSESSING EVIDENCE FOR NURSING PRACTICE

NINTH EDITION

Denise F. Polit, PhD, FAAN
President
Humanalysis, Inc.
Saratoga Springs, New York, *and*
Professor
Griffith University School of Nursing
Gold Coast, Australia
(www.denisepolit.com)

Cheryl Tatano Beck, DNSc, CNM, FAAN
Distinguished Professor
School of Nursing
University of Connecticut
Storrs, Connecticut

 Wolters Kluwer | Lippincott Williams & Wilkins
Health
Philadelphia · Baltimore · New York · London
Buenos Aires · Hong Kong · Sydney · Tokyo

Acquisitions Editor: Hilarie Surrena
Product Manager: Mary Kinsella
Editorial Assistant: Amanda Jordan
Design Coordinator: Joan Wendt
Manufacturing Coordinator: Karin Duffield
Prepress Vendor: Aptara, Inc.

Ninth edition

ISBN-13: 978-1-60547-782-4

9 8 7 6

Printed in the United States

Care has been taken to confirm the accuracy of the information presented and to describe generally accepted practices. However, the author(s), editors, and publisher are not responsible for errors or omissions or for any consequences from application of the information in this book and make no warranty, expressed or implied, with respect to the currency, completeness, or accuracy of the contents of the publication. Application of this information in a particular situation remains the professional responsibility of the practitioner; the clinical treatments described and recommended may not be considered absolute and universal recommendations.

The author(s), editors, and publisher have exerted every effort to ensure that drug selection and dosage set forth in this text are in accordance with the current recommendations and practice at the time of publication. However, in view of ongoing research, changes in government regulations, and the constant flow of information relating to drug therapy and drug reactions, the reader is urged to check the package insert for each drug for any change in indications and dosage and for added warnings and precautions. This is particularly important when the recommended agent is a new or infrequently employed drug.

Some drugs and medical devices presented in this publication have Food and Drug Administration (FDA) clearance for limited use in restricted research settings. It is the responsibility of the health care provider to ascertain the FDA status of each drug or device planned for use in his or her clinical practice.

DRC0915

Preface

This *Resource Manual* for the 9th edition of *Nursing Research: Generating and Assessing Evidence for Nursing Practice* complements and strengthens the textbook in important ways. The manual provides opportunities to reinforce the acquisition of basic research skills through systematic learning exercises, and we have placed particular emphasis on exercises that involve careful reading and critiquing of actual studies. Critiquing skills are increasingly important in an environment that promotes evidence-based nursing practice. Moreover, the ability to think critically about research decisions is fundamental to being able to design and plan one's own study.

Full research reports and a grant application are included in 13 appendices to this *Resource Manual*. These reports, which represent a rich array of research endeavors, form the basis for exercises in each chapter. There are reports of quantitative and qualitative studies, an evidence-based practice project report, an instrument development paper, a meta-analysis, and a metasynthesis. We are particularly excited about being able to include a full grant application that was funded by the National Institute of Nursing Research, together with the Study Section's summary sheet. We firmly believe that nothing is more illuminating than a good model when it comes to research communication.

A relatively new feature of this *Resource Manual*—added in the 8th edition—is the Toolkit, which offers important research resources to beginning and advanced researchers. Our mission was to include easily adaptable tools for a broad range of research situations. In our own careers as researchers, we have found that adapting existing forms, manuals, or protocols is far more efficient and productive than "starting from scratch." By making these tools available as Word files, we have made it possible for you to adapt tools to meet your specific needs, without the tedium of having to re-type basic information. We wish we had had this Toolkit in our early years as researchers! We think seasoned researchers are likely to find parts of the Toolkit useful as well.

The *Resource Manual* consists of 29 chapters—one chapter corresponding to every chapter in the textbook. Each chapter has relevant resources and exercises and answers to exercises for which there are objective answers are included at the back of the book in Appendix N. Each of the 29 chapters consists of four components:

- *A Crossword Puzzle*. Terms and concepts presented in the textbook are reinforced in an entertaining and challenging fashion through crossword puzzles.
- *Study Questions*. Each chapter contains several short individual exercises relevant to the materials in the textbook.
- *Application Exercises*. These exercises are geared to helping you to read, comprehend, and critique nursing studies. These exercises focus on studies in the appendices and ask questions that are relevant to the content covered in the textbook. There are two

sets of questions—*Questions of Fact* and *Questions for Discussion*. The Questions of Fact will help you to read the report and find specific types of information related to the content covered in the textbook. For these questions, there are "right" and "wrong" answers. For example, for the chapter on sampling, a question might ask: How many people participated in this study? The Questions for Discussion, by contrast, require an assessment of the merits of various features of the study. For example, a question might ask: Was there a *sufficient number* of study participants in this study? The second set of questions can be the basis for classroom discussions.

• *Toolkit* ✪. This section, on the accompanying CD-ROM, includes tools and resources that can save you time—and that will hopefully result in higher-quality tools than might otherwise have been the case. Each chapter has tools appropriate for the content covered in the textbook.

   We hope that you will find these resources rewarding, enjoyable, and useful in your effort to develop and hone skills needed in critiquing and doing research.

Contents

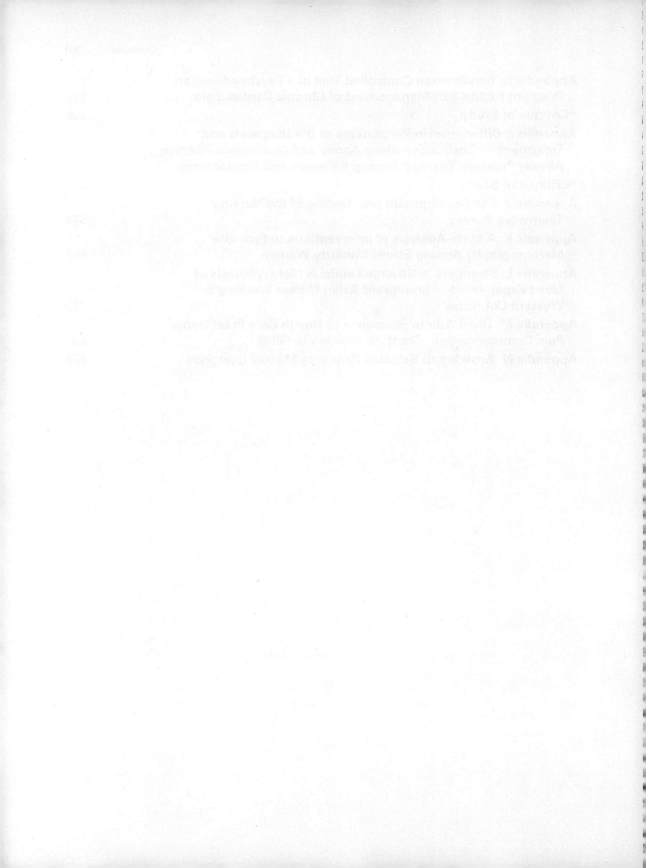

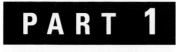

PART 1

Foundations of
Nursing Research

CHAPTER 1

Introduction to Nursing Research in an Evidence-Based Practice Environment

■ A. Crossword Puzzle

Complete the crossword puzzle below, which uses terms and concepts presented in Chapter 1. (Puzzles may be removed for easier viewing.)

Note that there is a crossword puzzle in many chapters of this *Resource Manual.* We hope they will be a "fun" way for you to review key terms used in each chapter. However, we are not professional puzzle designers and so there are some oddities about the puzzles. These oddities are not intended to be trick questions, but rather represent liberties we took in trying to get as many terms as possible into the puzzle. So, for example, there are a lot of acronyms (e.g., evidence-based practice = EBP) and abbreviations (e.g., evidence = evid), and even a few words that are written backwards (e.g., evidence = ecnedive). Two-word answers sometimes appear with a space (e.g., evidence-based) and sometimes they are just run together (e.g., evidencebased). The crossword puzzle answers are at the back of this *Resource Manual,* in case our intent is too obscure!

ACROSS

1. Nurses are increasingly encouraged to develop a practice that is _____ (hyphenated).
3. The clinical learning strategy developed at the McMaster School of Medicine (acronym)
4. A world view, a way of looking at natural phenomena
7. The world view that holds that there are multiple interpretations of reality, an alternative name for constructivist (abbr.)
10. The world view that assumes that there is an orderly reality that can be studied objectively
12. The precursor to the National Institute of Nursing Research (acronym)
13. Successively trying alternative solutions is known as _____ and error.
14. Research designed to solve a pressing practical problem is _____ research (abbr.).
16. Nurses get together in practice settings to critique studies in the context of journal _____.
17. Research designed to guide nursing practice is referred to as _____ nursing research (abbr.).
19. The U.S. agency that promotes and sponsors nursing research (acronym)
22. A source of knowledge or information reflecting ingrained customs
23. The _____ of nursing research began with Florence Nightingale.
24. The degree to which research findings can be applied to people who did not participate in a study (abbr.)
25. The type of reasoning that involves developing specific predictions from general principles (abbr.)

DOWN

1. Evidence that is rooted in objective reality and gathered through the senses
2. The assumption that phenomena are not random, but rather have antecedent causes
5. The repeating of a study to determine if findings can be upheld with a new group of people

6. A purpose of doing research, involving a portrayal of phenomena as they exist
8. A scheme for ordering the utility of evidence for practice is an evidence _____.
9. A purpose of doing research, often linked to theory
11. The techniques used by researchers to structure a study are called research _____ (abbr.).
15. The type of research that analyzes narrative, subjective materials is _____ research (abbr.).
18. The use of findings from research in a practice setting is called research _____ (abbr.).
20. Naturalistic inquiry typically takes place in the _____.
21. The U.S. agency charged with supporting research designed to improve the quality of healthcare and reduce health costs (acronym)

■ B. Study Questions

1. Why is it important for nurses who will never conduct their own research to understand research methods?

2. What are some potential consequences to the nursing profession if nurses stopped conducting their own research?

3. What are some of the current changes occurring in the healthcare delivery system, and how could these changes influence nursing research and the use of research findings?

4. Below are descriptions of several research problems. Indicate whether you think the problem is best suited to a qualitative or quantitative approach, and explain your rationale.
   a. What is the decision-making process of patients with prostate cancer weighing treatment options?
   b. What effect does room temperature have on the colonization rate of bacteria in urinary catheters?
   c. What are sources of stress among nursing home residents?
   d. Does therapeutic touch affect the vital signs of hospitalized patients?
   e. What is the meaning of *hope* among Stage IV cancer patients?
   f. What are the effects of prenatal instruction on the labor and delivery outcomes of pregnant women?
   g. What are the healthcare needs of the homeless, and what barriers do they face in having those needs met?

5. What are some of the limitations of quantitative research? What are some of the limitations of qualitative research? Which approach seems best suited to address problems in which you might be interested? Why is that?

6. Scan through the titles in the table of contents of a recent issue of a nursing research journal (e.g., *Nursing Research, Research in Nursing & Health, Journal of Advanced Nursing)*. Find the title of a study that you think is basic research and another that you think is applied research. Read the abstracts for these studies to see if you can determine whether your original supposition was correct.

7. Apply the questions from Box 1.1 of the textbook (available as a Word document in the Toolkit ✪ on the accompanying CD-ROM) to one or both of the following studies:

   • Dulko, D., & Mooney, K. (2010). Effect of an audit and feedback intervention on hospitalized oncology patients' perception of nurse practitioner care. *Journal of Nursing Care Quality, 25,* 22–30.
   • Kelly, J., D'Cruz, G., & Wright, D. (2010). Patients with dysphagia: Experiences of taking medications. *Journal of Advanced Nursing, 66,* 82–91.

8. Consider the nursing research priorities identified by the National Institute of Nursing Research or Sigma Theta Tau International, as identified in the book or on the websites of those organizations. Which priority resonates with *you*? Why?

■ C. Application Exercises

EXERCISE 1: STUDY IN APPENDIX A

Read the abstract and introduction to the report by Kennedy and Chen ("Changes in childhood risk taking") in Appendix A. Then answer the following questions:

Questions of Fact*

a. Is this report an example of "disciplined research"?
b. Is this a qualitative or quantitative study?
c. What is the underlying paradigm of the study?
d. Does the study involve the collection of empirical evidence?
e. Is the purpose of this study identification, description, exploration, explanation, and/or prediction and control?
f. Is this study applied or basic research?
g. Does this study address an EBP-focused question, such as a question about treatment, diagnosis, prognosis, harm and etiology, or meaning and process?

Questions for Discussion

a. How relevant is this study to the actual practice of nursing?
b. Could this study have been conducted as *either* a quantitative or qualitative study? Why or why not?

---

*Refer to Appendix N for answers and comments to the "Questions of Fact" in each chapter.

EXERCISE 2: STUDY IN APPENDIX B

Read the abstract and introduction to the report by Cricco-Lizza ("Rooting for the breast") in Appendix B. Then answer the following questions:

Questions of Fact

a. Is this report an example of "disciplined research"?
b. Is this a qualitative or quantitative study?
c. What is the underlying paradigm of the research?
d. Does the study involve the collection of empirical evidence?
e. Is the purpose of this study identification, description, exploration, explanation, and/or prediction and control?
f. Is this study applied or basic research?
g. Does this study address an EBP-focused question, such as a question about treatment, diagnosis, prognosis, harm and etiology, or meaning and process?

Questions for Discussion

a. How relevant is this study to the actual practice of nursing?
b. Could this study have been conducted as *either* a quantitative or qualitative study? Why or why not?
c. Which of the two studies cited in these exercises (the one in Appendix A or Appendix B) is of greater interest and/or relevance to you personally? Why?

■ D. The Toolkit

For Chapter 1, the Toolkit on the accompanying CD-ROM contains the following:

- Questions for a Preliminary Review of a Research Report (Box 1.1 of the textbook)
- Useful Websites for Chapter 1: Resources for an Introduction to Nursing Research

CHAPTER 2

Evidence-Based Nursing: Translating Research Evidence into Practice

■ A. Crossword Puzzle

Complete the crossword puzzle below, which uses terms and concepts presented in Chapter 2. (Puzzles may be removed for easier viewing.)

ACROSS

5. A clinical practice _____ based on rigorous systematic evidence is an important tool for evidence-based care.
8. An important database for finding clinical guidelines (UK-based) is the _____ database.
10. Environmental readiness for an innovation often involves assessments of implementation _____ in a given setting.
11. _____ reviews of RCTs are at the pinnacle of most evidence hierarchies.
14. The Cochrane Collaboration is a cornerstone of the EBP _ _ vement.
16. _ _ _ _ ground questions are ones that can be answered based on current best research evidence.
19. Are case reports of individual patients at the top of the evidence hierarchy?
21. Evidence-based decision making should integrate best research evidence with clinical _____.
24. Researchers can compute indices called _____ as estimates of the absolute magnitude of an effect (acronym).
25. _____ questions are foundational questions for a clinical problem, answers to which may be found, for example, in textbooks (abbr.).
27. In assessing whether an innovation is appropriate in a given setting, a _____ ratio should be estimated.
29. An index called _____ concerns the relative magnitude of an effect.
30. There is abundant evidence that nurses face several _____ to using research in their practice.

DOWN

1. A widely used tool for evaluating clinical guidelines is called the _____ instrument.
2. An important model for research utilization is called _____ of Innovations Theory.
3. Evidence-based practice involves the conscientious use of current _____ (evaluative) evidence.
4. The journal *Evidence-Based Nursing* presents _____ summaries of studies and systematic reviews from more than 150 journals.
6. Acronym describing main focus of the chapter
7. RU/EBP models are intended to serve as a guide for the _ _ _ _ _ _ entation of an innovation.
9. Research utilization is narrower in meaning than evidence-based _____.
12. Two of the most prominent _____ of EBP are Iowa and Stetler.
13. In a systematic review, evidence from multiple studies on the same _____ is integrated.
15. One trigger in the Iowa model, which involves an origin in the research literature, is called _____-focused.
17. The originator of a prominent theory on how new ideas are diffused and adopted
18. An arrangement of the worth of various types of evidence

20. The earliest model of research utilization in nursing was developed by _____.
22. Acronym for the five-component scheme for asking EBP questions
23. One trigger in the Iowa model, stemming from practice issues, is called _____-focused (abbr.).
26. A statistical method of combining evidence in a systematic review is _____-analysis.
28. The type of study at the second level of an evidence hierarchy focusing on intervention questions (acronym and backwards)

■ B. Study Questions

1. Identify the factors in your own practice setting that you think facilitate or inhibit research utilization and evidence-based practice (or, in an educational setting, the factors that promote or inhibit a climate in which EBP is valued). For any barriers, what steps might be taken to address those barriers?

2. Think about a nursing procedure that you have learned. What is the basis for this procedure? Determine whether the procedure is based on scientific evidence indicating that the procedure is effective. If it is not based on scientific evidence, on what is it based, and why do you think scientific evidence was not used?

3. Read one of the following articles and identify the steps of the Iowa Model (or an alternative model of EBP) that are represented in the RU/EBP projects described.
   a. Clarke, H. F., Bradley, C., Whytock, S., Handfield, S., van der Wal, R., & Gundry, S. (2005). Pressure ulcers: Implementation of evidence-based nursing practice. *Journal of Advanced Nursing, 49(6)*, 578–590.
   b. Doran, D., Mylopoulos, J., Kushniruk, A., Nagle, L., Laurie-Shaw, Sidani, S., Tourangeau, A. E., Lefebre, N., Reid-Haughian, C., Carryer, J. R., Cranley, L. A., & McArthur, G. (2007). Evidence in the palm of your hand: Development of an outcomes-focused knowledge translation intervention. *Worldviews of Evidence-Based Nursing, 4*, 69–77.
   c. Capasso, V., Collins, J., Griffith, C., Lasala, C., Kilroy, S., Martin, A., Pedro, J., & Wood, S. L. (2009). Outcomes of a clinical nurse specialist-initiated wound care education program: Using the promoting action on research implementation in health services framework. *Clinical Nurse Specialist, 23*, 252–257.
   d. Long, L., Burkett, K., & McGee, S. (2009). Promotion of safe outcomes: Incorporating evidence into policies and procedures. *Nursing Clinics of North America, 44*, 57–70.

4. Select a clinical study from the nursing research literature. Using the criteria indicated in the Worksheet for Evaluating Implementation Potential in the Toolkit ✖ in the accompanying CD-ROM, assess the potential for using the study results in your practice setting. If the study meets the three major classes of criteria for implementation potential, develop a utilization plan.

10 PART 1 ■ **Foundations of Nursing Research**

5. Compare the Iowa Model, as described in the textbook to an alternative model of evidence-based practice, as identified in Box 2.1. What are the main areas of similarity and difference in the models? Which model would work best in your setting?

■ C. Application Exercises

EXERCISE 1: STUDY IN APPENDIX C

Read the abstract and introduction to the report by Yackel and colleagues ("Nurse-Facilitated Depression Screening Program") in Appendix C. Then answer the following questions:

Questions of Fact

a. What was the purpose of this EBP project?
b. What was the setting for implementing this project?
c. Which EBP model was used as a framework for this project?
d. Did the project have a problem-focused or knowledge-focused trigger?
e. Who were the team members in this study, and what were their affiliations?
f. What, if anything, did the report say about the implementation potential of this project?
g. Was a pilot study undertaken?
h. Did this project involve an evaluation of the project's success?

Questions for Discussion

a. What might be a clinical foreground question that was used in seeking relevant evidence in preparing for this project? Identify components of the question (e.g., population, intervention, etc.).
b. What are some of the praiseworthy aspects of this project? What could the team members have done differently to improve the project?

EXERCISE 2: STUDY IN APPENDIX K

Read the abstract and introduction (from the beginning to the "Methods" section) of the report by Han and colleagues ("Interventions to Promote Mammography") in Appendix K. Then answer the following questions:

Questions of Fact

a. Does this report summarize a systematic review? If yes, what type of systematic review was it? Is this an example of preappraised evidence?
b. Where on the evidence hierarchy shown in Figure 2.1 of the textbook would this study belong?
c. What is the stated purpose of this study?

Copyright © 2012 Wolters Kluwer Health I Lippincott Williams & Wilkins. Polit & Beck: *Resource Manual for Nursing Research: Generating and Assessing Evidence for Nursing Practice* (9th ed.)

Questions for Discussion

a. What might be the clinical foreground question that guided this study? Identify components of the question (e.g., population, intervention, etc.).
b. What are some of the steps you would need to undertake if you were interested in using this study as a basis for an EBP project in your own practice setting?

■ D. The Toolkit

For Chapter 2, the Toolkit on the accompanying CD-ROM contains the following:

- Question Templates for Selected Clinical Foreground Questions (based on Table 2.1 of the textbook)
- Questions for Appraising the Evidence (Box 2.2 of the textbook)
- Worksheet: Questions for Evaluating the Implementation Potential of an Innovation under Scrutiny*
- Useful Websites for Chapter 2: Resources for Evidence-Based Practice

---

*This item does not appear in the textbook.

CHAPTER 3

Key Concepts and Steps in Qualitative and Quantitative Research

■ A. Crossword Puzzle

Complete the crossword puzzle below, which uses terms and concepts presented in Chapter 3. (Puzzles may be removed for easier viewing.)

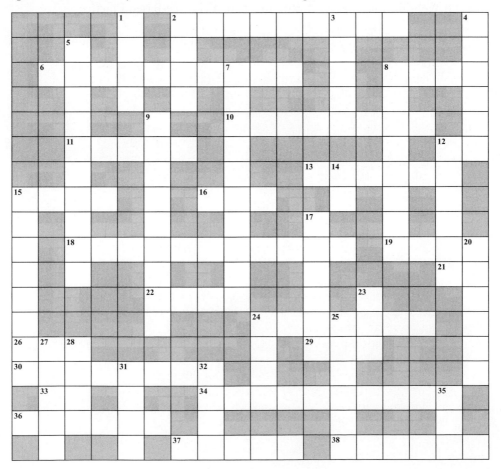

ACROSS

2. Another name for outcome variable is _____ variable.
6. An individual with whom a researcher must negotiate to gain entrée into a site
8. Two operationalizations of weight involve the pound system and the _____ system.
10. A step in experimental research involves the development of an intervention _____.
11. In "What is the effect of radon on health?" the independent variable is _____.
12. Acronym for a being from another planet (and name of a famous movie)
13. If the probability of a statistical test were .001, the results would be highly statistically _____ (abbr.).
15. Pieces of information gathered in a study
16. Data that are in the exact same form as when they were collected are _____ data.
18. The _____ definition indicates how a variable will be measured or observed.
19. A variable that has only two values or categories (abbr.)
21. A systematic, abstract explanation of phenomena (first and last letters)
22. A type of fieldwork done to enhance the value of a study for practicing nurses (abbr.)
24. The type of tests used by quantitative researchers to assess the reliability of their results (abbr.)
26. One _____ offered in the textbook was to always select a research problem in which there is a strong personal interest.
29. Some qualitative researchers do not undertake an upfront _____ review, so as to avoid having their conceptualization influenced by the work of others (abbr.).
30. The type of design used in qualitative studies
33. A bond or connection between phenomena (first two letters)
34. The type of research that tests an intervention
36. Terminology that often makes research reports difficult to read
37. A research investigation
38. The procedure of translating data into numerical values (backwards!)

DOWN

1. The qualitative research tradition that focuses on lived experiences (abbr.)
2. The independent variable in: "What is the effect of diet on cancer?"
3. The qualitative tradition that focuses on the study of cultures (abbr.)
4. In a qualitative analysis, researchers often search for these (backwards).
5. A principle used to decide when to stop sampling in a qualitative study
7. The entire aggregate of units in which a researcher is interested
8. A qualitative tradition that focuses on social psychological processes within a social setting is _____ theory.
9. A somewhat more complex abstraction than a concept
12. If the independent variable is the cause, the dependent variable is the _____.
14. The variable that is the cause of another variable (acronym)
15. A variable with a finite number of values between two points
17. A relationship in which one variable directly results in changes in another is a _____ relationship.

20. Quantitative researchers formulate _____, which state expectations about how variables are related (abbr.).
23. Quantitative researchers develop a knowledge context by doing a _____ review early in the project (abbr.).
24. The first _____ in a project involves formulating a research problem.
25. In terms of _____, the independent variable occurs before the dependent variable.
27. The type of format used to structure most research reports (acronym)
28. The type of reviewers who typically make recommendations about reports published in journals
31. A _____ sample is one that is representative of the population.
32. Quantitative researchers use a statistical _____ to analyze their data and test their hypotheses.
35. A relationship expresses a bond between at least _____ variables.

▪ B. Study Questions

1. Suggest operational definitions for the following concepts.
   a. Stress:
   b. Prematurity of infants:
   c. Fatigue:
   d. Pain:
   e. Obesity:
   f. Prolonged labor:
   g. Smoking behavior:

2. In each of the following research questions, identify the independent and dependent variables.
   a. Does assertiveness training improve the effectiveness of psychiatric nurses?
      Independent: _____
      Dependent: _____

   b. Does the postural positioning of patients affect their respiratory function?
      Independent: _____
      Dependent: _____

   c. Is patients' anxiety affected by the amount of touch received from nursing staff?
      Independent: _____
      Dependent: _____

   d. Is the incidence of decubitus ulcers reduced by more frequent turnings of patients?
      Independent: _____
      Dependent: _____

e. Are people who were abused as children more likely than others to abuse their own children?
Independent: _____
Dependent: _____

f. Is tolerance for pain related to a patient's age and gender?
Independent: _____
Dependent: _____

g. Are the number of prenatal visits of pregnant women associated with labor and delivery outcomes?
Independent: _____
Dependent: _____

h. Are levels of depression higher among children with a chronic illness than among other children?
Independent: _____
Dependent: _____

i. Is compliance with a medical regimen higher among women than among men?
Independent: _____
Dependent: _____

j. Does participating in a support group enhance coping among family caregivers of AIDS patients?
Independent: _____
Dependent: _____

k. Is hearing acuity of the elderly different at different times of day?
Independent: _____
Dependent: _____

l. Does home birth affect the parents' satisfaction with the childbirth experience?
Independent: _____
Dependent: _____

m. Does a neutropenic diet in the outpatient setting decrease the positive blood cultures associated with chemotherapy-induced neutropenia?
Independent: _____
Dependent: _____

3. Below is a list of variables. For each, think of a research question for which the variable would be the independent variable, and a second for which it would be the dependent variable. For example, take the variable "birth weight of infants." We might ask, "Does the age of the mother affect the birth weight of her infant?" (dependent variable). Alternatively, our research question might be, "Does the birth weight of infants (independent variable) affect their sensorimotor development at 6 months of age?" HINT: For the dependent variable problem, ask yourself, what

factors might affect, influence, or cause this variable? For the independent variable, ask yourself, what factors does *this* variable influence, cause, or affect?

a. Body temperature
   Independent: _____
   Dependent: _____

b. Amount of sleep
   Independent: _____
   Dependent: _____

c. Frequency of practicing breast self-examination
   Independent: _____
   Dependent: _____

d. Level of hopefulness in cancer patients
   Independent: _____
   Dependent: _____

e. Stress among victims of domestic violence
   Independent: _____
   Dependent: _____

4. Look at the table of contents of a recent issue of *Nursing Research* or *Research in Nursing & Health* (or another research-focused journal). Pick out a study title (not looking at the abstract) that implies that a relationship between variables was scrutinized. Indicate what you think the independent and dependent variable might be, and what the title suggests about the nature of the relationship (i.e., causal or not).

5. Describe what is wrong with the following statements:
   a. Opitz's experimental study was conducted within the ethnographic tradition.
   b. Brusser's experimental study examined the effect of relaxation therapy (the dependent variable) on pain (the independent variable) in cancer patients.
   c. In her grounded theory study of the caregiving process for caregivers of patients with dementia, Gabris explored the lived experience of caregiving.
   d. In Lace's phenomenological study of the meaning of futility among AIDS patients, subjects received an intervention designed to sustain hope.
   e. In her experimental study, Giblin developed her data collection plan after she introduced her intervention to a group of patients.

6. Read the following report of a qualitative study and identify segments of *raw data*:
   • Adams, J., & Neville, S. (2009). Men who have sex with men account for nonuse of condoms. *Qualitative Health Research, 19,* 1669–1677.

   Describe the effect that removal of the raw data would have on the report.

7. Apply the questions from Box 3.3 of the textbook (available as a Word document in the Toolkit ✪ on the accompanying CD-ROM) to one or both of the following studies:

   a. Fitzgerald, L., Kehoe, P., & Sinha, K. (2009). Hypothalamic-pituitary-adrenal axis dysregulation in women with irritable bowel syndrome in response to acute physical stress. *Western Journal of Nursing Research, 31,* 818–836.

   b. Rice, E. (2009). Schizophrenia and violence: Accepting and forsaking. *Qualitative Health Research, 19,* 840–849.

■ C. Application Exercises

EXERCISE 1: STUDY IN APPENDIX D

Read the abstract and introduction (the material before the method section) to the report by Whittemore and colleagues ("Diabetes Prevention Program") in Appendix D. Then answer the following questions:

Questions of Fact

a. Who were the lead researchers, and what are their credentials and affiliations?
b. Altogether, how many people were on the research team? (This information appears at the end of the article).
c. Did the researcher receive funding that supported this research? (See the end of the paper.)
d. Who were the study participants?
e. What is the independent variable (or variables) in this study? Is this variable *inherently* an independent variable?
f. What is the dependent variable (or variables) in this study? Is this variable *inherently* a dependent variable?
g. Did the introduction actually use the terms "independent variable" or "dependent variable"?
h. Were the data in this study quantitative or qualitative?
i. Were any relationships under investigation? What type of relationship?
j. Is this an experimental or nonexperimental study?
k. Was there any intervention? If so, what is it?
l. Did the study involve statistical analysis of data? Did it involve the qualitative analysis of data?
m. Does the report follow the IMRAD format?

Questions for Discussion

a. How relevant is this study to the actual practice of nursing?
b. Could this study have been conducted as *either* a quantitative or qualitative study? Why or why not?
c. How good a job did the researchers do in summarizing their study in the abstract?
d. How long do you estimate it took for this study to be completed?

EXERCISE 2: STUDY IN APPENDIX E

Read the abstract and introduction to the report by Beck ("The Arm") in Appendix E. Then answer the following questions:

Questions of Fact

a. Who was the researcher and what are her credentials and affiliation?
b. Did the researcher receive funding that supported this research?
c. Who were the study participants?
d. What were the key concepts in this study?
e. Were the data in this study quantitative or qualitative?
f. Were any relationships under investigation?
g. Could the study be described as an ethnographic, phenomenological, or grounded theory study?
h. Is this an experimental or nonexperimental study?
i. Does the report describe an intervention? If so, what is it?
j. Did the report provide information about how key study variables were measured?
k. Did the study involve statistical analysis of data? Did the study involve qualitative analysis of data?
l. Does the report follow the IMRAD format?

Questions for Discussion

a. How relevant is this study to the actual practice of nursing?
b. Could this study have been conducted as *either* a quantitative or qualitative study? Why or why not?
c. How good a job did the researcher do in summarizing her study in the abstract?
d. How long do you estimate it took for this study to be completed?
e. Which of the two studies cited in these exercises (the one in Appendix E or Appendix D) is of greater interest and/or relevance to you personally? Why?

EXERCISE 3: TRANSLATION EXERCISE

Below is an example of summary of a fictitious study, written in the style typically found in research journal articles. Terms that can be looked up in the glossary of the textbook are underlined. Then, a "translation" of this summary is presented, recasting the research information into language that is more digestible. Study this example and then use it as a model for "translating" the abstracts of one of the studies in the appendices of this book.

> **Summary of Fictitious Study.** The potentially negative sequelae of having an abortion on the psychological adjustment of adolescents have not been adequately studied. The present study sought to determine whether alternative pregnancy resolution decisions have different long-term effects on the psychological functioning of young women.

Three groups of low-income pregnant teenagers attending an inner-city clinic were the <u>subjects</u> in this study: those who delivered and kept the baby, those who delivered and relinquished the baby for adoption, and those who had an abortion. There were 25 subjects in each group. The study <u>instruments</u> included a self-administered <u>questionnaire</u> and a battery of psychological tests measuring depression, anxiety, and psychosomatic symptoms. The instruments were administered upon entry into the study (when the subjects first came to the clinic) and then 1 year after termination of the pregnancy.

The <u>data</u> were analyzed using <u>analysis of variance (ANOVA)</u>. The ANOVA tests indicated that the three groups did not differ significantly in terms of depression, anxiety, or psychosomatic symptoms at the initial testing. At the <u>posttest</u>, however, the abortion group had significantly higher scores on the depression scale, and these girls were significantly more likely than the two delivery groups to report severe tension headaches. There were no <u>significant</u> differences on any of the <u>dependent variables</u> for the two delivery groups.

The results of this study suggest that young women who elect to have an abortion may experience a number of long-term negative consequences. It would appear that appropriate efforts should be made to follow-up abortion patients to determine their need for suitable treatment.

Translated Version. As researchers, we wondered whether young women who had an abortion had any emotional problems in the long run. It seemed to us that not enough research had been done to know whether any psychological harm resulted from an abortion.

We decided to study this question ourselves by comparing the experiences of three types of teenagers who became pregnant—first, girls who delivered and kept their babies; second, those who delivered the babies but gave them up for adoption; and third, those who elected to have an abortion. All teenagers in the sample were poor, and all were patients at an inner-city clinic. Altogether, we studied 75 girls—25 in each of the three groups. We evaluated the teenagers' emotional states by asking them to fill out a questionnaire and to take several psychological tests. These tests allowed us to assess things such as the girls' degree of depression and anxiety and whether they had any complaints of a psychosomatic nature. We asked them to fill out the forms twice: once when they came into the clinic, and then again a year after the abortion or the delivery.

We learned that the three groups of teenagers looked pretty much alike in terms of their emotional states when they first filled out the forms. But when we compared how the three groups looked a year later, we found that the teenagers who had abortions were more depressed and were more likely to say they had severe tension headaches than teenagers in the other two groups. The teenagers who kept their babies and those who gave their babies up for adoption looked pretty similar 1 year after their babies were born, at least in terms of depression, anxiety, and psychosomatic complaints.

Thus, it seems that we might be right in having some concerns about the emotional effects of having an abortion. Nurses should be aware of these long-term emotional effects, and it even may be advisable to institute some type of follow-up procedure to find out if these young women need additional help.

■ D. The Toolkit

For Chapter 3, the Toolkit on the accompanying CD-ROM contains the following:

- Additional Questions for a Preliminary Review of a Study (Box 3.3 of the textbook)

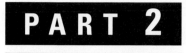

PART 2

Conceptualizing and Planning a Study to Generate Evidence for Nursing

CHAPTER 4

Research Problems, Research Questions, and Hypotheses

■ A. Crossword Puzzle

Complete the crossword puzzle below, which uses terms and concepts presented in Chapter 4. (Puzzles may be removed for easier viewing.)

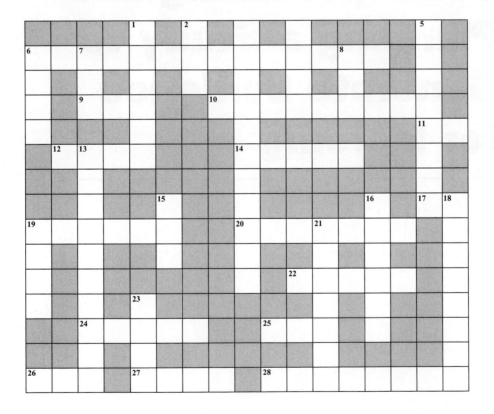

ACROSS

6. A hypothesis in which the specific nature of the predicted relationship is not stipulated.
9. A statement of purpose in a quantitative study indicates the key study variables and the _____ of interest (abbr.).
10. Researchers express the disturbing situation in need of study in their problem _____ .
11. A hypothesis stipulates the expected relationship between a(n) _____ and a DV (abbr.).
12. One phrase that indicates the relational aspect of a hypothesis is: _____ than.
14. One aspect of a problem statement concerns the _____ of the problem (e.g., how many people are affected?).
17. The name of a long-running television series based on a hospital drama
19. One source of research problems, especially for hypothesis-testing research.
20. A hypothesis with two or more independent and/or dependent variables.
22. The results of hypothesis testing never constitute _____ that the hypotheses are or are not correct.
24. The purpose of a study is often conveyed through the judicious choice of _____ .
25. A hypothesis almost always involves at least _____ variables.
26. In the question, "What is the effect of daily exercise on mood and weight?" mood and weight are the _____ (acronym).
27. A statement of purpose indicating that the intent of the study was to *prove* or *demonstrate* something suggests a _____ .
28. A research _____ is what researchers wish to answer through systematic study.

DOWN

1. A hypothesis with one independent and one dependent variable
2. The *actual* hypothesis of an investigator is the _____ hypothesis (abbr.).
3. Another name for *null* hypothesis
4. A practical consideration in assessing feasibility concerns the _____ of undertaking the study.
5. In complex hypotheses, there are _____ independent or dependent variables.
6. The hypothesis that posits no relationship between variables
7. The independent variable in the research question, "Does a midafternoon _____ improve evening mood state in the elderly?"
8. An intention of what to accomplish in a study
13. The researcher's overall goals of undertaking a study
15. A statement of the researcher's prediction about associations between variables (abbr.)

16. The study hypotheses should be stated _____ collecting the research data.
18. Hypotheses must predict a _____ between the independent and dependent variables (abbr.).
19. Hypotheses are typically put to a statistical _____.
21. A statement of _____ is a declaration that summarizes the general direction of the inquiry.
23. A research _____ is an enigmatic or troubling condition (abbr.).

■ B. Study Questions

1. Below is a list of topics that could be studied. Develop at least one research question for each, making sure that some questions could be addressed through qualitative research and others could be addressed through quantitative research. It will likely be helpful to use the question template in the accompanying Toolkit. ✖ (HINT: For quantitative research questions, think of these concepts as potential independent or dependent variables, then ask, "What might cause or affect this variable?" and "What might be the consequences or effects of this variable?" This should lead to some ideas for research questions.)

   a. Patient comfort
   b. Psychiatric patients' readmission rates
   c. Anxiety in hospitalized children
   d. Elevated blood pressure
   e. Incidence of sexually transmitted diseases (STDs)
   f. Patient cooperativeness in the recovery room
   g. Caregiver stress
   h. Mother–infant bonding
   i. Menstrual irregularities

2. Below are five nondirectional hypotheses. Restate each one as a directional hypothesis.

   a. Tactile stimulation and verbal stimulation are associated with physiological arousal among infants with congenital heart disease.
   b. The risk of hypoglycemia in term newborns is related to the infant's birth weight.
   c. The use of isotonic sodium chloride solution before endotracheal suctioning is related to oxygen saturation.
   d. Fluid balance is related to degree of success in weaning older adults from mechanical ventilation.
   e. Nurses administer different amounts of narcotic analgesics to male and female patients.

3. Below are five simple hypotheses. Change each one to a complex hypothesis by adding either a dependent or independent variable.

   a. First-time blood donors experience greater stress during the donation than donors who have given blood previously.
   b. Nurses who initiate more conversation with patients are rated as more effective in their nursing care by patients than those who initiate less conversation.
   c. Surgical patients who give high ratings to the informativeness of nursing communications experience less preoperative stress than do patients who give low ratings.
   d. Appendectomy patients whose peritoneums are drained with a Jackson-Pratt drain will experience more peritoneal infection than patients who are not drained.
   e. Women who give birth by cesarean delivery are more likely to experience postpartum depression than women who give birth vaginally.

4. In study questions 2 and 3 above, 10 research hypotheses were provided. Identify the independent and dependent variables in each.

5. Below are five statements that are *not* research hypotheses as currently stated. Suggest modifications to these statements that would make them testable research hypotheses.

   a. Relaxation therapy is effective in reducing hypertension.
   b. The use of bilingual healthcare staff produces high utilization rates of healthcare facilities by ethnic minorities.
   c. Nursing students are affected in their choice of clinical specialization by interactions with nursing faculty.
   d. Sexually active teenagers have a high rate of using male methods of contraception.
   e. In-use intravenous solutions become contaminated within 48 hours.

6. Examine a recent issue of a nursing research journal. Find an article that does not present a well-articulated statement of purpose. Write a statement of purpose for that study.

7. Read the introduction of one of the following reports. Use the critiquing guidelines in Box 4.3 of the textbook (available as a Word document in the Toolkit) ✖ to assess the study's problem statement, purpose statement, research questions, and/or hypotheses:

   • Sorensen, E., Seebeck, E., Scherb, C., Specht, J., & Loes, J. (2009). The relationship between RN job satisfaction and accountability. *Western Journal of Nursing Research, 31,* 872–888.
   • McCormack, A. (2010). Individuals with eating disorders and the use of online support groups as a form of social support. *CIN: Computers, Informatics, Nursing, 28,* 12–19.

■ C. Application Exercises

EXERCISE 1: STUDY IN APPENDIX F

Read the abstract and introduction to the report by Jurgens and colleagues ("Responding to Heart Failure Symptoms") in Appendix F. Then answer the following questions:

Questions of Fact

a. In which paragraph(s) of this report is the research problem stated?
b. Does this report present a statement of purpose? If so, what *verb* do the researchers use in the statement, and is that verb consistent with the type of research that was undertaken?
c. Does the report specify a research question? If so, was it well-stated? If not, indicate what the question was.
d. Does the report specify hypotheses? If there are hypotheses, were they appropriately worded? Are they directional or nondirectional? Simple or complex? Research or null?
e. If no hypotheses were stated, what would one be?
f. Were hypotheses tested?

Questions for Discussion

a. Did the researchers do an adequate job of describing the research problem? Describe in two to three sentences what the problem is.
b. Comment on the significance of the study's research problem for nursing.
c. Did the researchers do an adequate job of explaining the study purpose, research questions, and/or hypotheses?

EXERCISE 2: STUDY IN APPENDIX B

Read the abstract and introduction to the by Cricco-Lizza ("Rooting for the breast") in Appendix B. Then answer the following questions:

Questions of Fact

a. In which paragraph(s) of this report is the research problem stated?
b. Does this report present a statement of purpose? If so, what *verb* do the researchers use in the statement, and is that verb consistent with the type of research that was undertaken?
c. Does the report specify a research question? If so, was it well-stated? If not, indicate what the question was.
d. Does the report specify hypotheses? If there are hypotheses, were they appropriately worded? Are they directional or nondirectional? Simple or complex? Research or null?
e. Were hypotheses tested?

Questions for Discussion

a. Did the researcher do an adequate job of describing the research problem? Describe in two to three sentences what the problem is.
b. Comment on the significance of the study's research problem for nursing.
c. Did the researcher do an adequate job of explaining the study purpose, research questions, and/or hypotheses?

■ D. The Toolkit

For Chapter 4, the Toolkit on the accompanying CD-ROM contains the following:

- Research Question Templates for Selected Clinical Problems*
- Worksheet: Key Components of a Problem Statement*
- Guidelines for Critiquing Research Problems, Research Questions, and Hypotheses (Box 4.3 of the textbook)
- Useful Websites for Chapter 4: Resources for Research Problems

---

*These items do not appear in the textbook.

CHAPTER 5

Literature Reviews: Finding and Critiquing Evidence

■ A. Crossword Puzzle

Complete the crossword puzzle below, which uses terms and concepts presented in Chapter 5. (Puzzles may be removed for easier viewing.)

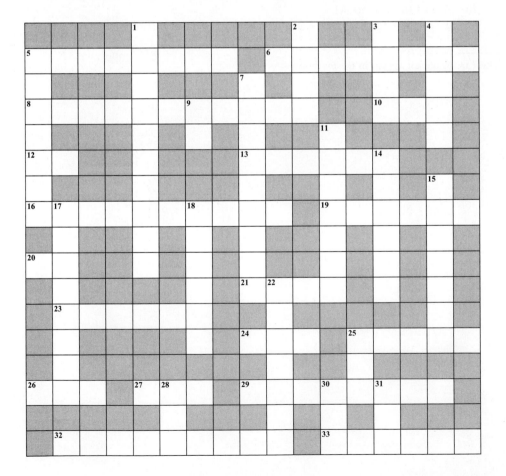

ACROSS

5. A good way to organize information when doing a complex literature review is to use one or more _____.
6. A careful appraisal of the strengths and weaknesses of a study
8. The _____ approach is a search strategy that involves finding a pivotal early study and then searching for subsequent citations to it.
10. A common abbreviation for "literature"
12. In a Results Matrix, the columns could be the _____ s (acronym).
13. The most important bibliographic database for nurses
16. The matrix to record assessments about prior studies is the _____ matrix.
19. The MEDLINE database can be accessed for free through _____.
20. A Boolean operator
21. In summarizing the literature, it is important to point out the _____ in the research literature that suggest the need for further research (backwards!).
23. If a researcher has been prominent in an area, it is useful to do a(n) _____ search.
24. In doing a computerized search, a match between a bibliographic entry and your search criteria is sometimes called a "_____."
25. In most databases, there are "wildcard codes" that can be used to extend a search to include all forms of truncated root _____.
26. A written lit _____ usually appears in the introduction of a research report (abbr.).
27. It is wise to _____ your search activities in a log book or a notebook to avoid unnecessary duplication of effort (abbr.).
29. The Cochrane _____ of Systematic Reviews is an excellent resource for locating earlier research reviews.
32. Descriptions of studies prepared by someone other than the investigators are _____ sources.
33. A _____ system that categorizes results in a systematic fashion is a good tool for organizing research results in a matrix.

DOWN

1. Qualitative researchers do not all agree about whether the _____ should be reviewed before undertaking a study.
2. Research reports with limited distribution are sometimes called the _____ literature.
3. A major resource for finding research reports are _____ databases (abbr.).
4. Reviewers should paraphrase and avoid a _____ from the literature if possible.
5. A very important bibliographic database for healthcare professionals
7. Research literature reviews should contain few (if any) clinical _____.
9. In a Results Matrix, the columns could be the _____ s (acronym).
11. A mechanism through which computer software translates topics into appropriate subject terms for a computerized literature search.

14. Literature searches can be done on one's own or with the assistance of a _____ (abbr.).
15. When doing a database search, one often begins with one _____ or more.
17. In launching a search, it might be best to conceptualize important _____s broadly, to avoid missing an important study.
18. An upfront literature review may not be undertaken by researchers doing a study within the grounded _____ tradition.
22. Findings from a report written by researchers who conducted a study are a _____ source in a research review.
25. The _____ of Knowledge is an important database, especially for its citation indexes.
28. In writing a review, reviewers should paraphrase information in their _____ words.
30. A search strategy sometimes called "footnote chasing" is the _____ approach (abbr.).
31. A Boolean operator

■ B. Study Questions

1. Below are several research questions. Indicate one or more keywords that you would use to begin a literature search on this topic.
   a. What is the lived experience of being a survivor of a suicide attempt?
   b. Does contingency contracting improve patient compliance with a treatment regimen?
   c. What is the decision-making process for a woman considering having an abortion?
   d. Is a special intervention for spinal cord injury patients effective in reducing the risk of pressure ulcers?
   e. Do children raised on vegetarian diets have different growth patterns than other children?
   f. What is the course of appetite loss among cancer patients undergoing chemotherapy?
   g. What is the effect of alcohol skin preparation before insulin injection on the incidence of local and systemic infection?
   h. Are bottle-fed babies introduced to solid foods sooner than breastfed babies?

2. Below are fictitious excerpts from research literature reviews. Each excerpt has a stylistic problem. Change each sentence to make it acceptable stylistically.
   a. Most elderly people do not eat a balanced diet.
   b. Patient characteristics have a significant impact on nursing workload.

c. A child's conception of appropriate sick role behavior changes as the child grows older.
d. Home birth poses many potential dangers.
e. Multiple sclerosis results in considerable anxiety to the family of the patients.
f. Studies have proved that most nurses prefer not to work the night shift.
g. Life changes are the major cause of stress in adults.
h. Stroke rehabilitation programs are most effective when they involve the patients' families.
i. It has been proved that psychiatric outpatients have higher than average rates of accidental deaths and suicides.
j. The traditional pelvic examination is sufficiently unpleasant to many women that they avoid having the examination.
k. It is known that most tonsillectomies performed three decades ago were unnecessary.
l. Few smokers seriously try to break the smoking habit.
m. Severe cutaneous burns often result in hemorrhagic gastric erosions.

3. Read the following research report (or another article of your choosing). Complete as much information as you can about this report using the protocol in Figure 5.5, which is included as a Word document in the Toolkit ✪ on the accompanying CD-ROM:

• Duncan, J. G., Bott, M. J., Thompson, S. A., & Gajewski, B. J. (2009). Symptom occurrence and associated clinical factors in nursing home residents with cancer. *Research in Nursing & Health, 32,* 453–464.

4. Read the literature review section from a research article appearing in a nursing journal in the early 1990s (some possibilities are suggested below). Search the literature for more recent research on the topic of the article and update the original researchers' review section. Use, among other search strategies, the descendancy approach. (Don't forget to incorporate in your review the findings from the cited research article itself.) Here are some possible articles:

• Long, K. A., & Boik, R. J. (1993). Predicting alcohol use in rural children. *Nursing Research, 42,* 79–86.
• Morse, J. M., & Hutchinson, E. (1991). Releasing restraints: Providing safe care for the elderly. *Research in Nursing & Health, 14,* 382–396.
• Quinn, M. M. (1991). Attachment between mothers and their Down syndrome infants. *Western Journal of Nursing Research, 13,* 382–396.
• Singer, N. (1995). Understanding sexual risk behavior from drug users' accounts of their life experiences. *Qualitative Health Research, 5,* 237–249.

5. Read the introduction/literature review section of one of the following reports. Use the critiquing guidelines in Box 5.4 of the textbook (available as a Word document in the Toolkit) ⊗ to assess the study's review of the literature, keeping journal page constraints in mind as you do so:

- Stark, M. A., & Miller, M. (2009). Barriers to the use of hydrotherapy in labor. *Journal of Obstetric, Gynecologic, & Neonatal Nursing, 38,* 667–675.
- Cantrell , M. A., & Conte, T. (2009). Between being cured and being healed: The paradox of childhood cancer survivorship. *Qualitative Health Research, 19,* 312–322.

■ C. Application Exercises

EXERCISE 1: STUDY IN APPENDIX K

Read the abstract, introduction, and the first subsection under "Methods" of the article by Han and colleagues ("Interventions to Promote Mammography") in Appendix K. Then answer the following questions:

Questions of Fact

a. What type of research review did the investigators undertake?
b. Did the researchers begin with a problem statement? Summarize the problem in a few sentences.
c. Did the researchers provide a statement of purpose? If so, what was it?
d. How many different databases did the researchers search? How many researchers were involved in the search? Were any manual methods used in the search?
e. What keywords were used in the search? Were the keywords related to the independent or dependent variable of interest?
f. Did the researchers restrict their search to English-language reports?
g. Did the researchers restrict their search to articles published after a certain date? If so, did the researchers state their rationale?
h. How many citations were initially identified by the search?
i. What are some of these reasons the researchers cited for eliminating some of the retrieved studies from further consideration?
j. How many studies ultimately were included in the review?
k. Were the studies included in the review qualitative, quantitative, or both?

Questions for Discussion

a. Did the researchers do an adequate job of explaining the problem and their purpose in undertaking the review?
b. Did the researchers appear to do a thorough job in their search for relevant studies?
c. Certain studies that were initially retrieved were eliminated. Did the researchers provide a sound rationale for their decisions?

EXERCISE 2: STUDY IN APPENDIX L

Read the abstract, introduction, and study design and method sections of the article by Xu ("Strangers in strange lands") in Appendix L. Then answer the following questions:

Questions of Fact

a. What type of research review did Xu undertake?
b. Did Xu begin with a problem statement? Did he articulate research questions? If yes, what were they?
c. How many different databases did Xu search? Were the searches of electronic databases? Were any manual methods used in the search?
d. What keywords were used in the search?
e. Did Xu restrict his search to English-language reports?
f. How many citations were initially identified by the search? How many studies were used in the review?
g. Were the studies included in the review qualitative, quantitative, or both?
h. Which qualitative research traditions were represented in the review?

EXERCISE 3: STUDY IN APPENDIX H

Read the article by McGillion and colleagues ("Chronic cardiac pain") in Appendix H and use the critiquing guidelines for a quantitative research report in Box 5.2 of the textbook (also in the accompanying Toolkit ✪) to answer as many questions as you can. Then read the critique of the study that is also included in Appendix H, making note of issues that are absent in your critique (or in ours).

EXERCISE 4: STUDY IN APPENDIX I

Read the article by Sawyer and colleagues ("Differences in Perceptions") in Appendix I and use the critiquing guidelines for a qualitative research report in Box 5.3 of the textbook (also in the accompanying Toolkit ✪) to answer as many questions as you can. Then read the critique of the study that is also included in Appendix I, making note of issues that are absent in your critique (or in ours!).

■ D. The Toolkit

For Chapter 5, the Toolkit on the accompanying CD-ROM contains a Word file with the following:

- Guide to an Overall Critique of a Quantitative Research Report (Box 5.2 of the textbook)
- Guide to an Overall Critique of a Qualitative Research Report (Box 5.3 of the textbook)

- Guidelines for Critiquing Literature Reviews (Box 5.4 of the textbook)
- Literature Review Protocol (Figure 5.5 of the textbook)
- Methodologic Matrix for Recording Key Methodologic Features of Studies for a Literature Review (Figure 5.6 of the textbook)
- Two Results Matrices for Recording Key Findings for a Literature Review (Figure 5.7 of the textbook)
- Evaluation Matrix for Recording Strengths and Weaknesses of Studies for a Literature Review (Figure 5.8 of the textbook)
- Log of Literature Search Activities in Bibliographic Databases*
- Useful Websites for Chapter 5: Resources for Literature Reviews

———————————

*This item does not appear in the textbook.

CHAPTER 6

Theoretical Frameworks

■ A. Crossword Puzzle

Complete the crossword puzzle below, which uses terms and concepts presented in Chapter 6. (Puzzles may be removed for easier viewing.)

ACROSS

4. The conceptual underpinnings of a study
5. The originator of the Health Promotion Model
10. One of the four elements in conceptual models of nursing (abbr.)
11. Abstractions assembled because of their relevance to a core concept form a _____ model.
13. Readings in the theoretical literature often give rise to a research _____.
14. Psychiatric nurse researchers sometimes obtain funding from an institute within the National Institutes of Health (NIH) with the acronym NI _ _.
16. A theory that focuses on a piece of human experience is sometimes called _____-range.
18. Another term for a schematic model is conceptual _____.
19. The originator of the Science of Unitary Human Beings
21. Roy conceptualized the _____ Model of nursing (abbr.)
22. The originator of the Theory of Uncertainty in Illness
23. The originator of the Theory of Human Becoming
24. A schematic _____ is a mechanism for representing concepts with a minimal use of words.
26. A construct that is a key mediator in many models of health behavior, such as the HPM and Social Cognitive Theory (acronym)
28. The mutually beneficial relationship between theory and research has been described as _____ (abbr.).
29. Concept analysis is sometimes used to develop conceptual _____ for frameworks (abbr.).
30. One of the originators of a theory of stress, with Lazarus
31. Orem's model of nursing focuses on _____, that is, what people do on their own behalf to maintain health and well-being.

DOWN

1. A theory aimed at explaining large segments of behavior or other phenomena
2. A theory that thoroughly accounts for or describes a phenomenon
3. A social psychological theory often used in nursing research is the Social _____ Theory (abbr.).
6. As classically defined, theories consist of concepts arranged in a logically interrelated _____ system, from which hypotheses can be generated.
7. The Theory of Planned Behavior is an extension of the Theory of _____ Action.
8. The acronym for Pender's model
9. A theory that focuses on a single piece of human experience is sometimes called middle- _____.
12. If a study is based on a theory, its framework is called the _____ framework.
15. The Stages of Change Model is also called the _ _ _ _ _theoretical Model.
16. A schematic model is also called a conceptual _____.
17. The originator of the Conservation Model of nursing

18. Another name for a grand theory is a _____ theory.
20. A type of theory originally from another discipline used productively by nurse researchers
24. The originator of the Model of Self-Care (backwards!)
25. A theory by two psychologists, often used by nurse researchers, is the Theory of Stress and Co _ _ _ _.
27. The originator of the social psychological theory focusing on a person's outcome expectations was _ _ _ dura.
28. Theories are built inductively from observations, which are often from disciplined _____ (abbr.).

■ B. Study Questions

1. Read some recent issues of a nursing research journal. Identify at least three different theories cited by nurse researchers in these research reports.

2. Choose one of the conceptual frameworks of nursing that were described in this chapter. Develop a research hypothesis based on this framework.

3. Select one of the research questions/problems listed below. Could the selected problem be developed within one of the models or theories discussed in this chapter? Defend your answer.
   a. How do men grapple with a diagnosis of prostate cancer?
   b. What are the factors contributing to perceptions of fatigue among patients with congestive heart failure?
   c. What effect does the presence of the father in the delivery room have on the mother's satisfaction with the childbirth experience?
   d. The purpose of the study is to explore why some women fail to perform breast self-examination regularly.
   e. What are the factors that lead to poorer health among low-income children than higher-income children?

4. Suggest an important outcome that could be studied using the Health Promotion Model (i.e., a health-promoting behavior). Identify another theory described in this chapter that could be used to explain or predict the same outcome. Which theory or model do you think would do a better job? Why?

5. Read one of the following articles, and then apply the criteria in Box 6.2 (available as a Word document in the Toolkit ❽ on the accompanying CD-ROM) to make a judgment about whether the study involved a *test* of a model or theory.
   • Bailey, D., Landerman, L., Barroso, J., Bixby, P., Mishel, M., Muir, A., Strickland, L., & Clipp, E. (2009). Uncertainty, symptoms, and quality of life in persons with chronic hepatitis C. *Psychosomatics, 50,* 138–146.
   • Peddle, C., Jones, L., Eves, N., Reiman, T., Sellar, C., Winton, T., & Courneya, K. S. (2009). Correlates of adherence to supervised exercise in patients awaiting surgical removal of malignant tumor lesions. *Oncology Nursing Forum, 36,* 287–295.

- Suliman, W., Welmann, E., Omer, T., & Thomas, L. (2009). Applying Watson's nursing theory to assess patient perceptions of being cared for in a multicultural environment. *Journal of Nursing Research, 17*, 293–297.

6. Read one of the following articles, and then apply the critiquing criteria in Box 6.3 (available as a Word document in the Toolkit ✪ on the accompanying CD-ROM) to evaluate the conceptual basis of the study.

- Duffett-Leger, L., Letourneau, N., & Croll, J. (2008). Cervical cancer screening practices among university women. *Journal of Obstetric, Gynecologic, & Neonatal Nursing, 37*, 572–581.
- Ip, W., Tang, C., & Goggins, W. (2009). An educational intervention to improve women's ability to cope with childbirth. *Journal of Clinical Nursing, 18*, 2125–2135.
- Hoffman, A., von Eye, A., Gift, A., Given, B., Given, C., & Rothert, M. (2009). Testing a theoretical model of perceived self-efficacy for cancer-related fatigue self-management and optimal physical functioning status. *Nursing Research, 58*, 32–41.

7. Read the following article, and then assess the following: (a) What evidence does the researcher offer to substantiate that her grounded theory is a good fit with her data? (b) To what extent is it clear or unclear in the article that symbolic interactionism was the theoretical underpinning of the study?

- Hamilton, R., Williams, J. K., Skirton, H., & Bowers, B. J. (2009). Living with genetic test results for hereditary breast and ovarian cancer. *Journal of Nursing Scholarship, 41*, 276–283.

■ C. Application Exercises

EXERCISE 1: STUDY IN APPENDIX F

Read the abstract and introduction (all of the material before the method section) of the article by Jurgens and colleagues ("Responding to Heart Failure Symptoms") in Appendix F. Then answer the following questions:

Questions of Fact

a. Does the study by Jurgens and colleagues involve a conceptual or theoretical framework? What is it called?
b. Is this framework one of the models of nursing cited in the textbook? Is it related to one of those models?
c. Does the report include a schematic model?
d. What are the key concepts in the model?
e. According to the framework, what factors *directly* affect the decision to seek care?
f. According to the framework, what factors *indirectly* affect the decision to seek care?
g. Did the report present conceptual definitions of key concepts?
h. Did the report explicitly present hypotheses deduced from the framework?

Questions for Discussion

a. Does the link between the problem and the framework seem contrived? Do the hypotheses (if any) naturally flow from the framework?
b. Do you think any aspects of the research would have been different without the framework?
c. Could the study have been undertaken using Pender's Health Promotion Model as its framework (see Figure 6.1 in the textbook)? Why or why not?
d. Would you describe this study as a model-testing inquiry or do you think the model was used more as an organizing framework?

EXERCISE 2: STUDY IN APPENDIX E

Read the abstract and introduction to the article by Beck ("The Arm") in Appendix E. Then answer the following questions:

Questions of Fact

a. Does Beck's study involve a conceptual or theoretical framework? What is it called?
b. Is this framework one of the models of nursing cited in the textbook? Is it related to one of those models?
c. Does the report include a schematic model? Was the model formulated prior to data collection?
d. What are the key concepts in the framework?
e. Did the report explicitly present hypotheses deduced from the framework?

Questions for Discussion

a. Does the link between the research problem in this study and the framework seem genuine?
b. Do you think any aspects of the research would have been different if Beck had conducted a straightforward descriptive study?
c. How helpful was the schematic model in communicating important features of the findings?
d. On the basis of your own personal and professional experience, how would you characterize the resulting model, in terms of its descriptive power and accuracy?

■ D. The Toolkit

For Chapter 6, the Toolkit on the accompanying CD-ROM contains a Word file with the following:

• Some Questions for a Preliminary Assessment of a Model or Theory (Box 6.1 of the textbook)

- Criteria to Determine if a Theory or Model is Being Tested in a Study (Box 6.2 of the textbook)
- Guidelines for Critiquing Theoretical and Conceptual Frameworks (Box 6.3 of the textbook)
- Useful Websites for Chapter 6: Resources for Theories and Conceptual Frameworks
- Selected Middle-Range Theories of Relevance for Nursing Research*

---

*This item does not appear in the textbook.

CHAPTER 7

Ethics in Nursing Research

■ A. Crossword Puzzle

Complete the crossword puzzle below, which uses terms and concepts presented in Chapter 7. (Puzzles may be removed for easier viewing.)

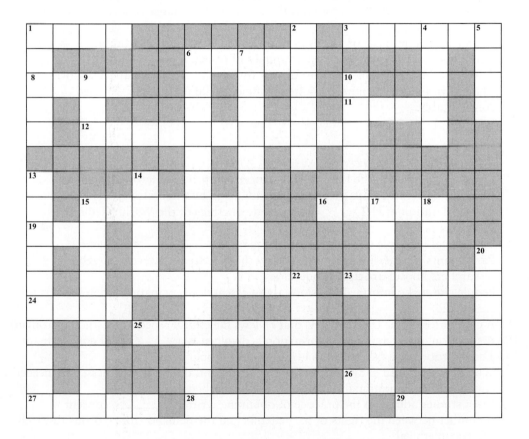

ACROSS

1. A fundamental right for study participants is freedom from _____.
3. Deliberately changing or omitting data or distorting results is _ _ _ _ _ _ ication.
6. Most disciplines have developed _____ of ethics.
8. Anonymity is a method of protecting participants' _ _ _ _ acy.
11. Researchers should conduct a _____-benefit assessment.
12. A major ethical principle concerning maximizing benefits of research
15. The type of consent procedure that may be required in qualitative research
16. A young _____ is usually considered a vulnerable subject.
19. Debriefings give participants an opportunity to _____ complaints.
21. A payment sometimes offered to participants as an incentive to take part in a study
23. Data collection without participants' awareness, using concealment
24. A procedure for collecting data without linking them to individual participants (abbr.)
25. The report that is the basis for ethical regulations for studies funded by the U.S. government
26. Numbers used in place of names to protect individual identities (abbr.)
27. Fraud and misrepresentations are examples of research _ _ _ _ _ nduct.
28. A major ethical principle involves respect for human _____ (backwards!).
29. The return of a questionnaire is often assumed to demonstrate _ _ _ _ ied consent (abbr.).

DOWN

1. Legislation passed in the U.S. in 1996 concerning privacy (acronym)
2. Informal agreement to participate in a study (e.g., by minors)
4. The Declaration of Hel _ _ _ _ _ is the code of ethics of the World Medical Association.
5. The ethical principle of *justice* includes the right to _____ treatment.
6. Participants' privacy is often protected by these procedures, even though the researchers know participants' identities.
7. People can make informed decisions about research participation when there is full _____.
9. A committee (in the United States) that reviews the ethical aspects of a study (acronym)
10. A situation in which private information is divulged is a _____ of confidentiality.
13. The appropriation of someone's ideas without proper credit
14. When short _____ are used to document consent, third-party witnesses are needed.
15. A vulnerable, institutionalized group with diminished autonomy.
17. Most studies adhere to the practice of obtaining written _____ consent.
18. A conflict between the rights of participants and the demands for rigorous research creates an ethical _____.
20. Research that adheres to _____ guidelines is designed to protect participants' rights.
22. Mismanagement of _____ can result in a type of research misconduct.
26. Numbers used in place of names to protect individual identities (abbr.)

■ B. Study Questions

1. Below are brief descriptions of several studies. Suggest some ethical dilemmas that are likely to emerge for each.
   a. A study of coping behaviors among rape victims
   b. An unobtrusive observational study of fathers' behaviors in the delivery room
   c. An interview study of the determinants of heroin addiction
   d. A study of pain assessment among mentally retarded children
   e. An investigation of verbal interactions among schizophrenic patients
   f. A study of the effects of a new treatment for adolescents with sickle cell disease
   g. A study of the relationship between sleeping patterns and acting-out behaviors in hospitalized psychiatric patients

2. Evaluate the ethical aspects of one or more of the following studies using the critiquing guidelines in Box 7.2 of the textbook (available as a Word document in the Toolkit ✪ of the accompanying CD-ROM), paying special attention (if relevant) to the manner in which the subjects' heightened vulnerability was handled.
   • Norris, J., Howell, E., Wydeven, M., & Kunes-Connell, M. (2009). Working with teen moms and babies at risk: The power of partnering. *MCN: The American Journal of Maternal/Child Nursing, 34,* 308–315.
   • Oliveria, J., & Burke, P. (2009). Lost in the shuffle: Culture of homeless adolescents. *Pediatric Nursing, 35,* 154–161.
   • Park, H., & Pringle-Specht, J. (2009). Effect of individualized music on agitation in individuals with dementia who live at home. *Journal of Gerontological Nursing, 35,* 47–55.

3. In the textbook, two studies with ethical problems were described in the historical background section (the study of syphilis among black men and the study in which mentally retarded children were deliberately infected with the hepatitis virus). Identify which ethical principles were transgressed in these studies.

4. In the following study, the authors indicated that informed consent was not required because there was "no deviation from the standard of care or risk to the subjects" (p. 108). Skim the introduction and method section of this paper and comment on the researchers' decision to not obtain informed consent:
   • Byers, J. F., Lowman, L. B., Francis, J., Kaigle, L., Lutz, N. H., Waddell, T., & Diaz, A. L. (2006). A quasi-experimental trial on individualized, developmentally supportive family-centered care. *Journal of Obstetric, Gynecologic, & Neonatal Nursing, 35*(1), 105–115.

5. Below is a brief description of the ethical aspects of a fictitious study, followed by a critique. Do you agree with the critique? Can you add other comments relevant to the ethical dimensions of the study?

Fictitious Study. Fortune conducted an in-depth study of nursing home residents to explore whether their perceptions about personal control over decision making differed from the perceptions of the nursing staff. The investigator studied 25 nurse–patient dyads to assess whether there were differing perceptions and experiences regarding control over activities of daily living such as arising, eating, and dressing. All of the nurses in the study were employed by the nursing home in which the patients resided. Because the nursing home had no IRB, and because Fortune's study was not funded by an organization that required IRB approval, the project was not formally reviewed. Fortune sought permission from the nursing home administrator to conduct the study. She also obtained the consent of the legal guardian or responsible family member of each patient. All study participants were fully informed about the nature of the study. The researcher assured the nurses and the legal guardians and family members of the patients of the confidentiality of the information and obtained their consent in writing. Data were gathered primarily through in-depth interviews with the patients and the nurses, at separate times. The researcher also observed interactions between the patients and nurses. The findings from the study suggested that patients perceived that they had more control over all aspects of the activities of daily living (except eating) than the nurses perceived that they had. Excerpts from the interviews were used verbatim in the research report, but Fortune did not divulge the location of the nursing home, and she used fictitious names for all participants.

Critique. Fortune did a reasonably good job of adhering to basic ethical principles in the conduct of her research. She obtained written permission to conduct the study from the nursing home administrator, and she obtained informed consent from the nurse participants and the legal guardians or family members of the patients. The study participants were not put at risk in any way, and the patients who participated may actually have enjoyed the opportunity to have a conversation with the researcher. Fortune also took appropriate steps to maintain the confidentiality of participants. It is still unclear, however, whether the patients knowingly and willingly participated in the research. Nursing home residents are a vulnerable group. They may not have been aware of their right to refuse to be interviewed without fear of repercussion. Fortune could have enhanced the ethical aspects of the study by taking more vigorous steps to obtain the informed, voluntary consent of the nursing home residents or to exclude patients who could not reasonably be expected to understand the researcher's request. Given the vulnerability of the group, Fortune probably should have established her own review panel composed of peers and interested lay people to review the ethical dimensions of her project. Debriefing sessions with study participants would also have been appropriate.

■ C. Application Exercises

EXERCISE 1: STUDY IN APPENDIX A

Read the first two subsections ("Participants" and "Procedures") in the method section of the article by Kennedy and Chen ("Changes in childhood risk taking") in Appendix A. Then answer the following questions:

Questions of Fact

a. Does the report indicate that the study procedures were reviewed by an IRB or other similar institutional ethical review committee?
b. Would the participants in this study be considered "vulnerable"?
c. Were participants subjected to any physical harm or discomfort or psychological distress as part of the study? What efforts did the researchers make to minimize harm and maximize good?
d. Were participants deceived in any way?
e. Were participants coerced into participating in the study?
f. Were appropriate informed consent procedures used? Was there full disclosure, and was participation voluntary?
g. Does the report discuss steps that were taken to protect the privacy and confidentiality of study participants?

Questions for Discussion

a. Do you think the benefits of this research outweighed the costs to participants—what is the overall risk/benefit ratio? Would you characterize the study as having *minimal risk*?
b. Do you consider that the researchers took adequate steps to protect the study participants? If not, what else could they have done?
c. The report indicates that the participants were paid a stipend. Comment on how appropriate you think this was.

EXERCISE 2: STUDY IN APPENDIX B

Read the method section of the article by Cricco-Lizza ("Rooting for the breast") in Appendix B. Then answer the following questions:

Questions of Fact

a. Does the report indicate that the study procedures were reviewed by an IRB or other similar institutional ethical review committee?
b. Would the study participants in this study be considered "vulnerable"?
c. Were participants subjected to any physical harm or discomfort or psychological distress as part of this study? What efforts did the researchers make to minimize harm and maximize good?
d. Were participants deceived in any way?
e. Were participants coerced into participating in the study?
f. Were appropriate informed consent procedures used? Was there full disclosure, and was participation voluntary?
g. Does the report discuss steps that were taken to protect the privacy and confidentiality of study participants?

Questions for Discussion

a. Do you think the benefits of this research outweighed the costs to participants—what is the overall risk/benefit ratio? Would you characterize the study as having *minimal risk*?

b. Do you consider that the researchers took adequate steps to protect the study participants? If not, what else could they have done?

c. Do you think that mothers and other family members should have been given an opportunity to opt out of the study? Should they have been asked to provide informed consent?

d. The report did not indicate that the study participants were paid a stipend. Do you think a stipend would have been necessary or appropriate in this study?

▪ D. The Toolkit

For Chapter 7, the Toolkit on the accompanying CD-ROM contains a Word file with the following:

- Worksheet for Assessing Potential Benefits and Risks of Research to Participants (Based on Box 7.1 of the textbook)
- Example of an Informed Consent Form for Participation in a Research Project, Example #1 (Figure 7.1 of the textbook)
- Example of an Informed Consent Form for Participation in a Research Project, Example #2*
- Fictitious Example of an Informed Assent Form for Children's Participation in a Research Project, Example #3*
- Simplifying Language in Informed Consent and Other Participant Forms: Selected Examples
- Checklist for De-Identifying Data to Comply with HIPAA Privacy Regulations*
- Example of an Authorization Form to Disclose Individually Identifiable Health Information, in Compliance with HIPAA Privacy Regulations*
- Fictitious Example of a Confidentiality Pledge for Project Staff*
- Guidelines for Critiquing the Ethical Aspects of a Study (Box 7.3 of the textbook)
- Useful Websites for Chapter 7: Resources for Ethics and Research

---

*These items do not appear in the textbook.

CHAPTER 8

Planning a Nursing Study

■ A. Crossword Puzzle

Complete the crossword puzzle below, which uses terms and concepts presented in Chapter 8. (Puzzles may be removed for easier viewing.)

ACROSS

1. The use of multiple sources or referents to draw conclusions about what constitutes the truth
7. Quantitative researchers aim to control _ _ _ _ _ eous variables (abbr.).
8. The type of design in which *different* people are compared is a _____-subjects design.
9. An important criterion for evaluating quantitative studies, referring broadly to the soundness of evidence
10. The extent to which qualitative study methods engender confidence in the truth of the data and interpretations (abbr.)
12. A type of study in which data are collected at a single point in time (acronym)
13. A bias that is _____ systematic bias is random bias.
14. One purpose of a pilot intervention study is to determine how large a "_____" of the intervention is appropriate.
15. When a researcher is not interested in studying change, data are usually collected at a _____ point in time.
16. A design involving comparisons of multiple age groups is a c _ _ _ _ _ comparison design.
18. Loss of participants from a study over time (abbr.)
19. A comparison based on relative rankings might involve asking whether, for example, those with high levels of pain have _____ levels of hopefulness than those with less pain.
23. When reflexivity is rigorously pursued, reflections and personal values are _____ in a journal or in memos.
24. A pilot study is undertaken to _____ the methods and procedures that would be used in a larger study.
26. A _____ study is sometimes called a feasibility study.
27. The accuracy and consistency of information obtained in a study (abbr.)
28. One type of longitudinal study is a follow-_____ study.
29. The process of pondering and thinking critically on the self

DOWN

1. A _____ study involves multiple points of data collection with different samples from the same population to detect patterns of change over time.
2. One critical design decision involves whether or not there will be a(n) _____, or whether the study will be nonexperimental.
3. The type of study that involves multiple points of data collection over an extended time
4. Gaining entrée is often an ongoing process of es _ _ _ _ _ _ _ ing relationships and rapport with gatekeepers.
5. The concept of _____ involves having certain features of the study established by chance.
6. Through self-reports, researchers can gather _____ data about events occurring in the past.
10. Another term for *extraneous* variable

11. An influence that distorts study results
14. In qualitative studies, a quality criterion that concerns whether evidence is believable and stable over time (abbr.)
17. In planning a study, it is useful to develop a _____ for major tasks.
20. Attrition is problematic because those who drop _____ of a study are rarely a random subset of all participants.
21. Research c _ _ _ _ _ _ is used to hold constant extraneous influences on the dependent variable.
22. Researchers chose from a myriad of methodologic _ _ _ _ ons in designing a study.
24. For gaining entrée, the establishment of _____ is a central issue.
25. Transferability is enhanced when qualitative researchers use _____ description in their reports.

■ B. Study Questions

1. A team of nurses wanted to assess whether a special intervention would lower the risk of bone mineral density loss among women undergoing chemotherapy for breast cancer. Think of how a study could be designed. Could the study be designed as any of the following—if yes, provide examples of how this could be designed:
   a. A within-group study?
   b. A between-group study?
   c. A cross sectional study?
   d. A longitudinal study?

2. Read one of the following studies. Point out instances of what you consider to be *thick description*.
   - Swift, M., & Scholten, I. (2010). Not feeding, not coming home: Parental experiences of infant feeding difficulties and family relationships in a neonatal unit. *Journal of Clinical Nursing, 19,* 249–258.
   - Woodgate, R., & Yanofsky, R. (2010). Parents' experiences in decision making with childhood cancer clinical trials. *Cancer Nursing, 33,* 11–18.

3. Read one of the following studies. Point out instances of what you consider to be *reflexivity*.
   - Huang, X., Sun, F., Yen, W., & Fu, C. (2008). The coping experiences of carers who live with someone who has schizophrenia. *Journal of Clinical Nursing, 17,* 817–826.
   - Martinsen, B., Harder, I., & Biering-Sorensen, F. (2009). Sensitive cooperation: A basis for assisted feeding. *Journal of Clinical Nursing, 18,* 708–715.
   - Ransom, J. E., Siler, B., Peters, R., & Maurer, M. J. (2005). Worry: women's experience of HIV testing. *Qualitative Health Research, 15,* 382–393.

4. Read the following article and identify important lessons learned in the pilot studies described: Heidrich, S., Brown, R. L., Egan, J. J., Perez, O. A., Phelan, C. H., Yeom, H., & Ward, S. E. (2009). An individualized representational intervention to improve

symptom management (IRIS) in older breast cancer survivors: Three pilot studies. *Oncology Nursing Forum, 36,* E133–143.

5. Read one of the following studies and try to estimate what a timeline for the study might have looked like. (If useful, use the timeline in the Toolkit ✪ on the accompanying CD-ROM.):

   • Bay, E., & Xie, Y. (2009). Pyschological and biological correlates of fatigue after mild-to-moderate traumatic brain injury. *Western Journal of Nursing Research, 31,* 731–747.
   • Renker, P., & Ronkin, P. (2006). Women's views of prenatal violence screening. *Obstetrics & Gynecology, 107,* 348–354.

6. Find a longitudinal study in a recent nursing journal. Could the study have been designed as a cross-sectional study? If not, why not? If yes, describe how the study could have been designed.

■ C. Application Exercises

EXERCISE 1: STUDY IN APPENDIX D

Read the introduction and method section of the article by Whittemore and colleagues ("Diabetes Prevention Program") in Appendix D. Then answer the following questions:

Questions of Fact

a. Did this study involve an intervention?
b. Was this study designed to make any comparisons? If so, what type of comparison was made?
c. Did this study use a within-subjects design, a between-subjects design, or a mixed design?
d. Was the study cross-sectional or longitudinal? How many times were data collected from study participants?
e. What was the location for this study?
f. What were the primary methods of data collection?
g. Was this a pilot study? If yes, what were the study objectives?

Questions for Discussion

a. Over how many months do you think this study was conducted?
b. Try to find an example of how the researchers controlled extraneous variables by "holding constant" possible confounding influences.
c. How would you rate the methods of data collection in terms of structure, researcher obtrusiveness, and objectivity? Discuss how appropriate the researchers' data collection decisions were.
d. Describe some of the things you might recommend doing in a larger scale study designed to assess the intervention. Do you think the intervention merits a larger, more rigorous study?

EXERCISE 2: STUDY IN APPENDIX I

Read the introduction and method section of the article by Sawyer and colleagues ("Differences in Perceptions") in Appendix I. Then answer the following questions:

Questions of Fact

a. Did this study involve an intervention?
b. Was this study designed to make any comparisons? If so, what type of comparison was made?
c. Was the study cross-sectional or longitudinal? How many times were data collected from study participants?
d. What was the location for this study?
e. What were the primary methods of data collection?
f. Was this a pilot study? If yes, what were the study objectives?

Questions for Discussion

a. How would you rate the methods of data collection in terms of structure, researcher obtrusiveness, and objectivity? Discuss how appropriate the researchers' data collection decisions were.
b. Discuss whether there is any evidence of reflexivity in this study.
c. Discuss aspects of this study that might bear on the issue of transferability.
d. Try to develop a timeline for the major activities in this study.

■ D. The Toolkit

For Chapter 8, the Toolkit on the accompanying CD-ROM contains the following:

• Sample Letter of Inquiry for Gaining Entrée into a Research Site (Fictitious) (Figure 8.2 of the textbook)
• Project Timeline, in Calendar Months, for a 24-Month Project (Figure 8.3 of the textbook)
• Worksheet for Documenting Design Decisions*

---

*This item does not appear in the textbook.

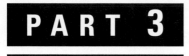

PART 3

Designing and Conducting Quantitative Studies to Generate Evidence for Nursing

CHAPTER 9

Quantitative Research Design

■ A. Crossword Puzzle

Complete the crossword puzzle below, which uses terms and concepts presented in Chapter 9. (Puzzles may be removed for easier viewing.)

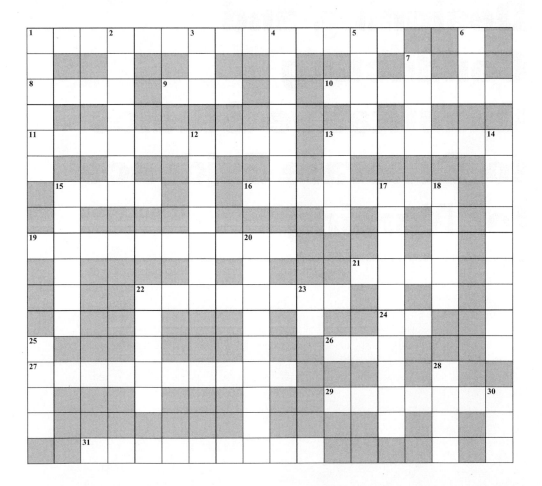

ACROSS

1. That against which the outcomes for an experimental group are compared
8. A type of control group in a quasi-experiment, using data from an earlier point in time (abbr.)
9. A type of control group used to offset the effect of special care to the experimental group (abbr.)
10. Randomization of people within specified subgroups (abbr.)
11. A _ _ _ _ _ _ _ _ _ ive design begins with the effect and looks back in time for a cause.
13. Another name for the "before" (preintervention) measures of the outcome variables
15. A major bias in research that does not involve random assignment is _____ selection.
16. A _ _ _ _ _ _ _ ive design begins with the cause and looks forward to an effect.
19. The number with a condition or disease at a fixed point, based on cross-sectional data from the population at risk, typically reported as a rate
21. A "box" is a diagram of a factorial design.
22. One criterion for causality is _____ plausibility.
24. The rate of new cases with a condition or disease for a fixed period of time (acronym)
26. In the medical literature, the term sometimes used for *group* or *condition*
27. To protect from possible bias, _____ concealment is recommended during randomization.
29. The Zelen design is often referred to as randomized _____.
31. The _____ effect is a bias, named after industrial experiments, that can arise from people's awareness of being studied.

DOWN

1. A(n) _____ design is the term used in the medical literature for a nonexperimental prospective study.
2. A(n) _____ experiment looks at the effects of an event that transpires in a fairly random fashion, such as a hurricane.
3. Another name for an experiment (acronym)
4. The type of randomization involving random assignment of large units (e.g., hospitals)
5. The _____-only design collects data from subjects following administration of the intervention only.
6. A type of intervention that is tailored to particular characteristics of people (acronym)
7. A _____-listed control group gets delayed treatment.
12. A pseudointervention
13. A _____ test is a measure of an outcome after the intervention has been administered.
14. Another term for an intervention
15. A type of quasi-experimental design involving multiple points of data collection before and after an intervention is a time _____.

17. The gold standard for inferring cause-and-effect relationships is a true _____.
18. One method of randomization involves use of a _____ of random numbers.
20. A type of design in which subjects serve as their own controls
22. When stratification is used prior to randomization, the design is called a randomized _____ design.
23. In an experiment, that which is manipulated (acronym)
25. Nonexperimental studies that test theory-driven causal linkages often use _____ analysis.
28. Randomization of a small number of subjects in small groupings of various sizes is called _____ block randomization (abbr.).
30. A factorial study involves at least _____ independent, manipulated variables.

■ B. Study Questions

1. Suppose you wanted to study self-efficacy among successful dieters who lost 20 or more pounds and maintained their weight loss for at least 6 months. Specify at least two different types of comparison strategies that might provide a useful comparative context for this study. Do your strategies lend themselves to experimental manipulation? If not, why not?

2. Below are 20 subjects who have volunteered for a study of the effects of noise on pulse rate. Ten must be assigned to the low-volume group and 10 to a high-volume group. Use the table of random numbers in Table 9.2 of the text (or in the tables of random numbers in the accompanying Toolkit ❌) to randomly assign subjects to groups.

L. Bentley	M. McGowan
L. Boehm	A. Messenger
D. Chorna	U. Moore
H. Dann	P. Morrill
L. Dansker	C. O'Dea
E. Gordon	A. Petty
R. Greenberg	D. Roberts
J. Harte	V. Rotan
S. Kulli	H. Seidler
P. Labovitz	R. Smalling

    Assume all participants in the first column above are in their 20s and all those in the second column are in their 30s. How good a job did your randomization do in terms of equalizing the two groups according to age? Add 10 more names to each age group and assign these additional 20 subjects. Now compare the low-volume and high-volume groups in terms of the age distribution. Did doubling the sample size improve the distribution of subjects' ages within the two volume-level groups?

3. A nurse researcher found a relationship between teenagers' level of knowledge about birth control and their level of sexual activity. That is, teenagers with higher levels of sexual activity knew more about birth control than teenagers with less sexual activity. Suggest at least three interpretations for this finding. Is this a research problem that is *inherently* nonexperimental? Why or why not?

4. The following study was described a double-blind experiment. Review the design for this study, and comment on the appropriateness of the blinding procedures. What biases were the researchers trying to avoid? Were they successful?

   • Schmelzer, M., Schiller, L., Meyer, R., Rugari, S., & Case, P. (2004). Safety and effectiveness of large-volume enema solutions. *Applied Nursing Research, 17*(4), 265–274.

5. Suppose that you were interested in testing the hypothesis that regular ingestion of aspirin reduced the risk of colon cancer. Describe how such a hypothesis could be tested using a retrospective case-control design. Now, describe a prospective cohort design for the same study. Compare the strengths and weaknesses of the two approaches.

6. Read the introduction and methods section of one of the following reports. Use the critiquing guidelines in Box 9.1 of the textbook (available as a Word document in the Toolkit ✪) to evaluate features of the research design:

   • Rice, V., Weqlicki, L., Templin, T., Jamil, H., & Hammad, A. (2010). Intervention effects on tobacco use in Arab and non-Arab American adolescents. *Addictive Behaviors, 35*, 46–48.
   • Sammarco, A., & Konecny, L. (2010). Quality of life, social support, and uncertainty among Latina and Caucasian breast cancer survivors. *Oncology Nursing Forum, 37*, 93–99.
   • Yang, M., Li, L., Zhu, H., Alexander, I., Liu, S., Zhou, W., & Ren, X. (2009). Music therapy to relieve anxiety in pregnant women on bedrest. *MCN: The American Journal of Maternal/Child Nursing, 34*, 316–323.

7. A nurse researcher is interested in studying the success of several different approaches to feeding patients with dysphagia. Can the researcher use a correlational design to examine this problem? Why or why not? Could an experimental or quasi-experimental approach be used? How?

■ C. Application Exercises

EXERCISE 1: STUDY IN APPENDIX A

Read the method section of the article by Kennedy and Chen ("Changes in childhood risk taking") in Appendix A. Then answer the following questions:

Questions of Fact

a. Was there an intervention in this study?
b. Is the design for this study experimental, quasi-experimental, or nonexperimental?
c. Was this a cause-probing study?
d. What were the independent and dependent variables?
e. Was randomization used? If yes, what method was used to assign subjects to groups?
f. In terms of the counterfactual strategies described in the textbook, what approach did the researchers use?
g. What is the specific name of the research design used in this study?
h. Is the overall design a within-subjects or between-subjects design?
i. Was any blinding (masking) used in this study?
j. Would this study be described as longitudinal? Would it be described as prospective?
k. Was this study based on an earlier pilot study?

Questions for Discussion

a. What was the intervention? Comment on how well the intervention was described, including a description of how it was developed and refined.
b. Comment on the researchers' counterfactual strategy. Could a more powerful or effective strategy have been used?
c. Discuss ways in which this study achieved or failed to achieve the criteria for making causal inferences.
d. Comment on the researchers' blinding strategy.
e. Comment on the timing of postintervention data collection.

EXERCISE 2: STUDY IN APPENDIX F

Read the method section of the article by Jurgens and colleagues ("Responding to Heart Failure Symptoms") in Appendix F. Then answer the following questions:

Questions of Fact

a. Was there an intervention in this study?
b. Is the design for this study experimental, quasi-experimental, or nonexperimental?
c. Was this a cause-probing study?
d. What were the independent and dependent variables in this study?
e. Was the independent variable amenable to manipulation?
f. Was randomization used? If yes, what method was used to assign subjects to groups?
g. What is the specific name of the research design used in this study?
h. Was any blinding (masking) used in this study?
i. Would this study be described as longitudinal? Would it be described as prospective?

Questions for Discussion

a. Comment on the researchers' comparison. Could a more powerful or effective strategy have been used?
b. Discuss ways in which this study achieved or failed to achieve the criteria for making causal inferences.
c. Comment on the timing of data collection.

▪ D. The Toolkit

For Chapter 9, the Toolkit on the accompanying CD-ROM contains a Word file with the following:

- Guidelines for Critiquing Research Designs in Quantitative Studies (Box 9.1 of the textbook)
- Table of Random Numbers: 2-Digit Numbers*
- Table of Random Numbers: 3-Digit Numbers*
- Procedures for Permuted Block Randomization*
- Situations that are Especially Conducive to a Randomized Experimental Design*
- Useful Websites for Chapter 9: Resources for Quantitative Research Design

---

*These items do not appear in the textbook.

CHAPTER 10

Rigor and Validity in Quantitative Research

■ A. Crossword Puzzle

Complete the crossword puzzle below, which uses terms and concepts presented in Chapter 10. (Puzzles may be removed for easier viewing.)

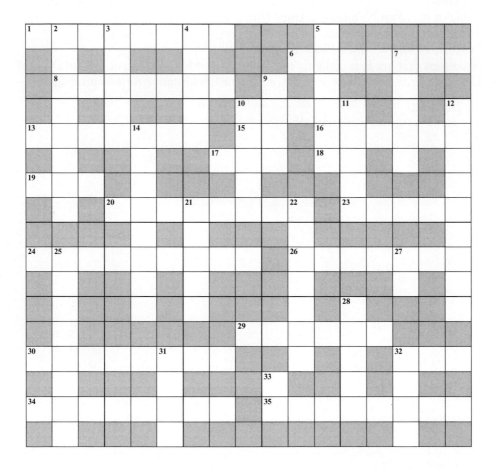

ACROSS

1. Intervention _____ concerns the faithfulness of implementing a treatment.
6. A construct validity threat that stems from what a researcher _____ can be addressed through blinding.
8. There is less extraneous variation in delivering a treatment when research personnel are well _____.
10. When statistical _____ is strengthened, statistical conclusion validity is enhanced.
13. The testing threat is the effect of a(n) _____ on subjects' performance on a posttest.
15. A professional credential of nurses
16. The _____ framework is a model for designing and testing interventions with strong internal and external validity (hyphenated).
17. The validity threat that involves changes occurring as a result of the passage of time is called _ _ _ uration.
18. In a nonexperimental study, there is no intervention and so the issue of treatment fidelity is _____ (widely used acronym).
19. In lieu of pair matching, researchers sometimes _ _ _ ance groups on confounding variables to achieve comparability.
20. Problems with construct validity involve a _____ (lack of congruence) between a higher order construct and its operationalization.
23. The principle of _ _ _ _ _ eneity, which constrains variation of extraneous variables, is a control mechanism that affects generalizability.
24. Attrition can result in the internal validity threat of _____.
26. The biggest threat to internal validity is _ _ _ _ _ _ _ on—that is, the risk of pre-existing differences between groups being compared.
29. Each _____ to validity can undermine researchers' ability to make appropriate inferences.
30. Standardization is enhanced when there is a formal _____ for delivering an intervention.
32. The type of study done in real-world clinical settings with efforts to bridge the gap between internal and external validity (acronym)
34. Internal validity can be enhanced through design decisions and through a(n) _____ of bias after the study is completed.
35. The "A" in the RE-AIM framework stands for this, referring to its degree of use.

DOWN

2. The type of validity that concerns inferences that study outcomes were caused by the independent variable rather than by other factors.
3. An aspect of intervention fidelity concerns whether or not those receiving the intervention actually _____ the skills and behaviors they learned during the intervention in real life.
4. An intention to _____ analysis involves analyzing outcomes for all people in their original treatment conditions.

5. The type of validity that concerns inferences about generalizability (abbr.)

7. One method of statistically controlling confounding variables is through analysis of _____ (abbr.).

9. If a control group member receives the intervention, this is _ _ _ _ amination of treatments.

10. Efforts to balance internal and external validity have given rise to _ _ _ _ _ical clinical trials that are conducted in real-world clinical settings (abbr.).

11. The "R" in the RE-AIM framework stands for this.

12. A threat to internal validity is temporal _____, which concerns questions about which came first, the independent or dependent variable.

14. Effectiveness trials focus on external validity issues, while _____ trials are more concerned with internal validity.

21. The "M" in the RE-AIM framework stands for _ _ _ _ _enance.

22. A threat to internal validity concerning the occurrence of events external to an independent variable that could affect outcomes

25. The bias that is of concern in crossover designs

27. Concerns inferences from the particular exemplars of a study to higher order constructs (acronym)

28. A _ _ _ _ _ulation check evaluates whether the treatment was in place as intended.

31. A potential _____ of enhancements to internal validity is that external validity could be lowered.

32. _____ matching involves one-to-one efforts to make subjects in different groups equivalent with regard to key confounding variables.

33. The best mechanism for controlling extraneous subject characteristics is _____ (acronym).

■ B. Study Questions

1. Suppose you wanted to compare the growth of infants whose mothers were heroin addicts with that of infants of nonaddicted mothers. Describe how you would design such a study, being careful to indicate what confounding variables you would need to control and how you would control them. Identify the major threats to the internal validity of your design.

2. A nurse researcher is interested in testing the effect of a special high-fiber diet on cardiovascular risk factors (e.g., cholesterol level) in adults with a family history of cardiovascular disease. Describe a design you would recommend for this problem, being careful to indicate what confounding variables you would need to control and how you would control them. Suggest methods of strengthening the power of the design. Identify possible threats to the internal validity of your design.

3. Read the method section of one of the following quasi-experimental studies. Identify one or more threats to the internal validity of the study. Then describe strategies that could be used to strengthen the study's internal validity.

- Metheny, N., Davis-Jackson, J., & Stewart, B. (2010). Effectiveness of an aspiration risk-reduction protocol. *Nursing Research, 59,* 18–25.
- Padula, C., Hughes, C., & Baumhover, L. (2009). Impact of a nurse-driven mobility protocol on functional decline in hospitalized older adults. *Journal of Nursing Care Quality, 24,* 325–331.
- Yuan, S., Chou, M., Hwu, L., Chang, Y., Hsu, W., & Kuo, H. W. (2009). An intervention program to promote health-related physical fitness in nurses. *Journal of Clinical Nursing, 18,* 1404–1411.

4. Suppose you were studying the effects of range-of-motion exercises on radical mastectomy patients. You start your experiment with 50 experimental subjects and 50 control subjects. Your intervention requires experimental subjects to come for daily sessions over a 2-week period, while control subjects come only once at the end of 2 weeks. Your final group sizes are 40 for the experimental group and 49 for the control group. The results of your study indicate that the experimental group did better in raising the arm of the affected side above head level. What effects, if any, do you think subject attrition might have had on the internal validity of your study?

5. For each of the following research questions, indicate the type of design you could use to best address it; indicate confounding variables that should be controlled and how your design would control them:

- What effect does the presence of the newborn's father in the delivery room have on the mother's subjective report of pain?
- What is the effect of different types of bowel evacuation regimes for quadriplegic patients?
- Does the inability to speak and understand English affect a person's access to hospice services?

6. Read the introduction and methods section of one of the following reports. Use the critiquing guidelines in Box 10.1 of the textbook (available as a Word document in the Toolkit ✪) to assess the study's validity:

- Baraz, S., Parvardeh, S., Mohammadi, E., & Broumand, B. (2010). Dietary and fluid compliance: An educational intervention for patients having haemodialysis. *Journal of Advanced Nursing, 66,* 60–68.
- Crilly, J., Chaboyer, W., Wallis, M., Thalib, L., & Polit, D.F. (2010). An outcomes evaluation of an Australian Hospital in the Nursing Home admission avoidance programme. *Journal of Clinical Nursing, 19,* 3010–3018.
- Rice, V., Weglicki, L., Templin, T., Jamil, H., & Hammad, A. (2010). Intervention effects on tobacco use in Arab and non-Arab adolescents. *Addictive Behaviors, 35,* 46–48.
- Wujcik, D., Shyr, Y., Li, M., Clayton, M., Ellington, L., Menon, U., & Mooney, K. (2009). Delay in diagnostic testing after abnormal mammography in low-income women. *Oncology Nursing Forum, 36,* 709–715.

■ C. Application Exercises

EXERCISE 1: STUDY IN APPENDIX A

Read the method section of the article by Kennedy and Chen ("Changes in childhood risk taking") in Appendix A. Then answer the following questions:

Questions of Fact

a. Which of the methods of research control described in this chapter were used to control confounding variables?
b. Could this study have been designed as a crossover study?
c. What confounding variables were controlled?
d. Was there any attrition in this study?
e. Was an intention-to-treat analysis performed?
f. Is there evidence that constancy of conditions was achieved?
g. Were group treatments as distinct as possible to maximize power? If not, why not?
h. Was selection a threat to the internal validity of this study?
i. Was mortality a threat to the internal validity of this study?

Questions for Discussion

a. Does this study seem strong in terms of statistical conclusion validity? How could statistical conclusion validity have been strengthened?
b. Discuss issues relating to the intervention fidelity in this study.
c. Is this study strong in internal validity? What, if any, are the threats to the internal validity of this study?
d. Is this study strong in construct validity? What, if any, are the threats to the construct validity of this study?
e. Is this study strong on external validity? What, if any, are the threats to the external validity of this study?
f. Consider the pros and cons of adding an attention control group in this study. What type of *attention* condition could have been used?

EXERCISE 2: STUDY IN APPENDIX D

Read the methods and results sections of the report by Whittemore and colleagues ("Diabetes prevention program") in Appendix D. Then answer the following questions:

Questions of Fact

a. Is the design for this study experimental, quasi-experimental, or nonexperimental?
b. What were the independent and dependent variables in this study?
c. Was randomization used? What was the unit of randomization? Why was this unit of randomization used?

d. Which of the methods of research control described in this chapter were used to control confounding variables?
e. What confounding variables were controlled?
f. Was there any attrition in this study?
g. Was an intention-to-treat analysis performed?
h. What did the researchers do to strengthen the external validity of this study?

Questions for Discussion

a. What was the intervention? Comment on how well the intervention was described, including the description of how it was developed and refined.
b. Comment on the researchers' counterfactual strategy. Could a more powerful or effective strategy have been used?
c. Does this study seem strong in terms of statistical conclusion validity? How could statistical conclusion validity have been strengthened?
d. Discuss issues relating to intervention fidelity in this study.
e. Is this study strong in internal validity? What, if any, are the threats to the internal validity of this study?
f. Is this study strong in construct validity? What, if any, are the threats to the construct validity of this study?
g. Is this study strong on external validity? What, if any, are the threats to the external validity of this study?

▪ D. The Toolkit

For Chapter 10, the Toolkit on the accompanying CD-ROM contains a Word file with the following:

- Guidelines for Critiquing Design Elements and Study Validity in Quantitative Studies (Box 10.1 of the textbook)
- Example of a Table of Contents for a Procedures Manual for an Intervention Study*
- Example of an Observational Checklist for Monitoring Delivery of an Intervention*
- Example of a Contact Information Form for a Longitudinal Study*
- Example of Methods to Enhance External Validity, and Potential Associated Costs to Internal (or Other) Validity*
- Matrix for Design Decisions and Possible Effects on Study Validity*
- Useful Websites for Chapter 10: Resources for Quantitative Research Design

---

*These items do not appear in the textbook.

CHAPTER 11

Specific Types of Quantitative Research

■ A. Crossword Puzzle

Complete the crossword puzzle below, which uses terms and concepts presented in Chapter 11. (Puzzles may be removed for easier viewing.)

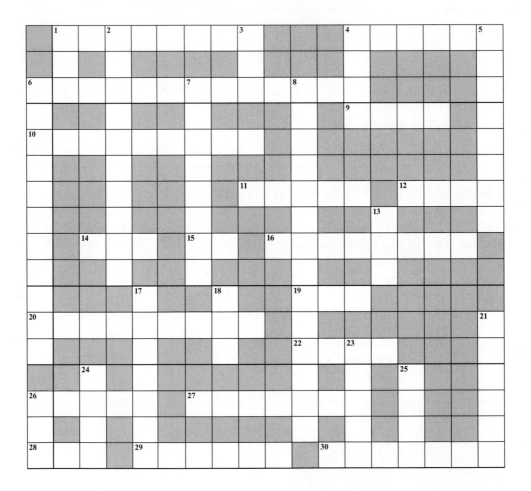

Copyright © 2012 Wolters Kluwer Health I Lippincott Williams & Wilkins. Polit & Beck: *Resource Manual for Nursing Research: Generating and Assessing Evidence for Nursing Practice* (9th ed.)

ACROSS

1. Interviews that are done face-to-face
4. A(n) _ _ _ _ _ _ive evaluation assesses the worth of a program or policy (abbr.).
6. A multiphase effort to refine and test the effectiveness of a clinical intervention (2 words)
9. Another term for interviews done in person is _____ to _____.
10. An analysis of data done with an existing dataset
11. Surveys can be done by distributing _ _ _ _ _ionnaires by mail (abbr.).
12. A(n) _ _ _ _id design is an effort to bridge the gap between efficacy and effectiveness studies.
14. An impact analysis provides information about the _____ effects of a program.
15. In a clinical trial, the phase sometimes called effectiveness research
16. _ _ _ _ _ _ _ _ _ic research focuses on improving research strategies (abbr.).
19. An alternative to in-person interviews is interviews by _ _ _ephone.
20. A method of collecting self-report data orally
22. A Phase II trial often involves a pilot _____ of a new treatment.
26. In clinical trials, an efficacy study is the third _____.
27. In evaluations, a(n) _____ analysis describes the extent to which a program is achieving certain goals.
28. The phase of a clinical trial that is an RCT
29. A Gallup poll is one of these.
30. A(n) _ _ _ _ _ _ _ _ors approach to needs assessments involves organizing existing information

DOWN

1. Findings from evaluations and outcomes research can be used in the formulation of local and national _ _ _icies.
2. A Phase III clinical trial is usually a(n) _____ controlled trial.
3. Personal interviews are an expensive approach to surveys because they require a _____ of personnel time.
4. Data collected by asking people questions in a survey is via _____ reports.
5. In the Donabedian framework, the three key factors are process, outcomes, and s_ _ _ _ _ _ _ _.
6. One type of evaluation of the economic effects of an intervention (2 words)
7. In a cost utility _____, quality-adjusted life year is often an important outcome.
8. An evaluation of the process of putting a new intervention into place is a(n) _____ analysis.
13. Acronym for an important classification system of outcomes for nurses
17. Another name for an implementation analysis is _____ analysis.
18. Sometimes surveys can be administered over the Inter _____.

21. The type of evaluation that uses an experimental design is a(n) _____ analysis.
23. A _____ assessment can use a survey or key informant approach (backwards!).
24. A new survey technology that gives respondents privacy in answering questions is audio-_____.
25. Large-scale telephone surveys increasingly rely on _____ technology.
26. The Del_ _ _ technique involves multiple rounds of questioning to achieve consensus.

■ B. Study Questions

1. Suppose you were interested in studying the research questions below by conducting a survey. For each, indicate whether you would recommend using a personal interview, a telephone interview, or a self-administered questionnaire to collect the data. What is your rationale?

   a. What are the health-related problems of military personnel returning from combat deployments?
   b. What strategies do emergency department nurses use to identify and correct medical errors?
   c. What type of nursing communications do presurgical patients find most helpful?
   d. What is the relationship between a teenager's health-risk appraisal and their risk-taking behavior (e.g., smoking, unprotected sex, drug use, etc.)?
   e. What are the health-promoting activities pursued by inner-city single mothers?
   f. How is employment of parents affected by the health problems or disability of a child?

2. Identify a nursing-sensitive outcome. Propose a research question that would use the outcome as the dependent variable. Would you consider the research to answer this question an example of outcomes research?

3. Read the introduction and method section of one of the following reports. Use the critiquing guidelines in Box 11.1 of the textbook (available as a Word document in the Toolkit ✖) to critique the study:

   • Kwekkeboom, K., Abbott-Anderson, K., & Wanta, B. (2010). Feasibility of a patient-controlled cognitive behavioral intervention for pain, fatigue, and sleep disturbance in cancer. *Oncology Nursing Forum, 37*(3), E151–159.
   • McIlrath, C., Keeney, S., McKenna, H., & McLaughlin, D. (2010). Benchmarks for effective primary care-based nursing services for adults with depression. *Journal of Advanced Nursing, 66*, 269–281.
   • Roche, M., Diers, D., Duffield, C., & Catling-Paul, C. (2010). Violence toward nurses, the work environment, and patient outcomes. *Journal of Nursing Scholarship, 42*, 13–22.

- York, N., & Lee, K. (2010). A baseline evaluation of casino air quality after enactment of Nevada's Clean Indoor Air Act. *Public Health Nursing, 27,* 158–163.

▪ C. Application Exercises

EXERCISE 1: STUDIES IN APPENDICES A, D, F, AND H

Which of the studies in the specified appendices of this *Resource Manual* (if any) could be considered:

a. A clinical trial?
b. Outcomes research?
c. Survey research?
d. A needs assessment?
e. A replication?
f. A secondary analysis?

EXERCISE 2: STUDY IN APPENDIX J

Read the first few sections (the sections before "Data Analysis") of the article by Kalisch and colleagues ("Nursing Teamwork Survey") in Appendix J. Then answer the following questions:

Questions of Fact

a. Was this study a clinical trial or nursing intervention research? If yes, what phase would this most likely be?
b. Was this study an evaluation? If yes, what type (process analysis, etc.)?
c. Was this outcomes research?
d. Was this study a survey?
e. Was this study an example of methodologic research?
f. What is the basic research design for this study (i.e., experimental, nonexperimental, etc.)?

Questions for Discussion

a. Comment on the adequacy and appropriateness of the use of various types of data in this study.
b. What are some of the uses to which the findings and product of this study could be put?

■ D. The Toolkit

For Chapter 11, the Toolkit on the accompanying CD-ROM contains a Word file with the following:

- Some Guidelines for Critiquing Studies Described in Chapter 11 (Box 11.1 of the textbook)
- Guidelines for Critiquing a Cost/Economic Analysis*
- Useful Websites for Chapter 11: Resources for Specific Types of Research

----

*This item does not appear in the textbook.

CHAPTER 12

Sampling in Quantitative Research

■ A. Crossword Puzzle

Complete the crossword puzzle below, which uses terms and concepts presented in Chapter 12. (Puzzles may be removed for easier viewing.)

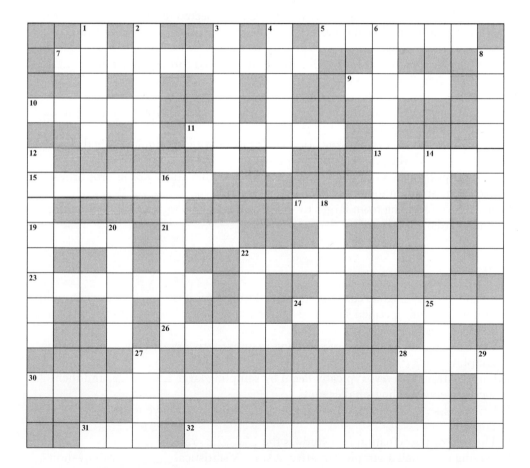

ACROSS

5. The _ _ _ _ _ _ible population is the one that is available to a researcher.
7. An aggregate set of individuals or objects with specified characteristics
9. Another name for purposive sampling is _ _ _ _mental sampling.
10. A sample is a s_ _ _ _ _ of a specified population.
11. An effect size summarizes the _ _ _ _ _ _th of a relationship between two variables.
13. Criteria designating characteristics a population does *not* have are _ _ _ _ _sion criteria.
15. The most basic unit of a population
17. A distortion that arises when a sample is not representative of the population reflects sampling _____.
19. A sampling approach in which participants are selected because of known attributes is called _ _ _ _osive sampling.
21. The bias arising when some potential respondents decline is _____ response bias.
22. In _ _ _ _ _ _atic sampling, every *k*th element is selected (abbr.).
23. A type of sampling based on referrals from participants is sometimes called _____ sampling.
24. The specific attributes of a population are designated through eligibility _____.
26. A strong sampling design can enhance the study's value for evidence-_____ practice.
28. A sampling method involving referrals from other people already in the sample is _ _ _ _ball sampling.
30. In quantitative studies, the key criterion for evaluating a sample is whether it is _____ of the population.
31. _ _ _proportionate sampling involves sampling within strata *not* in proportion to the size of the strata in the population.
32. Successive sampling from larger to smaller units occurs in _____ sampling (backwards!).

DOWN

1. Sampling every eligible case for a specified time period is _ _ _ _ _cutive sampling.
2. Sampling within specified subgroups of the population, using nonprobability sampling
3. Subdivisions of a population
4. The most widely used type of sampling in quantitative research is _ _ _ _ _ _ience sampling.
6. Large national surveys typically begin by sampling large _____, and then successively sampling smaller units.
8. Criteria specifying characteristics that participants *must* have to be included in the sample
12. The rate of participation in a study is the _____ rate.
14. Having too small a sample can affect a study's statistical _ _ _ _ _usion validity.

16. Sampling methods in which not every element of a population has an equal chance of being selected (abbr.)
18. The sampling _ _ _ _ _ _ al is the standard distance between elements in a systematic sample.
20. _____ analysis is used by quantitative researchers to estimate the number of subjects needed in a study.
22. The total number of participants in a study is the sample _____.
25. A probability sample involves selection of elements at _____.
27. A stratified random sample is _____ likely to be biased than a quota sample.
29. When disproportionate sampling is used, _ _ _ _ hting is necessary to arrive at estimates of overall population values.

■ B. Study Questions

1. Draw a simple random sample of 15 people from the sampling frame of Table 12.3 of the textbook, using the table of random numbers that appears in Table 9.2. Begin your selection by blindly placing your finger at some point on the table.

2. Suppose you have decided to use a systematic sampling design for a study. The known population size is 5,000, and the sample size desired is 250. What is the sampling interval? If the first element selected is 23, what would be the second, third, and fourth elements selected?

3. Suppose you were interested in studying the attitude of clinical specialists toward autonomy in work situations. Suggest a possible target and accessible population. What strata might be identified if quota sampling were used?

4. Identify the type of quantitative sampling design used in the following examples:
   a. One hundred inmates randomly sampled from a random selection of five federal penitentiaries
   b. All the oncology nurses participating in a continuing education seminar
   c. Every 20th patient admitted to the emergency room between January and June
   d. The first 20 male and the first 20 female patients admitted to the hospital with hypothermia
   e. A sample of 250 members randomly selected from a roster of American Nurses' Association members
   f. 25 experts in critical care nursing

5. Nurse A is planning to study the effects of maternal stress, maternal depression, maternal age, and family economic resources on a child's socioemotional development among both intact and mother-headed families. Nurse B is planning to study body position on patients' respiratory functioning. Describe the kinds of samples that the two nurses would need to use. Which nurse would need the larger sample? Defend your answer.

6. Read the introduction and method section of one of the following articles. Use the guidelines in Box 12.1 of the textbook (available as a Word document in the Toolkit ✪) to critique the sampling plan:

- Chuang, C., Chang, P., Chen, Y., Hsieh, W., Lin, S., & Chen, P. (2010). Maternal return to work and breastfeeding: A population-based cohort study. *International Journal of Nursing Studies, 47,* 461–474.
- Clark, M., & Diamond, P. (2010). Depression in family caregivers of elders: A theoretical model of caregiver burden, sociotropy, and autonomy. *Research in Nursing & Health, 33,* 20–34.
- Ridner, S. L., Walker, K., Hart, J., & Myers, J. (2010). Smoking identities and behavior: Evidence of discrepancies, issues for measurement and intervention. *Western Journal of Nursing Research, 32,* 434–446.

■ C. Application Exercises

EXERCISE 1: STUDIES IN APPENDICES A, C, D, H, AND J

a. Which of the studies in the selected appendices of this *Resource Manual* (if any) used a probability sample?
b. Which of the studies in the selected appendices of this *Resource Manual* (if any) used convenience sampling?
c. Which of the studies in the selected appendices of this *Resource Manual* (if any) used quota sampling?

EXERCISE 2: STUDY IN APPENDIX F

Read the method sections of the article by Jurgens and colleagues ("Responding to heart failure symptoms") in Appendix F. Then answer the following questions:

Questions of Fact

a. What was the target population of this study? How would you describe the accessible population?
b. What were the eligibility criteria for the study?
c. Was the sampling method probability or nonprobability? What specific sampling method was used?
d. How were study participants recruited?
e. What efforts did the researchers make to ensure a diverse (and hence more representative) sample?
f. What was the sample size that the research team achieved?
g. Was a power analysis used to determine sample size needs? If yes, what number of subjects did the power analysis estimate as the minimum needed number?

Questions for Discussion

a. Comment on the adequacy of the researchers' sampling plan and recruitment strategy. How representativeness was the sample of the target population? What types of sampling biases might be of special concern?
b. Do you think the sample size was adequate? Why or why not?

■ D. The Toolkit

For Chapter 12, the Toolkit on the accompanying CD-ROM contains a Word file with the following:

- Guidelines for Critiquing Quantitative Sampling Designs (Box 12.1 of the textbook)
- Useful Websites for Chapter 12: Resources for Sampling

Data Collection in Quantitative Research

■ A. Crossword Puzzle

Complete the crossword puzzle below, which uses terms and concepts presented in Chapter 13. (Puzzles may be removed for easier viewing.)

ACROSS

1. In structured observation, a(n) _____ is used with a category system to record the incidence of observed events or behaviors.
5. A tool that yields a score placing people on a continuum with regard to an attribute
7. In observation studies, the instruments should be tested by having two or more _ _ _ependent observers code or rate the event and then comparing results.
9. One method of recording observations is to have observers use _____ scales to provide judgments about the behavioral construct along a continuum.
11. The type of question most prevalent in self-administered questionnaires (2 words)
14. Respondents rate concepts on a series of bipolar rating scales in a(n) _ _ _ _ _ _ic differential.
15. A description of a situation or person designed to elicit study participants' reactions
19. A _____ card is presented to respondents in interviews when response options are complex or multiple questions have the same options.
21. The tendency to distort self-report information in characteristic ways is a response _____ bias.
22. The two _____ alternatives to "What is your gender?" are "male" and "female."
23. One advantage of using questionnaires is the absence of any interviewer _____.
26. A(n) _ _ _ _ _ _iew is a type of self-report that typically yields better quality data than a self-administered questionnaire.
30. One type of observational bias is the bias toward central _____, which distorts observations toward a middle ground.
33. The error of _____ occurs when observers characteristically rate things positively.
34. A Likert-type scale may also be referred to as a _ _ _ _ated rating scale.
35. The type of question that forces respondents to select one of two competing alternatives (2 words)

DOWN

1. A(n) _ _ _egory system is used to organize observational events or occurrences.
2. A type of summated rating scale used to measure agreement or disagreement with statements
3. Extracting biophysiologic material from people yields _____ vitro measures.
4. On an agreement continuum, the most extreme negative response option (acronym)
6. In Q-sorts, the objects being sorted are _____.
8. One advantage of questionnaires is that responses can be _ _ _ _ ymous, which ensures privacy.
10. The type of observational sampling approach used to select periods when observations are made
12. The type of observational sampling involving integral episodes
13. A bias stemming from people's wanting to "look good" is called a social _____ bias.
15. A questioning method to measure clinical symptoms along a 100-mm continuum is a _____ analog scale.

16. A self-report approach involving the sorting of statements into different piles along a continuum.
17. On a 5-point Likert scale, if SD were scored 5, SA would be scored _____.
18. The error of _____ occurs when observers characteristically rate things too harshly.
20. Self-report instruments can be administered as _____-based surveys over the Internet.
24. Filter questions often involve the use of _____ patterns to route people appropriately through a self-report instrument.
25. A rating scale along the continuum "exhausted" to "energized" is using _____ adjectives.
27. If both positive and negative items were included in a scale, the researcher would need to _____ the scoring of one type or the other before summing item scores.
28. The question "What is it like to be a cancer survivor?" is _____ ended.
29. The most widely used method of data collection by nurse researchers is by _____-report.
31. The number of piles in a Q-sort is typically _____ or eleven.
32. Many psychosocial scales are called _ _ _ _ osite scales because they are a combination of multiple items.

■ B. Study Questions

1. Suppose you were interested in studying attitudes toward risky behavior (e.g., unsafe sex, drug use, speeding) among adolescents. Develop the following types of questions designed to measure these attitudes.
   a. A forced-choice item
   b. A Likert-type item
   c. An open-ended question

2. Below are hypothetical responses for Respondent Y and Respondent Z to the statements on the Likert scale presented in Table 13.2 of the textbook. What would the total score for both of these respondents be, using the scoring rules described in Chapter 13?

Item No.	Respondent Y	Respondent Z
1	D	SA
2	A	D
3	SA	D
4	?	A
5	D	SA
6	SA	D
TOTAL SCORE:	___	___

3. Below are hypothetical responses for Respondents A, B, C, and D to the Likert statements presented in Table 13.2 of the text. Three of these four sets of responses contain some indication of a possible response-set bias. Identify *which* three, and identify the types of bias.

Item No.	Respondent A	Respondent B	Respondent C	Respondent D
1	A	SA	SD	D
2	A	SD	SA	SD
3	SA	D	SA	D
4	A	A	SD	SD
5	SA	A	SD	SD
6	SA	SD	SA	D
Bias:	_____	_____	_____	_____

4. Identify five constructs of clinical relevance that would be appropriate for measurement using a visual analog scale (VAS).

5. Suggest response alternatives for the following questions that might appear in a questionnaire.
   a. In a typical month, how frequently do you practice breast self-examination?
   b. When was the last time you had your blood pressure tested?
   c. Which of the following statements best describes your attitude toward nurse practitioners?
   d. What is your marital status?
   e. How would you rate your nursing research instruction in terms of overall quality of teaching?
   f. How often do you skip breakfast?
   g. How important is it to you to avoid a pregnancy at this time?
   h. How many cigarettes do you smoke in a typical day?
   i. From which of the following sources have you learned about the dangers of smoking?
   j. Which of the following statements best describes the physical pain you experienced during labor and delivery?

6. Hall administered a survey to high school students to learn about their eating patterns, particularly focusing on their consumption of high-fat foods. She distributed questionnaires that were accompanied with a cover letter that follows. Review and critique this cover letter, analyzing its tone, wording, and content.

   Dear Student:
   This questionnaire is part of a study to learn about some health-related issues among high school students. Through this study, we hope to have a better understanding of young people in America. Students from 25 high schools in the United States are being asked to help us in this effort. Your high school was selected at random.

Your responses to this questionnaire are completely anonymous. No one will know your answers, and so, even though some of the questions are personal, we hope that you will answer honestly. The quality of the picture we will have of high school students today depends on your willingness to provide thorough and honest answers.

Please answer every question. When you are through, please turn the questionnaire in to your homeroom teacher.

Your cooperation in completing this questionnaire is deeply appreciated.

Sincerely,
Liz Hall, R.N.

7. Construct a VAS to measure fatigue. Administer the VAS two ways: (1) to yourself at 10 different times of the day and (2) to 10 different people at the same time of day. For the two types of administrations, is there similarity in scores, or is there a wide range of responses? Which of the two yields scores with a wider range?

8. Below is a list of five variables. Indicate briefly how you would operationalize each using structured observational procedures.
   a. Fear in hospitalized children
   b. Pain during childbirth
   c. Dependency in psychiatric patients
   d. Empathy in nursing students
   e. Cooperativeness in chemotherapy patients

9. Three nurse researchers were collaborating on a study of the effect of preoperative visits to surgical patients by operating room nurses on the stress levels of those patients just before surgery. One researcher wanted to use the patients' self-reports to measure stress; the second suggested using pulse rate and the Palmer Sweat Index; the third recommended using an observational measure of stress. Which measure do you think would be the most appropriate for this research problem? Can you suggest other possible measures of stress that might be even more appropriate? Justify your response.

10. Read the introduction and methods section of one of the following reports. Use the critiquing guidelines in Boxes 13.3 and 13.4 of the textbook (available as Word documents in the Toolkit ❌) to critique the data collection aspects of the study:
    • Pressler, S., Subramanian, U., Kareken, D., Perkins, S., Gradus-Pizlo, I, Sauvé, M. J., Ding, Y., Kim, J., Sloan, R., Jaynes, H., & Shaw, R. M. (2010). Cognitive deficits in chronic heart failure. *Nursing Research, 59,* 127–139.
    • Stewart, J., Mishel, M., Lynn, M., & Terhorst, L. (2010). Test of a conceptual model of uncertainty in children and adolescents with cancer. *Research in Nursing & Health, 33,* 179–191.
    • Swenson, K., Nissen, M., & Henly, S. (2010). Physical activity in women receiving chemotherapy for breast cancer. *Oncology Nursing Forum, 37,* 321–330.

■ C. Application Exercises

EXERCISE 1: STUDY IN APPENDIX C

Read the method section of the article by Yackel and colleagues ("Nurse-facilitated depression screening program") in Appendix C. What types of data did the researchers collect in this EBP project? Comment on the data collection plan, and the specific methods used to collect data. What recommendations would you make for supplementary data, keeping in mind the practical constraints of this practice project?

EXERCISE 2: STUDY IN APPENDIX D

Read the method section of the article by Whittemore and colleagues ("Diabetes prevention program") in Appendix D. Then answer the following questions, focusing in particular on what the researchers did to collect data on program efficacy:

Questions of Fact

a. Did this study use any self-report measures? What variables were measured by self-report?

b. Were examples of specific questions included in the report?

c. Did the researchers' instruments include both open-ended and closed-ended questions? Did the report mention the use of any specific types of self-reports, such as visual analog scales, forced-choice questions, event calendar questions, and so on?

d. Were any composite scales used? If yes, were they of the Likert type?

e. Was self-report data gathered by interview or by self-administered questionnaires (or both)?

f. Did the researchers develop their own self-report measures, or did they use instruments or scales that had been developed by others?

g. Did the researchers describe the criteria they used in selecting instruments? If so, what were they?

h. Did the report mention anything about the readability level of self-report instruments?

i. Did the report describe how long it took, on average, for respondents to complete the self-report instrument?

j. Did the researchers collect any data through observation? If no, could observation have been used to measure key concepts? If yes, what variables were measured through observation?

k. Did the researchers collect any biophysiologic measures? If yes, what variables were measured through biophysiologic methods?

l. Does the report describe the procedures for using biophysiologic measurements? Were procedures standardized?

m. Who gathered the data in this study? How were the data collectors trained?

Questions for Discussion

a. Comment on the adequacy of the researchers' description of their data collection approaches and procedures.

b. Do you think that Whittemore and colleagues operationalized their outcome measures in the best possible manner? Could different or supplementary measures have been used to enhance the quality of the study's evidence?

c. Comment on the procedures used to collect data in this study. Were adequate steps taken to ensure the highest possible quality data?

■ D. The Toolkit

For Chapter 13, the Toolkit on the accompanying CD-ROM contains a Word file with the following:

- Guidelines for Critiquing Data Collection Plans (Box 13.3 of the textbook)
- Guidelines for Critiquing Structured Data Collection Methods (Box 13.4 of the textbook)
- Data Collection Flow Chart*
- Example of a Cover Letter for a Mailed Questionnaire (Figure 13.4 of the textbook)
- Example of a Visual Analog Scale
- Example of a Show Card for a Personal Interview*
- Example of a Reminder Postcard for a Mailed Questionnaire*
- Example of an Event History Calendar*
- Example of a Data Matrix for Recording Data Decisions*
- Example of a Table of Contents for an Interviewer Training Manual*
- Model Sections for an Interviewer Training Manual*
  - Answering Respondents' Questions
  - Avoiding Interviewer Bias
  - Probing and Obtaining Full Responses
- Annotated Guidelines Relating to Key Demographic Questions*
- Basic Demographic Questionnaire*
- Example of a Letter Requesting Permission to Use an Instrument*
- Useful Websites for Chapter 13: Resources for Structured Data Collection

---

*These items do not appear in the textbook.

CHAPTER **14**

Measurement and Data Quality

■ A. Crossword Puzzle

Complete the crossword puzzle below, which uses terms and concepts presented in Chapter 14. (Puzzles may be removed for easier viewing.)

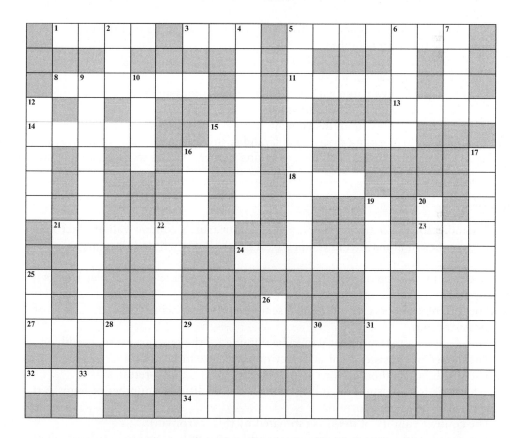

ACROSS

1. The type of validity involving the extent to which a measure "looks" valid
3. Sensitivity is plotted against specificity in a(n) _ _ _ curve (acronym).
5. The type of validity concerned with adequate representation of all facets of a concept's domain
8. Predictive validity and concurrent validity are aspects of _ _ _ _ _ _ ion-related validity.
11. An unreliable instrument could _____ be valid.
13. A receiver _ _ _ _ ating curve can be used to determine the best dividing point for cases and noncases in a screening instrument.
14. Measurement involves assigning numbers according to established _____.
15. The kappa statistic can be used to estimate inter-_____ reliability.
18. One means of assessing construct validity is through the known _____ technique (abbr.).
21. The ability of an instrument to differentiate the construct being measured from other similar concepts (abbr.)
23. An index relating to specificity and sensitivity that captures proportion of area and indicates degree of accuracy (acronym)
24. The most widely evaluated aspect of reliability is a measure's _____ consistency.
27. A thorough evaluation of an instrument involves a(n) _____ assessment.
31. To assess the stability of an instrument, it must be administered _____.
32. An approach to assessing discriminant validity involves _____ trait measurement.
34. To _____ an attribute involves assigning numeric values to designate its quantity.

DOWN

2. The indicator summarizing assessments of a measure's content validity (acronym)
4. The coefficient alpha was developed by a psychologist whose last name was _____.
5. Evidence that different methods of measuring an attribute yield similar results supports _____ validity.
6. The difference between an obtained score and the true score is the _____ of measurement.
7. The score on a measure that would be obtained if the measure were infallible
9. The degree of consistency or accuracy of a measure indicates its _____.
10. The reliability method used to assess stability is _____–retest.
12. A formula for adjusting reliability coefficients for different number of items is the Spearman-_____ formula.
16. The content validity of *items* is estimated by this (acronym).
17. The correlation between an instrument and a currently measured criterion gives an estimate of _____ validity.

19. An instrument's ability to identify a case correctly is its _ _ _ _ _ _ _ _ ity.
20. A criterion for assessing the extent to which an instrument measures what it purports to measure
22. A likelihood _____ summarizes the relationship between specificity and sensitivity in a single number.
25. The proportion of people with a positive result who have the target outcome or disease (backwards acronym)
26. An alternative to classical measurement theory (acronym)
28. In screening instruments, "cases" are separated from "noncases" at the _____ off point.
29. A complex technique for exploring construct validity with multiple measures of multiple constructs (acronym)
30. The _____ coefficient is an index used to summarize the magnitude and direction of relationships between variables (abbr.).
33. The ratio of true-positive results to false-positive results is the _ _+.

▪ B. Study Questions

1. The reliability of measures of which of the following attributes would *not* be appropriately assessed using a test–retest procedure with 1 month between administrations. Why?
   a. Attitudes toward abortion:
   b. Stress:
   c. Achievement motivation:
   d. Nursing effectiveness:
   e. Depression:

2. Comment on the meaning and implications of the following statement:

   A researcher found that the internal consistency of her 20-item scale measuring attitudes toward nurse–midwives was .74, using the Cronbach alpha formula.

3. In the following situation, what might be some of the sources of measurement error?

   One hundred nurses who worked in a large metropolitan hospital were asked to complete a 10-item Likert scale designed to measure job satisfaction. The questionnaires were distributed by nursing supervisors at the end of shifts. The staff nurses were asked to complete the forms and return them immediately to their supervisors.

4. Identify what is incorrect about the following statements:
   a. "My scale is highly reliable, so it must be valid."
   b. "My instrument yielded an internal consistency coefficient of .80, so it must be stable."
   c. "The validity coefficient between my scale and a criterion measure was .40; therefore, my scale must be of low validity."

    d. "My scale had a reliability coefficient of .80. Therefore, an obtained score of 20 is indicative of a true score of 16."

    e. "The validation study proved that my measure has construct validity."

    f. "My advisor examined my new measure of dependence in nursing home residents and, based on its content, assured me the measure was valid."

5. An instructor has developed an instrument to measure knowledge of research terminology. Would you say that more reliable measurements would be yielded before or after a year of instruction on research methodology, using the exact same test, or would there be no difference? Why?

6. What types of groups do you feel might be useful for a known-groups approach assessing contrast validity for a measure of the following?

    a. Emotional maturity

    b. Attitudes toward alcoholics

    c. Territorial aggressiveness

    d. Job motivation

    e. Subjective pain

7. Read the introduction and method section of one of the following reports. Use the critiquing guidelines in Box 14.1 of the textbook (available as a Word document in the Toolkit ✖) to critique the measurement and data quality aspects of the study:

    • Larrabee, J., Wu, Y., Persily, C., Simoni, P., Johnston, P., Marcischak, T., Mott, C. L., & Gladden, S. D. (2010). Influence of stress resiliency on RN job satisfaction and intent to stay. *Western Journal of Nursing Research, 32,* 81–102.

    • Sammarco, A., & Konecny, L. (2010). Quality of life, social support, and uncertainty among Latina and Caucasian breast cancer survivors: A comparative study. *Oncology Nursing Forum, 37,* 93–99.

    • Sutton, D., & Raines, D. (2010). Health-related quality of life following a surgical weight loss intervention. *Applied Nursing Research, 23,* 52–56.

■ C. Application Exercise

Read the method section of the article by Kennedy and Chen ("Changes in childhood risk taking") in Appendix A—paying special attention to the subsections labeled "Measures." Then answer the following questions:

Questions of Fact

a. Where was information about the psychometric properties of the instruments used in this study presented?

b. Was information about internal consistency reliability (as found in previous studies) reported for all of the instruments used in the study? If not, for which scales was internal consistency not reported?

c. Were any of the Cronbach alphas reported less than .70? If yes, for which scales or subscales?

d. Was stability assessed for any of the scales? If yes, which ones? What was the interval used in these scales for assessing stability? Were any of the stability coefficients less than .70?

e. What approach to validity was reported as having been used for the following scales:
   - Self-Perception Profile
   - Child's Health Self-Concept Scale
   - Short Acculturation Scale
   - Injury Behavior Checklist?

f. Did Kennedy and Chen rely on assessments of reliability from other researchers, or did they perform any reliability assessments themselves?

g. Was information about the specificity or sensitivity of any of the instruments provided in the report?

Questions for Discussion

a. Describe what some of the sources of measurement error might have been in this study. Did the researchers take adequate steps to minimize measurement error?

b. For scales without information on test–retest reliability, do you think that stability is an important aspect of capturing the construct reliably?

c. Comment on the adequacy of information in the report about efforts to select or develop high-quality instruments.

d. Comment on the quality of the measures that Kennedy and Chen used in their study. Do you feel confident that instruments yielded adequately reliable and valid measures of the key constructs?

■ D. The Toolkit

For Chapter 14, the Toolkit on the accompanying CD-ROM contains a Word file with the following:

- Guidelines for Critiquing Data Quality in Quantitative Studies (Box 14.1 of the textbook)
- Suggestions for Enhancing Data Quality and Minimizing Measurement Error in Quantitative Studies*
- Useful Websites for Chapter 14: Resources for Measurement and Data Quality

---

*This item does not appear in the textbook.

CHAPTER 15

Developing and Testing Self-Report Scales

■ A. Crossword Puzzle

Complete the crossword puzzle below, which uses terms and concepts presented in Chapter 15. (Puzzles may be removed for easier viewing.)

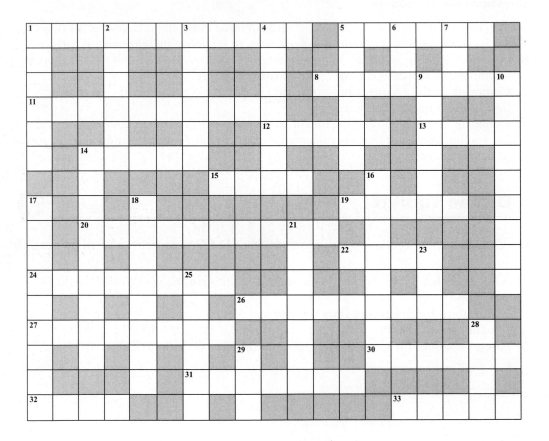

ACROSS

1. The type of factor analysis that stipulates no a priori hypotheses about the dimensionality of a set of items
5. _____ analysis is used to shed light on the dimensionality of a set of items.
8. In translations, _____ equivalence concerns the extent to which the meaning of items is the same in the target language as it was in the source.
11. In principal components analysis, a(n) _____ is equal to the sum of squared weights for a factor.
12. When item difficulty is the only parameter being considered in an IRT analysis, it is said to be a _____ model.
13. Developing a pool of items is often best done as a _____ effort.
14. Initially, it is best to develop 3 to 4 times as many _____ as are believed to be needed for a scale.
15. On a Likert-type scale, each item consists of a declarative _____ and a set of response options.
19. In confirmatory factor analysis, the first phase involves testing of a measurement _____.
20. In EFA, the first phase is called factor _____.
22. One index of readability is the reading _____ score.
24. Most Likert-type scales have five or seven _____ options.
26. The most widely used factor extraction method is _____ components analysis.
27. The purpose of a scale is not to place participants into a(n) _____ but rather to array them along a continuum.
30. In scale development, a(n) _____ sampling model is often assumed—random sampling of a set of items from a hypothetical universe of items (backwards!).
31. One source of items for a new scale is from a _____ analysis.
32. In item response theory, items with different levels of _ _ _ _iculty are sought.
33. Development of a high-quality multi-item _____ is a challenging, labor-intensive activity.

DOWN

1. In content validation work, it is necessary to establish a(n) _____ panel to review items.
2. The underlying construct in a scale is sometimes referred to as the _____ variable.
3. In wording items, double negatives should _____ be avoided.
4. If there are negative and positive items on a scale, some have to be _____-scored.
5. The _____-Kinkaid grade level is one of several indexes of readability.
6. The type of factor analysis undertaken to test and confirm hypotheses about items and scales (acronym)
7. One purpose of a panel of content experts is to weed _____ faulty or weak items.
9. Translations are typically done into the _____ tongue of the translator.
10. Translations and back translations typically involve the use of a(n) _____ to arrive at a consensus.

14. For a traditional Likert-type scale, item _____ should be comparable across items.
16. In exploratory factor analysis, the second phase involves factor _____.
17. In computing item–scale correlations, the preferred approach is the _____ approach, which removes the item from the calculation of the total scale score.
18. In a Likert scale, items should be fairly _____ worded so that differences of opinion can be elicited.
21. Factor rotation can be orthogonal or _____.
23. The type of factor analysis that does not have a priori hypotheses (acronym)
25. CFA is a subset of an advanced class of statistical techniques called _____ equation modeling (abbr.).
28. One of the first tasks in scale construction is the development of a(n) _____ of items.
29. A good scale must be _ _ _ -dimensional and internally consistent.

■ B. Study Questions

1. Below are 15 attitudinal items that are intended to represent a first draft for a scale on mammography attitudes. Read the items and then do the following: (1) Make any revisions you think are appropriate to strengthen each item and the overall scale, including deleting, replacing, or adding items; remember that the scale should be unidimensional, or there should be multiple subscales. (2) Indicate what response options you would recommend for this scale. (3) Calculate what the possible range of responses would be on the scale, as you have revised it. (4) Order the items in a manner you feel would be appropriate.

    a. Having a mammogram will help me detect breast cancer early.
    b. If I find a lump early through a mammogram, I will have a better chance of surviving breast cancer.
    c. Having a mammogram is a good way to find a very small breast lump.
    d. Having a mammogram means I don't have to bother with breast self-examination.
    e. Having a mammogram will decrease my risk of dying from breast cancer.
    f. If I have a mammogram, I will be doing something to take care of myself.
    g. I am afraid to have a mammogram because I might find out something bad.
    h. Having a mammogram would be embarrassing.
    i. I avoid having mammograms because they are too painful.
    j. I just don't have time for a mammogram.
    k. Having a mammogram would expose me to unnecessary radiation.
    l. I can't afford the expense of having a mammogram.
    m. I have other health problems that are more important than getting a mammogram.
    n. I don't need to have a mammogram because no one in my family has had breast cancer.
    o. Having a mammogram isn't necessary for women who examine their own breasts.

2. Administer the revised scale to a small pretest sample (10 to 15 women). Use cognitive questioning to help you better understand how the items are interpreted by respondents. Make revisions as appropriate. If others in your class have completed these two study questions, compare your scales.

3. Read the introduction, method, and results sections of one of the following reports. Use the critiquing guidelines in Box 15.1 of the textbook (available as a Word document in the Toolkit ✖) to critique the study:

   • Cunqueiro, M., Comeche, M., & Docampo, D. (2009). Childbirth Self-Efficacy Inventory: Psychometric testing of the Spanish version. *Journal of Advanced Nursing, 65*, 2710–2718.
   • Dougherty, M., & Larson, E. (2010). The nurse–nurse collaboration scale. *Journal of Nursing Administration, 40*, 17–25.
   • Wood, K., Stewart, A., Drew, B., Shceinman, M., & Frolicher, E. (2009). Development and initial psychometric evaluation of the Patient Perspective of Arrythmia Questionnaire. *Research in Nursing & Health, 32*, 504–516.

■ C. Application Exercise

Read the report by Kalisch and colleagues ("Nursing Teamwork Survey") in Appendix J. Then answer the following questions:

Questions of Fact

a. Was the instrument described in this paper based on a theoretical model? If so, what is its name? Who developed the model?
b. Did the authors claim that there were no existing scales to measure teamwork?
c. How were items for the Nursing Teamwork Survey (NTS) developed?
d. How many items were initially developed? How many items were on the final scale?
e. What were the response options for the items on the scale?
f. What do higher scores on the scale represent?
g. Was the readability of the items assessed? If yes, what was the reading level?
h. Was the instrument pretested with the target population? Was cognitive questioning used?
i. Was there a content validation effort for this scale? How many experts were on the panel? What were their qualifications? Was a CVI computed? If so, what was its value? How was the scale-CVI computed?
j. What are the characteristics of sample members in the psychometric study? How many people participated?
k. Was the internal consistency of the scale assessed? If yes, what was the value of the alpha coefficient for the final version of the total scale?
l. Was the test–retest reliability of the scale assessed? If yes, what was the time interval between testings and who was in the sample? What was the value of the reliability coefficient for the total scale?

m. Was exploratory factor analysis undertaken? If yes, what factor extraction method was used? How many factors emerged? Was this consistent with the original conceptualization? What were the eigenvalues of the factors? Was orthogonal or oblique rotation used? What names were given to the factors? How many items were associated with the factors? Did any items have factor loadings that were considered too low?

n. Did the researchers compute inter-item correlations? If so, what were the values obtained?

o. Was confirmatory factor analysis performed? If so, what were the findings?

p. What other steps were taken to evaluate the validity of the scale?

Questions for Discussion

a. Comment on the adequacy of the scale development process.

b. Comment on the researchers' choice of response options.

c. How effective was the researchers' efforts to establish the content validity of the instrument?

d. Comment on the sampling plan for the psychometric assessment, in terms of both size and sampling method. Overall, how adequate was the sample that was used?

e. How thorough do you think the researchers were in their efforts to assess the psychometric properties of the instrument? What other types of evidence do you think the researchers should have collected?

f. How much confidence would you have in the NTS instrument? Do you feel that the evidence supporting its high quality is persuasive?

▪ D. The Toolkit

For Chapter 15, the Toolkit on the accompanying CD-ROM contains a Word file with the following:

- Guidelines for Critiquing Scale Development and Validation Reports (Box 15.1 of textbook)
- Example of Cognitive Questioning*
- Example of a Cover Letter for Expert Content Validity Panel*
- Example of Part of a Content Validity Questionnaire (Figure 15.1 of textbook)
- Example of a Query Letter for Commercial Publication of an Instrument*
- Example of a Table Of Contents for an Instrument Manual*
- Useful Websites for Chapter 15: Resources for Scale Development

---

*These items do not appear in the textbook.

CHAPTER 16

Descriptive Statistics

■ A. Crossword Puzzle

Complete the crossword puzzle below, which uses terms and concepts presented in Chapter 16. (Puzzles may be removed for easier viewing.)

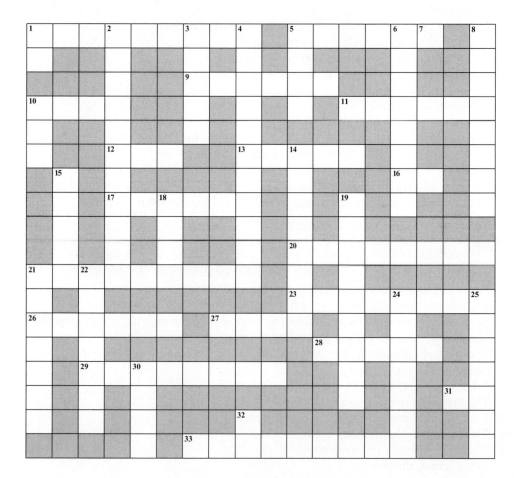

ACROSS

1. Frequency distributions that have a peak in the center and each half mirrors the other
5. Intercorrelations among key variables are frequently displayed in a correlation _____.
9. A unimodal, symmetric distribution that is not too peaked or too flat
10. The ratio of two probabilities (the probability of an event occurring to the probability that it will not occur) is the _____ ratio.
11. Distributions whose peaks are "off center"
12. A correlation index for ordinal-level data
13. Each variable can be described in terms of its _____ of measurement, which affects appropriate mathematic operations.
16. A common risk index—the simple proportion of people who experienced an undesirable outcome (acronym)
17. The most common correlation index: the Pearson product–_____ coefficient
20. Interval measures provide no information about _____ magnitude.
21. A way to display a bivariate distribution is in a(n) _ _ _ _ _ _ _ _ _cy table.
23. Another name for a bivariate display (abbr.) (See 21 across)
26. In nominal measurement, the _____ used to code a variable has no inherent quantitative meaning.
27. A measure of central tendency indicating the most "popular" value
28. The number needed to _____ is an estimate of how many people would need to receive an intervention to prevent an undesirable outcome.
29. When the tail of a frequency distribution points to the left, the skew is _____.
31. An index of central tendency that indicates the midpoint of a distribution (abbr.)
33. An index of a sample is a statistic; an index of a population is a(n) _____.

DOWN

1. The most frequently used index of variability or dispersion (acronym)
2. There are four levels of _____ for research variables.
3. A crude index of variability—the highest value minus the lowest
4. Relationships between two variables can be described through _____ procedures.
5. The sum of all data values, divided by the number of cases
6. The level of measurement in which distances between values are equal, but there is no rational zero
7. A bar over this is used as a symbol for the mean.
8. The mean is the most commonly used index of central _____.
10. The _ _ _inal measurement scale rank orders values.
14. The standard deviation squared
15. The highest level of measurement
18. In lay terms, the *average*
19. One type of graphic display of frequency distribution data
21. A distribution of data can be described by its shape, _____ tendency, and variability.
22. The variable *gender* is measured on this level.

24. Bivariate relationships can be graphed on a _____ plot.
25. A distribution that has two peaks
30. Another name for a bell-shaped curve is a _ _ _ _ sian distribution.
32. A commonly reported risk index in nursing journals (acronym)

■ B. Study Questions

1. For each of the following variables, specify the <u>highest</u> possible level of measurement that you think a researcher could attain.
   a. Attitudes toward the mentally handicapped
   b. Birth order
   c. Length of time in labor
   d. White blood cell count
   e. Blood type
   f. Tidal volume
   g. Degrees Celsius
   h. Unit assignment for nursing staff
   i. Scores on a fear of death scale
   j. Amount of sputum

2. Prepare a frequency distribution and histogram for the following set of data values, which represent the ages of 30 women receiving estrogen replacement therapy:

   47 50 51 50 48 51 50 51 49 51

   54 49 49 53 51 52 51 52 50 53

   49 51 52 51 50 55 48 54 53 52

   Describe the resulting distribution in terms of its symmetry and modality.

3. Calculate the mean, median, and mode for the following pulse rates:

   78 84 69 98 102 72 87 75 79 84 88 84 83 71 73

4. On page 96 there is a contingency table from an SPSS printout. The table presents data from a study of sexually active teenagers in which both males and females were asked how old they were when they first had sexual intercourse. Each row in the table indicates the ages specified by the respondents. The last row contains the code for respondents who could not remember how old they were, coded 88. Answer the following questions about this contingency table:
   a. How many males were included in the study?
   b. How many females first had sexual intercourse at age 14?
   c. What percentage of respondents were 16 years of age when they first had sexual intercourse?
   d. What percentage of males did not know at what age they first had sexual intercourse?

e. Of those respondents who were 13 years of age when they first had sexual intercourse, what percentage was female?

AGE * GENDER Crosstabulation

			GENDER		
			Male	**Female**	**Total**
AGE	13	Count	1	2	3
		% within AGE	33.3%	66.7%	100.0%
		% within GENDER	2.2%	4.4%	3.3%
		% of Total	1.1%	2.2%	3.3%
	14	Count	6	3	9
		% within AGE	66.7%	33.3%	100.0%
		% within GENDER	13.3%	6.7%	10.0%
		% of Total	6.7%	3.3%	10.0%
	15	Count	9	6	15
		% within AGE	60.0%	40.0%	100.0%
		% within GENDER	20.0%	13.3%	16.7%
		% of Total	10.0%	6.7%	16.7%
	16	Count	15	10	25
		% within AGE	60.0%	40.0%	100.0%
		% within GENDER	33.3%	22.2%	27.8%
		% of Total	16.7%	11.1%	27.8%
	17	Count	11	14	25
		% within AGE	44.0%	56.0%	100.0%
		% within GENDER	24.4%	31.1%	27.8%
		% of Total	12.2%	15.6%	27.8%
	18	Count	2	8	10
		% within AGE	20.0%	80.0%	100.0%
		% within GENDER	4.4%	17.8%	11.1%
		% of Total	2.2%	8.9%	11.1%
	88 Don't remember	Count	1	2	3
		% within AGE	33.3%	66.7%	100.0%
		% within GENDER	2.2%	4.4%	3.3%
		% of Total	1.1%	2.2%	3.3%
Total		Count	45	45	90
		% within AGE	50.0%	50.0%	100.0%
		% within GENDER	100.0%	100.0%	100.0%
		% of Total	50.0%	50.0%	100.0%

5. Suppose a researcher has conducted a study concerning lactose intolerance in children. The data reveal that 12 boys and 16 girls have lactose intolerance, out of a sample of 60 children of each gender. Construct a contingency table and calculate the row, column, and total percentages for each cell in the table. Discuss the meaning of these statistics.

6. Ask 25 friends, classmates, or colleagues the following four questions:
   - How many brothers and sisters do you have?
   - How many children do you expect to have in total?
   - Would you describe your family during your childhood as "close" or "not very close"?
   - On your 14th birthday, were you living with both biologic parents, primarily with one biologic parent, or with neither biologic parent?

   When you have gathered your data, calculate and present several statistics that describe the information you obtained.

7. Suppose that 400 participants (200 per group) were in the intervention study described in connection with Table 16.7 in the textbook, and that 60% of those in the experimental group and 90% of those in the control group continued smoking. Compute the various risk indexes in this scenario.

8. Read one of the following research reports and use the critiquing guidelines in Box 16.1 (available as a Word document in the Toolkit for this chapter ✖) to critique the researchers' analyses, ignoring at this point discussions of inferential statistics and statistical tests:
   - Lamp, J., & Macke, J. (2010). Relationships among intrapartum maternal fluid intake, birth type, neonatal output, and neonatal weight loss during the first 48 hours after birth. *Journal of Obstetric, Neonatal, & Gynecologic Nursing, 39,* 169–177.
   - Park, H. J., Jarrett, M., & Heitkemper, M. (2010). Quality of life and sugar and fiber intake in women with irritable bowel syndrome. *Western Journal of Nursing Research, 32,* 218–232.
   - Schell, K., Morse, K., & Waterhouse, J. (2010). Forearm and upper-arm oscillometric blood pressure comparison in acutely ill adults. *Western Journal of Nursing Research, 32,* 322–340.

■ C. Application Exercises

EXERCISE 1: STUDY IN APPENDIX F

Read the results section of the article by Jurgens and colleagues ("Responding to heart failure symptoms") in Appendix F. Then answer the following questions:

Questions of Fact

a. Did Jurgens and her colleagues present descriptive statistics describing characteristics of the sample? If yes, where were they presented, in the table or in the text?

b. Referring to Table 2, answer the following questions:
   - Which variables described in the tables, if any, were measured as nominal-level variables?
   - Which variables described in the tables, if any, were measured as ordinal-level variables?
   - Which variables described in the tables, if any, were measured as interval-level variables?
   - Which variables described in the tables, if any, were measured as ratio-level variables?
   - State in one sentence what the "typical" participant was like demographically.
   - What percentage of the sample had a household income less than $25,000 in the prior year?

c. Referring to Table 3, answer the following questions:
   - Which descriptive statistics are presented in this table?
   - Why did the researchers use the particular measure of central tendency that they selected?
   - Which symptom was experienced by the most study participants?
   - Which symptom had the longest duration?

d. Referring to Table 4, answer the following questions:
   - Which descriptive statistics are presented in this table?
   - What was the level of measurement of the variables in this table?
   - What was the average score of participants on the scale measuring seriousness of symptoms?

Questions for Discussion

a. Discuss the effectiveness of the presentation of information in the tables. What, if anything, could be done to make the tables more informative, more comprehensible, or more efficient? Should there have been additional tables?

b. Did Jurgens and colleagues use the appropriate statistics to describe their data? For example, did the statistics correspond to the levels of measurement of the variables? Could additional descriptive statistics been used to more fully describe the data?

EXERCISE 2: STUDY IN APPENDIX H

Read the results section of the article by McGillion and colleagues ("Chronic cardiac pain") in Appendix H. Then answer the following questions:

Questions of Fact

a. Did McGillion and his colleagues present descriptive statistics describing characteristics of the sample? If yes, where were they presented, in the table or in the text?

b. Referring to Tables 1 and 2, answer the following questions:
  • Which variable described in the tables, if any, was measured as a nominal-level variable?
  • Which variable described in the tables, if any, was measured as an ordinal-level variable?
  • Which variable described in the tables, if any, was measured as an interval-level variable?
  • Which variable described in the tables, if any, was measured as a ratio-level variable?

c. Referring to Tables 1 and 2, answer the following questions:
  • Which descriptive statistics are presented in these two tables?
  • What was the mean age of subjects in the treatment group?
  • What percentage of subjects in the control group had thyroid problems as a comorbidity?
  • Which group was more variable in terms of the length of time they had lived with angina?
  • With regard to which comorbid condition was there the biggest difference in incidence between the two groups?

Questions for Discussion

a. Discuss the effectiveness of the presentation of information in the tables. What, if anything, could be done to make the tables more informative, more comprehensible, or more efficient? Should there have been other tables?

b. Did McGillion and colleagues use the appropriate statistics to describe their data? For example, did the statistics correspond to the levels of measurement of the variables? Could additional descriptive statistics been used to more fully describe the data?

▪ D. The Toolkit

For Chapter 16, the Toolkit on the accompanying CD-ROM contains a Word file with the following:

  • Guidelines for Critiquing Descriptive Statistics (Box 16.1 of the textbook)
  • Table Templates for Presenting Descriptive Statistics*
    • Table Template 1: Sample Description Table
    • Table Template 2: Contingency Table
    • Table Template 3: Correlation Matrix
  • Useful Websites for Chapter 16: Resources for Descriptive Statistics

---

*These items do not appear in the textbook.

CHAPTER 17

Inferential Statistics

■ A. Crossword Puzzle

Complete the crossword puzzle below, which uses terms and concepts presented in Chapter 17. (Puzzles may be removed for easier viewing.)

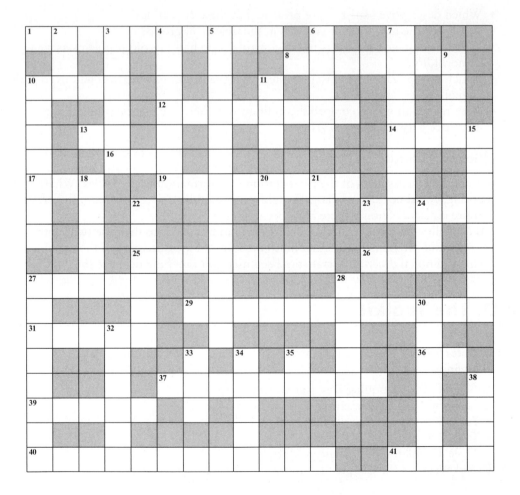

ACROSS

1. A(n) _____ interval indicates degree of precision in parameter estimation.
8. One of the two broad approaches in statistical inference is hypothesis _____.
10. The probability of committing a Type II error
12. Data from a design in which there are multiple measurements of a continuous outcome variable can be analyzed using a(n) _____-measures ANOVA.
13. In statistical testing, the error that reflects a false negative is a Type _____ error.
14. A nonparametric analog to a *t*-test is the _____-Whitney *U* test.
16. A test comparing the means of three groups is a _____-way analysis of variance.
17. An ES index in an ANOVA situation is _____-squared.
19. The _____ error of the mean is the SD of a theoretical distribution of means.
23. A Bonferroni correction involves a correction to _____ to reflect multiple tests with the same data.
25. The _____ region of a theoretical distribution indicates whether the null hypothesis is *improbable*.
26. The test most often used when a hypothesis concerns differences in proportions is _____-squared.
27. When sample sizes are very small, Fisher's _____ test should be used to test differences in proportions.
29. By convention, the standard criterion for statistical _____ is an alpha of .05.
31. A(n) _____ analysis can be used during the planning of a study to estimate sample size needs.
36. If the computer indicated that $p = .15$, this would indicate the relationship being tested was _____ (acronym).
37. Even though researchers often have directional hypotheses, they most often report the results of _____-_____ tests.
39. In statistical testing, a false positive is a(n) _____ error.
40. A sampling _____ is theoretical, not based on actual data values.
41. Most statistical _ _ _ _ yses involve inferential statistics.

DOWN

2. If both tails of the sampling distribution are not used to test the null hypothesis, the test is called _____ tailed.
3. The statistic computed in analysis of variance
4. Each statistical analysis is associated with certain _____ of freedom that usually reflect sample size.
5. The class of statistics that is also called distribution-free and that has less restrictive assumptions about how variables are distributed
6. An alpha of .01 is a more stringent _____ of significance than an alpha of .05.

7. For dichotomous variables, the sampling distribution is called a(n) _____ distribution.
9. In an ANOVA context, the overall mean for an entire sample, with all groups combined, is the _ _ _ _ d mean.
10. An independent groups statistical test is used for _____-subjects designs.
11. With ordinal data, one correlation index is Kendall's _____.
15. When the null hypothesis is not rejected, results are sometimes described as _____.
18. The analysis used to compare 3+ group means (acronym)
20. The number of observations free to vary about a parameter (acronym)
21. An extension of a paired *t*-test to 3 time periods would call for _ _ -ANOVA (acronym).
22. In a repeated measures analysis, the within-subjects analysis effect involves a time _____.
24. An index describing the relationship between two dichotomous variables
27. In an analysis of contingency table data, observed frequencies are contrasted with _____ frequencies.
28. The nonparametric analog of a paired *t*-test is the Wilcoxon _____ rank test.
30. A(n) _____ result indicates that the null hypothesis cannot be rejected (abbr.).
32. Cohen's *d* is an index used to estimate _____ size in a two-group mean difference situation.
33. The simplest type of multifactor ANOVA is a _____-way ANOVA.
34. Two group means can be compared using a(n) _____-_____.
35. The following might be the information for a 95% _____: (−1.25, .78).
38. In hypothesis testing, researchers typically seek to reject the _____ hypothesis.

■ B. Study Questions

1. A research team measured the amount of time (in minutes) spent in recreational activities by a sample of 200 hospitalized paraplegic patients. They compared male and female patients, as well as those 50 years of age and younger versus those over 50 years of age. The four group means were as follows:

	Male	Female
≤ 50	98.2 (*n* = 50)	70.1 (*n* = 50)
> 50	50.8 (*n* = 50)	68.3 (*n* = 50)

A two-way ANOVA yielded the following results:

	F	df	p
Gender	3.61	1,196	>.05
Age group	5.87	1,196	<.05
Gender x Age group	6.96	1,196	<.01

Discuss the meaning of these results.

2. The correlation between the number of days absent per year and annual salary in a sample of 100 employees of an insurance company was found to be −.23 (p = .02). Discuss this result in terms of significance levels and meaning.

3. Indicate which bivariate statistical test(s) you would use to analyze data for the following variables:

   a. Variable 1 is psychiatric patients' gender; variable 2 is whether or not the patient has attempted suicide in the past 12 months.
   b. Variable 1 is the participation versus nonparticipation of patients with a pulmonary embolus in a special intervention; variable 2 is the pH of the patients' arterial blood gases.
   c. Variable 1 is serum creatinine concentration levels; variable 2 is daily urine output.
   d. Variable 1 is the number of patients' comorbidities—0, 1, or 2 or more; variable 2 is the patients' degrees of self-reported depression on a 30-item depression scale.

4. On the next page is a correlation matrix produced in SPSS, based on real data from a study of low-income mothers. Answer the following questions with respect to this matrix:

   a. How many respondents completed the SF-12 scale?
   b. What is the correlation between body mass index (BMI) and scores on the physical health subscale of the SF12?
   c. Is the correlation between physical health and mental health subscale scores significant at conventional levels?
   d. What is the probability that the correlation between BMI and number of doctor visits in the previous year is simply a function of chance?
   e. To which variable(s) is BMI value related at or below the .01 level of significance?
   f. Explain what is meant by the correlation between the physical and mental health scale scores.

		Number of Doctor Visits, Past 12 mo	Body Mass Index	SF12: Physical Health Component Score	SF12: Mental Health Component Score
Correlations					
Number of doctor visits, past 12 mo	Pearson Correlation	1.000	.131[**]	−.316[**]	−.133[**]
	Sig. (2-tailed)		.000	.000	.000
	N	997	967	890	890
Body Mass Index	Pearson Correlation	.131[**]	1.000	−.134[**]	−.078[*]
	Sig. (2-tailed)	.000		.000	.022
	N	967	970	866	866
SF12: Physical Health Component Score	Pearson Correlation	−.316[**]	−.134[**]	1.000	.168[**]
	Sig. (2-tailed)	.000	.000		.000
	N	890	866	893	893
SF12: Mental Health Component Score	Pearson Correlation	−.133[**]	−.078[*]	.168[**]	1.000
	Sig. (2-tailed)	.000	.022	.000	
	N	890	866	893	893

[**]Correlation is significant at the 0.01 level (2-tailed).
[*]Correlation is significant at the 0.05 level (2-tailed).

5. Below is a list of variables. Assume that you have data from 500 nurses on these variables. Develop two or three hypotheses regarding the relationships among these variables, and indicate what statistical tests you would use to test your hypotheses.

   • Number of years of nursing experience
   • Type of employment setting (hospital, nursing school, public school system, industry)
   • Salary
   • Marital status (never married, currently married, divorced or separated, widowed)
   • Job satisfaction (dissatisfied, neither dissatisfied nor satisfied, or satisfied)
   • Number of children under 18 years of age
   • Gender
   • Intent to remain in nursing (from 0, highly unlikely to 10, definitely)

6. Estimate the required total sample sizes for the following situations:
   a. Comparison of two group means: $\alpha = .05$; power $= .90$; ES $= .35$.
   b. Correlation of two variables: $\alpha = .05$; power $= .80$; $\rho = .20$.

7. Read one of the following research reports and use the critiquing guidelines in Box 17.1 (available as a Word document in the Toolkit for this chapter ✖) to critique the researchers' analyses, ignoring at this point discussions of multivariate statistics such as multiple regression:

- Ahn, Y., Sohn, M., & Yoo, E. (2010). Breast functions perceived by Korean mothers: Infant nutrition and female sexuality. *Western Journal of Nursing Research, 32*, 363–378.
- Friend, D., & Chertok, I. (2009). Evaluation of an educational intervention to promote breast pump use among women with infants in a special nursery in Kenya. *Public Health Nursing, 26*, 339–345.
- Kelly, M., Johnson, E., Lee, V., Massey, L., Purser, D., Ring, K., Sanderson, S., Styles, J., & Wood, D. (2010). Delayed versus immediate pushing in second stage of labor. *MCN: The American Journal of Maternal/Child Nursing, 35*, 81–88.

■ C. Application Exercises

EXERCISE 1: STUDY IN APPENDIX D

Read the results section of the article by Whittemore and colleagues ("Diabetes prevention program") in Appendix D. Then answer the following questions:

Questions of Fact

a. Which bivariate statistical tests discussed in Chapter 17 did Whittemore and colleagues use in their analyses presented in Table 2?
b. What is the independent variable in the analyses presented in Table 2? What are the dependent variables?
c. What was the purpose of the tests presented in Table 2?
d. For each of the following characteristics shown in Table 2, indicate the null hypothesis, the test used, whether the null hypothesis was rejected, and what the probability level was.

- Age
- Race
- BMI
- Physical activity

e. For the first characteristic in question c (age), state a sentence describing the result of the test that could be reported in a research article.
f. What percent of participants in the treatment group had income less than $20,000? What percent of control group members had incomes less than $20,000? Were income differences between the two groups statistically significant?
g. Overall, how many tests in Table 2 were statistically significant at conventional levels?
h. Did the report indicate that a power analysis was done while planning the study to estimate sample size needs?

Questions for Discussion

a. Discuss the effectiveness of the presentation of information in Table 2. What, if anything, could be done to make this table more informative, more comprehensible, or more efficient?

b. Did Whittemore and colleagues use the appropriate statistical tests to analyze their data? If not, what tests should have been performed?

c. Did the researchers present a sufficient amount of information about their statistical tests? What additional information would have been helpful?

EXERCISE 2: STUDY IN APPENDIX H

Read the results section of the article by McGillion and colleagues ("Chronic cardiac pain") in Appendix H. Then answer the following questions:

Questions of Fact

a. According to the text of this article, the researchers tested the initial comparability of the treatment and control groups with regard to baseline characteristics. Answer the following questions about that statement:

- Which bivariate statistical tests discussed in Chapter 17 would have been used to compare the two groups?
- Were probability levels for these tests shown in the tables?
- What did the article state about the results from these tests?

b. Which bivariate statistic described in Chapter 17 was presented in Tables 3 and 4?

c. In Tables 3 and 4, what was the independent variable? What were the dependent variables?

d. Did the report indicate that a power analysis was done while planning the study to estimate sample size needs?

Questions for Discussion

a. Discuss the effectiveness of the presentation of information in the tables. What, if anything, could be done to make the tables more informative, more comprehensible, or more efficient? Should there have been other tables?

b. Did McGillion and colleagues use the appropriate statistical tests to analyze their data? If not, what tests should have been performed?

c. Did the researchers present a sufficient amount of information about their statistical tests? What additional information would have been helpful?

■ D. The Toolkit

For Chapter 17, the Toolkit on the accompanying CD-ROM contains a Word file with the following:

- Guidelines for Critiquing Bivariate Inferential Analyses (Box 17.1 of the textbook)
- Table Templates for Selected Bivariate Analyses*
  - Table Template 1A: Independent *t*-Tests
  - Table Template 1B: Independent *t*-Tests (Alternative Format)
  - Table Template 2: Paired *t*-Tests
  - Table Template 3: One-Way ANOVA
  - Table Template 4: RM-ANOVA
  - Table Template 5A: Chi-Squared Tests (For Two-Group Comparisons)
  - Table Template 5B: Chi-Squared Tests (For 2+ Group Comparisons)
- Useful Websites for Chapter 17: Resources for Inferential Statistics

---

*These items do not appear in the textbook.

CHAPTER 18

Multivariate Statistics

■ A. Crossword Puzzle

Complete the crossword puzzle below, which uses terms and concepts presented in Chapter 18. (Puzzles may be removed for easier viewing.)

ACROSS

1. Analyses to test causal pathways with nonexperimental data use _____ equations.
6. OLS is an acronym for an estimation procedure in which the "O" stands for _____.
8. Multiple regression uses a(n) _____-squares criterion to solve equations.
11. A model in which the flow of causation is presumed to be in one direction
13. A key index in logistic regression is the _____ ratio.
14. Another name for a z-score is a(n) _____ score.
20. In ANCOVA, the variables that are statistically controlled
22. The general _____ model is a broad class of procedures that encompasses ANOVA and multiple regression.
23. A(n) _____ of prediction almost always occurs in regression, because correlations between predictors and outcome variables are not perfect.
24. An alternative to OLS estimation is _____ likelihood estimation.
26. The _____ statistic is used to test the significance of individual predictors in logistic regression.
28. Causal models can be tested using _____ analysis.
30. A statistical index used to test the overall fit of a causal model (acronym)
31. The likelihood ratio test in logistic regression is sometimes called a goodness-of-_____ test.
32. Logistic regression uses a different _____ procedure than standard multiple regression (MLE).
33. ANCOVA can yield information about _____ means that remove the effects of covariates.
34. In regression analyses, an independent variable is often called a(n) _____ variable.

DOWN

1. A regression approach that uses a statistical criterion to enter predictors into the model.
2. Error terms in regression are sometimes called the _____.
3. When multicollinearity is present, the results tend to be uns _ _ _ _ _.
4. When the dependent variable is dichotomous, a common analytic approach is to use _____ regression.
5. The analysis used to compare groups when there are 2+ dependent variables and confounders need to be controlled (acronym)
7. When RM-ANOVA is used to compare experimental and control group subjects at multiple points in time, it is the _ _ _ _raction that is of greatest interest.
9. The R _____ statistic indicates the proportion of variance of a dependent variable explained by all predictors (abbr.).
10. The _____-Lemeshow test is one approach to testing an overall logistic regression model.

12. The class of statistical analysis involving multiple variables is called multi _ _ _ _ _ _ _ statistics.
15. A least-squares approach to making predictions about group membership (categorical dependent variables) is _____ analysis.
16. An approach to regression that involves entry of predictors in a researcher-determined sequence is called _ _ _ _ archical regression.
17. Regression analysis that predicts a continuous outcome with at least two predictors is called _____ regression.
18. Acronym for a key statistical index in logistic regression
19. Simple regression involves _____ predictor variable.
21. A procedure for testing causal models (acronym)
25. A group _____ can be adjusted to reflect net effects after statistically controlling one or more variables.
26. A standardized regression coefficient is called a beta _____.
27. A dichotomous variable coded as 1 versus 0, used in regression analyses, is called a _____ variable.
29. A(n) _____ design includes both a within-subject factor and a between-subject factor.

■ B. Study Questions

1. Examine the correlation matrix below and explain the various entries. Explain why the *multiple* correlation coefficient between variables B through E and Satisfaction with Nursing Care (variable A) is .54. Could it be smaller? How could it be made larger? What is the R^2 for the correlation between Satisfaction with Nursing Care and the other variables? What does this mean?

	A Satisfaction with Nursing Care	B Age	C Depression Scores	D Length of Stay	E Educational Level
Variable A	1.00				
Variable B	−.26	1.00			
Variable C	−.48	.29	1.00		
Variable D	−.19	.22	.68	1.00	
Variable E	.10	−.07	−.17	−.24	1.00

2. In the following examples, which multivariate procedure is most appropriate for analyzing the data?

   a. A researcher is testing the effect of verbal expressiveness, self-esteem, age, and the availability of family supports among a group of recently discharged psychiatric patients on recidivism (i.e., whether they will be readmitted within 12 months after discharge).

   b. A researcher is comparing the bereavement and coping processes (as measured on an interval-level scale) of recently widowed versus recently divorced individuals, controlling for their age and length of marriage.

   c. A researcher wants to test the effects of (a) two drug treatments and (b) two dosages of each drug on (a) blood pressure and (b) the pH and Po_2 levels of arterial blood gases.

   d. A researcher wants to predict hospital staff absentee rates based on staff rank, shift, number of years with the hospital, and marital status.

   e. A researcher wants to test the effects of two alternative diets on blood sugar levels measured at baseline, and then 1, 3, and 6 months later.

3. Below is a list of variables that a nurse researcher might be interested in predicting. For each, suggest at least three independent variables that could be used in a multiple regression analysis.

   a. Amount of time spent exercising weekly among teenagers
   b. Nurses' frequency of administering pain medication
   c. Body mass index (as a measure of obesity)
   d. Patients' level of fatigue
   e. Anxiety levels of prostatectomy patients

4. Wang and colleagues, in their 2001 study (*Clinical Nursing Research, 10*, 29–38), used a series of *t*-tests and chi-squared tests to compare two groups of patients who underwent cardiac catheterization with regard to measures of safety, comfort, and satisfaction: those with 4 hours versus 6 hours of bed rest. Identify two or three multivariate procedures that could have been used to analyze the data, being as specific as possible (e.g., if you suggest ANCOVA, identify appropriate covariates).

5. Read one of the following studies and use the critiquing guidelines in Box 17.1 of the textbook (available as a Word document in the Toolkit for the previous chapter ✪) to evaluate the multivariate statistical analyses:

   • Blacklock, R., Rhodes, R., Blanchard, C., & Gaul, C. (2010). Effects of exercise intensity and self-efficacy on state anxiety with breast cancer survivors. *Oncology Nursing Forum, 37*, 206–212.

   • Edwards, Q., Li, A., Pike, M., Kolonel, L., Henderson, B., & McKean-Cowdin, R. (2010). Patterns of regular use of mammography—body weight and ethnicity. *Journal of the American Academy of Nurse Practitioners, 22*, 162–169.

   • Mulder, P., Johnson, T., & Baker, L. (2010). Excessive weight loss in breastfed infants during the postpartum hospitalization. *Journal of Obstetric, Gynecologic, & Neonatal Nursing, 39*, 15–26.

■ C. Application Exercises

EXERCISE 1: STUDY IN APPENDICES A, D, AND H

Skim the method and results sections of the reports in Appendices A, D, and H. Then answer the following questions:

Questions of Fact

a. Did any of these studies use multiple regression analysis? If yes, what were the dependent variables and what were the predictors?
b. Did any of these studies use ANCOVA? If yes, what groups were being compared? What were the dependent variables and what were the covariates?
c. Did any of these studies use other types of multivariate analyses discussed in this chapter? If yes, which ones?
d. Did any of these studies report confidence intervals?
e. Did any of these studies report effect size estimates?

Question for Discussion

Did the researchers in these studies use the most powerful and appropriate statistical analyses possible? What type of analyses might have been better?

EXERCISE 2: STUDY IN APPENDIX F

Read the method (data analysis) and results section of the article by Jurgens and colleagues ("Responding to heart failure symptoms") in Appendix F. Then answer the following questions:

Questions of Fact

a. What approach to entering variables into the multiple regression equation was used in this study?
b. In what order were predictor variables entered into the regression model?
c. Referring to Table 5 and the accompanying text, answer the following questions:
   • What was the dependent variable in the multiple regression analysis?
   • How many predictors were significantly associated with the dependent variable in this analysis?
   • While controlling other predictors, which predictor variable was most strongly predictive of the dependent variable?
   • What was the value of R^2?
   • Did the table provide information that could be used by others to predict the dependent variable (i.e., the regression equation)?
   • Is the overall regression equation statistically significant?
d. Did the authors assess the risk of multicollinearity for their regression analysis? If yes, what did they conclude?

Questions for Discussion

a. Comment on the researchers' strategy for entering variables into the regression equation. Would you recommend an alternative approach?

b. Were there other multivariate analyses that the researchers could have used but did not? Would you recommend the use of such analyses? Why or why not?

■ D. The Toolkit

For Chapter 18, the Toolkit on the accompanying CD-ROM contains a Word file with the following:

- Table Templates for Presenting Selected Multivariate Analyses*
  - Table Template 1: Simultaneous Multiple Regression
  - Table Template 2: Hierarchical Multiple Regression
  - Table Template 3: ANCOVA
  - Table Template 4: Logistic Regression
- Useful Websites for Chapter 18: Resources for Multivariate Statistics

_____

*These items do not appear in the textbook.

CHAPTER 19

Processes of Quantitative Data Analysis and Interpretation

■ A. Crossword Puzzle

Complete the crossword puzzle below, which uses terms and concepts presented in Chapter 19. (Puzzles may be removed for easier viewing.)

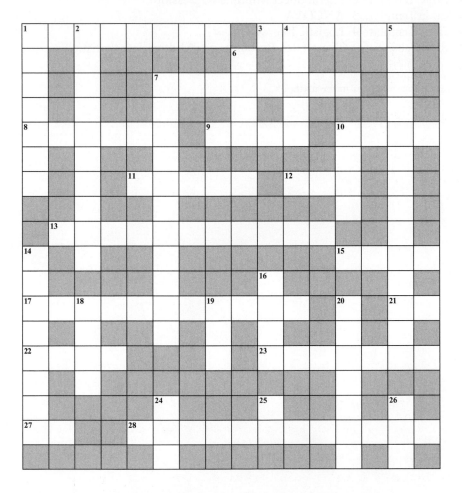

ACROSS

1. The deletion of cases with missing data on an analysis-by-analysis basis
3. To understand the magnitude and importance of results, it is useful to compute _____ sizes.
7. Coding decisions are documented in a _____.
8. When sample _____ extends over a long period of time, tests for cohort effects are advisable.
9. A pattern of missingness in which the value of the missing information is correlated with it being missing (acronym)
10. When there are missing items on a scale, _____ mean substitution involves using the mean item score for that person on other items on the scale.
11. When some hypotheses are upheld and others are not, results are said to be _____.
12. A pattern of missingness in which the value of the missing number is correlated with another measured variable but not with the missing information itself _____ (acronym)
13. Data cleaning includes _____ checks, which examine whether there are any contradictions in the data within individual cases.
15. Before the principal analyses are undertaken, researchers should test for various types of _____.
17. To test for the robustness of results, researchers sometimes undertake _____ analyses.
21. Each case in a data set should be assigned a(n) _____ number.
22. A coded value that is impossible within the coding scheme is a(n) _____ code.
23. Refusals and skipped questions require special _____ values codes.
27. An imputation approach in which an iterative procedure with a maximum-likelihood-based algorithm is used to produce the best parameter estimates (acronym).
28. One strategy for resolving missing values is to use mean _____.

DOWN

1. When there are multiple sites, it is useful to test whether _____ across sites is appropriate.
2. One broad missing values strategy involves the _____ of values to estimate those that are missing.
4. A(n) _____ effect can occur if there is insufficient possibility for variation in low scores.
5. Researchers often need to do a data _____ to get coded values into a form appropriate for analysis.
6. After drawing conclusions about the accuracy of their findings, researchers need to interpret what they _____.
7. The first step in doing an interpretation involves establishing the _____ of the findings.
10. In nonexperimental studies, an important maxim to remember is that _____ does not prove causation (abbr.).

14. _____ deletion is sometimes called complete case analysis.
16. In preparing to compute scale values, a procedure called _____ reversal is sometimes necessary to ensure scoring in a consistent direction.
18. It is tricky to use traditional hypothesis testing to test a hypothesis that is actually the _____ (absence of a relationship).
19. Sometimes a transformation involves creating a dummy _ _ _iable for multivariate analysis.
20. The findings of a study are also called the _____.
24. An extreme value outside the normal range is called a(n) _ _ _lier.
25. The "gold standard" approach to imputation (acronym)
26. A type of transformation that can render skewed data more normal (abbr.)

■ B. Study Questions

1. Read the following study, and (a) indicate which steps in the process shown in Figure 19.1 were described in the report and (b) comment on whether the absence of other information affected the quality of the research evidence: McDaniel, J., Ahijevych, K., & Belury, M. (2010). Effect of n-3 oral supplements on the n-6/n-3 ratio in young adults. *Western Journal of Nursing Research, 32,* 64–80.

2. Read the following study, which involved some data transformations. Comment on the researchers' decision to use transformations and the results that were achieved: Fernandes, C., Worster, A., Eva, K., Hill, S., & McCallum, C. (2006). Pneumatic tube delivery system for blood samples reduces turnaround times without affecting sample quality. *Journal of Emergency Nursing, 32,* 139–143.

3. Read one of the following studies, and evaluate the extent to which the researchers assessed possible biases. Can you think of analyses that could have been performed to strengthen the credibility of the results?
   • Nyamathi, A., Sinha, K., Greengold, B., Cohen, A., & Marfisee, M. (2010). Predictors of HAV/HBV vaccination completion among methadone maintenance clients. *Research in Nursing & Health, 33,* 120–132.
   • Oh, P. J., & Kim, S. H. (2010). Effects of a brief psychosocial intervention in patients with cancer receiving adjuvant therapy. *Oncology Nursing Forum, 37,* E98–104.

4. In the following research article, a team of researchers reported that they obtained some nonsignificant results that were not consistent with expectations. Review and critique the researchers' interpretation of the findings and suggest some possible alternatives: McDonald, D., Martin, D., Foley, D., Baker, L., Hintz, D., Faure, L., Erman, N., Palozie, J., Lundquist, K., O'Brien, K., Prior, L., Songco, N., Muscillo, G., Graziani, D., Tomczyk, M., & Price, S. (2010). Motivating people to learn cardiopulmonary resuscitation and use of automated external defibrillators. *Journal of Cardiovascular Nursing, 25,* 69–74.

■ C. Application Exercises

EXERCISE 1: STUDY IN APPENDIX A

Read the method, results, and discussion sections of the article by Kennedy and Chen ("Changes in childhood risk taking") in Appendix A. Then answer the following questions:

Questions of Fact

a. Did the report provide information about how missing data were handled?
b. Did the report indicate that tests were performed to assess the degree to which their data met assumptions for parametric tests such as regression analysis?
c. Did the researchers provide evidence about the success of randomization—that is, whether participants in the experimental and control groups were equivalent at the outset and, thus, selection biases were absent?
d. Did any study participants withdraw from the study? What was the rate of attrition in the two groups? Did the researchers report an analysis of attrition biases?
e. Was the analysis an intention-to-treat analysis?
f. In the discussion section, was there any explicit discussion about the study's internal validity, external validity, or statistical conclusion validity?
g. Did the discussion section link study findings to findings from prior research—that is, did the authors place their findings into a broader context?
h. Did the discussion section explicitly mention any study limitations?

Questions for Discussion

a. Discuss the thoroughness of the researchers' description about their analytic and data management strategy.
b. Do you agree with the researchers' interpretations of their results? Why or why not?
c. Discuss the extent to which the discussion included all important results.
d. To what extent do you think the researchers' adequately described the study's limitations and strengths?
e. Discuss the extent to which the results as described in this report would facilitate an EBP-type assessment of the evidence.

EXERCISE 2: STUDY IN APPENDIX D

Read the method, results, and discussion sections of the article by Whittemore and colleagues ("Diabetes prevention program") in Appendix D. Then answer the following questions:

Questions of Fact

a. Did the report provide information about how missing data were handled?
b. Did the report mention any transformations? If yes, what was transformed?
c. Did all study participants fully complete the intervention? What was the rate of attrition? Did the researchers report an analysis of attrition biases?
d. Was an intention-to-treat analysis used?
e. Did the discussion section link study findings to findings from prior research?
f. Did the discussion section explicitly mention any "lessons learned" in this pilot study?

Questions for Discussion

a. Discuss the thoroughness of the researchers' description about their analytic and data management strategy.
b. Do you agree with the researchers interpretations of their results? Why or why not?
c. To what extent do you think the researchers' adequately described the study's limitations and strengths?

▪ D. The Toolkit

For Chapter 19, the Toolkit on the accompanying CD-ROM contains a Word file with the following:

- Guidelines for Critiquing Interpretations in Discussion Sections of Quantitative Research Reports (Box 19.1 of the textbook)
- Data Transformations for Distribution Problems*
- Supplementary Table of Research Biases*
- Useful Websites for Chapter 19: Resources for Analysis and Interpretation

---

*These items do not appear in the textbook.

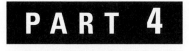

PART 4

Designing and Conducting Qualitative Studies to Generate Evidence for Nursing

CHAPTER 20

Qualitative Research Design and Approaches

■ A. Crossword Puzzle

Complete the crossword puzzle below, which uses terms and concepts presented in Chapter 20. (Puzzles may be removed for easier viewing.)

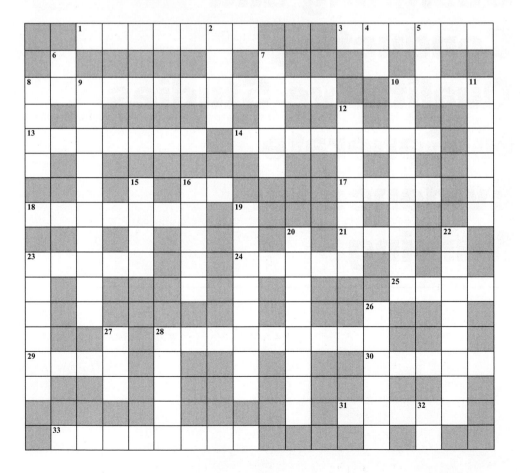

ACROSS

1. A(n) _____ aid is a resource that tells researchers what is in an archive.
3. A(n) _____ case study design is appropriate when an exemplar represents an extreme or unique case.
8. Leininger's phrase for research at the interface between culture and nursing
10. The type of phenomenology that includes the step of bracketing is _ _ _ _riptive.
13. Another term for auto-ethnography is _____ ethnography.
14. Research that focuses on gender discrimination
16. _ _ternal criticism concerns the authenticity of historical evidence.
17. A type of psychological research that studies the environment's influence on behavior (abbr.)
18. One of the two originators of grounded theory
21. A type of action research (acronym)
23. Knowledge that is so embedded in a culture that people do not talk about it
24. A type of phenomenology sometimes called hermeneutics is _ _ _ _ _pretive.
25. The perspective that is the outsider's view
28. Qualitative researchers' ability to derive information from a wide array of sources
29. Traditional qualitative research does not adopt a strong political or _ _ _ _logical perspective.
30. Qualitative research design decisions typically unfold while researchers are in the _____.
31. Qualitative research that is not done within any specific tradition is often called _ _ _ _ _iptive qualitative.
33. Qualitative research design is typically a(n) _____ design.

DOWN

2. _ _ _ _ative analysis focuses on *story* as the object of inquiry.
4. _ _ ternal criticism concerns an assessment of the worth of historical evidence.
5. _____ developed a linguistic approach for narrative analysis.
6. A qualitative tradition concerned with theory development about social processes (acronym)
7. Phenomenologists study _____ experiences.
8. The perspective that is the insider's view
9. The systematic collection and analysis of materials relating to the past is _____ research.
10. The type of analysis designed to understand the rules and structure of conversations
11. The nurse researcher who worked with an originator of grounded theory to develop an alternative approach
12. A type of phenomenology focusing on the *meaning* of experiences (abbr.)
15. The second step in descriptive phenomenology is to in_ _ _ _.
16. A phenomenological question is: What is the _ _ _ _ _ce of this phenomenon?
19. Research that involves a critique of society is based on _____ theory.

20. The biology of human behavior
22. An aspect of experience that phenomenologists study is relationality or lived human
    _____ (backward!).
23. An approach to classifying qualitative research design is according to a qualitative
    _ _ _ _ _ _ion.
26. Qualitative researchers often maintain a(n) _ _ _ _ _ _ive journal to record their own
    presuppositions and biases.
27. Qualitative designs are _____ experimental.
28. The phenomenological concept _____-in-the-world acknowledges people's
    physical ties to their world.
32. An analytic procedure in grounded theory research used to develop and refine
    categories (acronym).

▪ B. Study Questions

1. For each of the research questions below, indicate what type of qualitative research
   tradition would likely guide the inquiry, and why you think that would be the case.
   a. What is the social psychological process through which couples deal with the
      sudden loss of an infant through SIDS?
   b. How does the culture of a suicide survivors' self-help group adapt to a successful
      suicide attempt by a former member?
   c. What are the power dynamics that arise in conversations between nurses and
      bed-ridden nursing home patients?
   d. What is the lived experience of the spousal caretaker of an Alzheimer patient?

2. Skim the following two studies, which are examples of ethnographic and
   phenomenological studies. What were the central phenomena under investigation?
   Compare and contrast the methods used in these two studies (e.g., how were data
   collected? How many study participants were there? To what extent did the design
   unfold while the researchers were in the field?)
   - *Ethnographic Study:* Murphy, F., & Philpin, S. (2010). Early miscarriage as
     "matter out of place": An ethnographic study of nursing practice in a hospital
     gynaecological unit. *International Journal of Nursing Studies, 47,* 534–541.
   - *Phenomenological Study:* Fries, K. (2010). African American women and
     unplanned cesarean birth. *MCN: The American Journal of Maternal/Child
     Nursing, 35,* 110–115.

3. Skim one of the following participatory action research (PAR) studies and comment
   on the roles of participants and researchers. In what ways would the study have
   been different if a participatory approach had not been used?
   - Austin, W., Goble, E., Strang, V., Mitchell, A., Thompson, E., Lantz, H., Balt, L.,
     Lemermeyer, G., & Vass, K. (2009). Supporting relationships between family and
     staff in continuing care settings. *Journal of Family Nursing, 15,* 360–383.

- Etowa, J., Keddy, B., Egbeyemi, J., & Eghan, F. (2007). Depression: The "invisible grey fog" influencing the midlife health of African Canadian women. *International Journal of Mental Health Nursing, 16,* 203–213.
- Harrison, A., & Branding, J. (2009). Improving mental health care for older people within a general hospital in the U.K. *Nursing & Health Sciences, 11,* 293–300.

4. Read one of the case studies suggested below and evaluate the extent to which the case study approach was appropriate. What were the drawbacks and benefits of using this approach? Was this a single or multiple case study? Would the design best be described as holistic or embedded?

- Mawn, B., Siquiera, E., Koren, A., Slatin, C., Devereux-Melillo, K., Pearce, C., & Hoff, L. (2010). Health disparities among health care workers. *Qualitative Health Research, 20,* 68–80.
- Nurjannah, I., Fitzgerald, M., & Foster, L. (2009). Patients' experiences of absconding from a psychiatric setting in Indonesia. *International Journal of Mental Health Nursing, 18,* 326–335.
- Sassi-Matthias, M., & Babrow, A. (2007). Problematic integration of uncertainty and desire in pregnancy. *Qualitative Health Research, 17,* 786–798.

5. Read one of the studies below, and evaluate the extent to which the problem was well suited to the grounded theory research tradition. Which of the schools of grounded theory thought was followed in this study? Does the report explicitly discuss how the constant comparative method was used?

- Kartalova-O'Doherty, Y., & Tedstone-Doherty, D. (2010). Recovering from recurrent mental health problems: Giving up and fighting to get better. *International Journal of Mental Health Nursing, 19,* 3–15.
- Law, R. (2009). "Bridging worlds": Meeting the emotional needs of dying patients. *Journal of Advanced Nursing, 65,* 2630–2641.
- McCreadie, M., & Wiggins, S. (2009). Reconciling the good patient persona with problematic and non-problematic humour: A grounded theory. *International Journal of Nursing Studies, 46,* 1079–1091.

6. Read one of the studies below, and think about how the researcher could have adopted a critical theory or feminist perspective. In what way would the methods for such a modification differ from the methods used?

- Greenslade, M., Elliott, B., & Mandville-Anstey, S. (2010). Same-day breast cancer surgery: A qualitative study of women's lived experiences. *Oncology Nursing Forum, 37,* E92–97.
- Pieters, H., & Heilerman, M. (2010). "I can't do it on my own": Motivation to enter therapy for depression among low-income, second generation, Latinas. *Issues in Mental Health Nursing, 31,* 279–287.
- Ohalete, N., Georges, J., & Doswell, W. (2010). Tales from the "hood": Placing reproductive health communication between African American fathers and children in context. *ABNF Journal, 21,* 14–20.

■ C. Application Exercises

EXERCISE 1: STUDY IN APPENDIX E

Read the abstract and introduction to the report by Beck ("The arm") in Appendix E. Then answer the following questions:

Questions of Fact

a. In which tradition was this study based? Did this study have an ideological perspective?
b. Was this a descriptive or interpretive study?
c. What is the central phenomenon under study?
d. Was the study longitudinal?
e. Is there evidence of bracketing?
f. Is the research question congruent with a qualitative approach and with the specific research tradition (i.e., is the domain of inquiry for the study congruent with the domain encompassed by the tradition)?

Questions for Discussion

a. How well is the research design described in the report? Are design decisions explained and justified?
b. Does it appear that Beck made all design decisions up front, or did the design emerge during data collection, allowing her to capitalize on early information?
c. Were there any elements of the design or methods that appear to be more appropriate for a qualitative tradition other than the one Beck identified as the underlying tradition?
d. Could this study have been undertaken within an ideological framework? If so, what changes to the research methods would be necessary?

EXERCISE 2: STUDY IN APPENDIX G

Read the design and method sections of the report by Rasmussen and colleagues ("Young Women with Type 1 Diabetes") in Appendix G. Then answer the following questions:

Questions of Fact

a. In which tradition was this study based?
b. Which specific approach was used—that of Glaser and Strauss, Strauss and Corbin, or Charmaz?
c. What is the central phenomenon under study?
d. Was the study longitudinal?
e. What was the setting for this research?
f. Did the report indicate or suggest that constant comparison was used?
g. Was a core variable or basic social process identified? If yes, what was it?

h. Is the research question congruent with a qualitative approach and with the specific research tradition (i.e., is the domain of inquiry for the study congruent with the domain encompassed by the tradition)?
i. Did the researchers use methods that were congruent with the qualitative research tradition?
j. Did this study have an ideological perspective? If so, which one?

Questions for Discussion

a. How well is the research approach described in the report? Were design decisions explained and justified?
b. Does it appear that the researchers made design decisions up front, or did the approach emerge during data collection, allowing them to capitalize on early information?
c. Were there any elements of the design or methods that appear to be more appropriate for a qualitative tradition other than the one the researchers identified as the underlying tradition?
d. Could this study have been undertaken within an ideological framework? If so, what changes to the research methods would be necessary?

■ D. The Toolkit

For Chapter 20, the Toolkit on the accompanying CD-ROM contains a Word file with the following:

- Guidelines for Critiquing Qualitative Designs (Box 20.1 of the textbook)
- Useful Websites for Chapter 20: Resources for Qualitative Research Design

CHAPTER 21

Sampling in Qualitative Research

■ A. Crossword Puzzle

Complete the crossword puzzle below, which uses terms and concepts presented in Chapter 21. (Puzzles may be removed for easier viewing.)

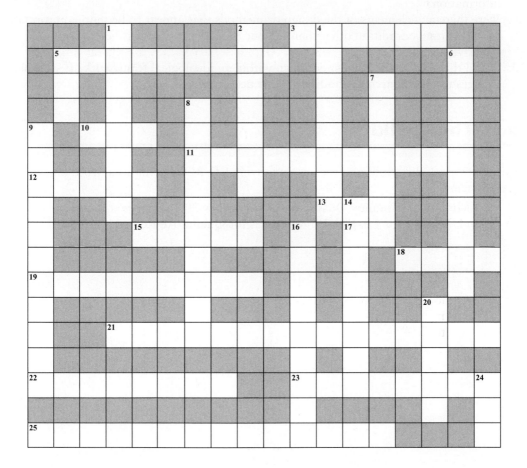

ACROSS

3. _ _ _ _ _ _ tory case sampling involves gaining access to a case representing a phenomenon previously inaccessible to scrutiny.
5. A widely used purposive sampling approach is maximum _____ sampling.
10. Ethnographers sometimes begin sampling by using a "_____ net" approach.
11. The type of sampling preferred by grounded theory researchers
12. A type of sampling that selects below average, average, and above average cases is _ _ _ _ _ified purposive.
13. In phenomenological research, the number of participants is usually fewer than _____.
15. Another name for snowball sampling is _____ sampling.
17. The symbol < stands for this (acronym).
18. The lower the _____ quality, the larger the sample usually must be.
19. Most often, qualitative researchers use a _____ approach to sampling, selecting specific types of participants who can best maximize information richness.
21. One of three models of generalization, sometimes called "reader generalizability"
22. _____ (or disconfirming) cases are sometimes sampled as a means of challenging researchers' interpretations.
23. _____ is a criterion for assessing a qualitative sampling strategy that concerns the sufficiency and quality of data the sample yielded.
25. Analytic _____ involves efforts to go from particulars of the sample and the data to a broader theory or conceptualization.

DOWN

1. _____ case sampling involves selecting important cases regarding the phenomenon of interest.
2. In _ _ _ _ _ _eous sampling, diversity is deliberately reduced to permit a more focused inquiry.
4. Sampling in qualitative studies often occurs in a(n) _____ manner, with decisions about who to sample and how many people to sample affected by what has already been learned.
5. Another term for convenience sample is _ _ _unteer sample.
6. The proximal _____ model involves developing a conception of the extent to which research contexts are comparable to contexts to which study results could be applied.
7. _____ case sampling is an approach in which the most unusual or extreme cases are selected.
8. The principle used by qualitative researchers to decide when to stop sampling
9. Qualitative researchers are encouraged to use thick _____ to enhance the ability of other people to assess congruence of contexts.
14. In phenomenological research, a participant must have experienced the phenomenon of interest in order to be _____ for the study.

16. Sampling of politically _____ cases is sometimes used to select or deselect cases for a study.

20. Ty _ _ _ _ _ case sampling involves selecting cases to highlight what is usual or normal.

24. Ethnographers rely on a sample of _____ informants (backwards!).

■ B. Study Questions

1. For each of the research questions below, indicate what type of qualitative sampling approach you would recommend, being as specific as you can about sampling approach and sample size.
   a. What is the process of adaptation and coping among the partners of AIDS patients?
   b. What is the lived experience of having a child who is diagnosed with leukemia?
   c. What rituals relating to dying are undertaken by nursing home residents and staff?
   d. What is the experience of waiting for service in a hospital emergency department?
   e. What is the process by which men and women come to terms with an unexpected diagnosis of pancreatic cancer?

2. Suppose a qualitative researcher wanted to study the life quality of cancer survivors. Suggest what the researcher might do to obtain a maximum variation sample, a typical case sample, a homogeneous sample, and an extreme case sample.

3. Read one of the following studies and identify specific examples of what could be called *thick description:*
   • Doherty, M. E. (2010). Voices of midwives: A tapestry of challenges and blessings. *MCN: American Journal of Maternal/Child Nursing, 35,* 96–101.
   • Swanlund, S. (2010). Successful cardiovascular medication management processes as perceived by community-dwelling adults over age 74. *Applied Nursing Research, 23,* 22–29.

4. Read the introduction and methods section of one of the following qualitative reports. Use the guidelines in Box 21.1 of the textbook (available as a Word document in the Toolkit ✪) to critique the sampling plan:
   • Anderberg, P., & Berglund, A. (2010). Elderly persons' experiences of striving to receive care on their own terms in nursing homes. *International Journal of Nursing Practice, 16,* 64–68.
   • Bratcher, J. R. (2010). How do critical care nurses define a "good death" in the intensive care unit? *Critical Care Nursing Quarterly, 33,* 87–99.
   • Fisher, S., & Colyer, H. (2009). Making decisions about care: What it means for hospice inpatients with terminal progressive disease. *International Journal of Palliative Nursing, 15,* 548–553.

■ C. Application Exercises

EXERCISE 1: STUDY IN APPENDIX B

Read the method section of the article by Cricco-Lizza ("Rooting for the breast") in Appendix B. Then answer the following questions:

Questions of Fact

a. What were the eligibility criteria for this study?
b. How were study participants recruited?
c. What type of sampling approach was used?
d. How many participants comprised the sample?
e. Was data saturation achieved?
f. Were sample characteristics described? If yes, what were those characteristics?

Questions for Discussion

a. Comment on the adequacy of the researcher's sampling plan and recruitment strategy for achieving the goals of the study.
b. Do you think Cricco-Lizza's sample size was adequate? Why or why not?
c. Cricco-Lizza used nurse experience as her dimension of variability in selecting key informants. What other dimensions might have been used productively?

EXERCISE 2: STUDY IN APPENDIX G

Read the method section of the article by Rasmussen and colleagues ("Young women with type I diabetes") in Appendix G. Then answer the following questions:

Questions of Fact

a. What were the eligibility criteria for this study?
b. How were study participants recruited?
c. What type of sampling approach was used?
d. How many study participants comprised the sample?
e. Was data saturation achieved?
f. Did the sampling strategy include confirming and disconfirming cases?
g. Were sample characteristics described? If yes, what were those characteristics?

Questions for Discussion

a. Comment on the adequacy of the researchers' sampling plan and recruitment strategy for achieving the goals of a grounded theory study.
b. Assume that you had no resource constraints to address the research questions in this study. What sampling plan would you recommend?

c. Do you think the sample size in this study was adequate? Why or why not?

d. Comment on issues relating to the transferability of findings from this study.

■ D. The Toolkit

For Chapter 21, the Toolkit on the accompanying CD-ROM contains a Word file with the following:

- Guidelines for Critiquing Qualitative Sampling Designs (Box 21.1 of the textbook)
- Useful Websites for Chapter 21: Resources for Qualitative Sampling

CHAPTER 22

Data Collection in Qualitative Research

■ A. Crossword Puzzle

Complete the crossword puzzle below, which uses terms and concepts presented in Chapter 22. (Puzzles may be removed for easier viewing.)

ACROSS

1. The type of interview in which the interviewer uses a list of questions that must be covered
6. Participants can be asked to maintain a journal or _____ that provides rich, ongoing data about aspects of ordinary life.
7. Observational data are maintained in _____ notes.
8. The type of observation often undertaken in qualitative studies to "get inside" a social situation is _____ observation.
13. Interviewers may benefit from a(n) _____ guide that specifies the question areas that must be covered.
14. Methodologic _____ document participant observers' thoughts about their strategies while in the field.
15. A chronology of daily events during field observations is maintained in _____.
16. _____ histories are used to gather personal recollections of events and their perceived causes or consequences.
18. The think-_____ method involves having people talk about decisions as they are making them.
19. The _ _ _ _rnet can yield rich qualitative data, for example, through postings in chat rooms.
21. A skilled interviewer must learn how to _____ effectively to elicit more detail (backwards!).
22. An unstructured interview often begins with a(n) _____ tour question.
23. Observational notes include descriptive and _ _ _ _ective notes.

DOWN

2. The person who leads a focus group session
3. Unstructured interviews cons_ _ _ _ _ neither the interviewers nor the participants.
4. Photo _____ is a technique that uses photographs to encourage participant narratives.
5. A visual record of an observational setting can be made by _____ taping it.
8. Observers have to make decisions about _____ themselves in the field so as best to capture the behaviors and events of interest.
9. The technique called _____ incidents focuses on the circumstances surrounding particularly notable incidents.
10. The best method to record unstructured interviews is to _____ tape them.
11. Researchers who tape their interviews must then _____ them so that the data can be read, re-read, and analyzed.
12. In a life _____ interview, participants are encouraged to provide a chronologic narration of life experiences.
17. Both semistructured and focus group interviews typically involve use of a topic _____.
20. Participant observers may often have to excuse themselves from a setting to briefly _____ down notes about what is transpiring.

■ B. Study Questions

1. Suppose you were interested in studying the frustrations of patients awaiting laboratory test results before a decision on postsurgical treatment for breast cancer can be made. Develop a topic guide for a focused interview on this topic.

2. Below are several research problems. Indicate which type of unstructured approach you might recommend using for each. Defend your response.

   a. By what process do older brothers and sisters of a handicapped child adapt to their sibling's disability?
   b. What is it like to have a persistent wound?
   c. What stresses does the spouse of a terminally ill patient experience?
   d. What type of information does a nurse draw on most heavily in formulating nursing diagnoses?
   e. What are the coping mechanisms and perceived barriers to coping among severely disfigured burn patients?

3. Develop a topic guide that focuses on nursing students' reasons for selecting nursing as a career and their satisfactions and dissatisfactions with their decision. Administer the topic guide to five first-year nursing students in a face-to-face interview situation. Now, administer the topic guide in a focus group setting with five nursing students. Compare the kinds of information that the two approaches yielded. What, if anything, did you learn in the group setting that did not emerge in the personal interviews (and vice versa)?

4. Would a psychiatric nurse researcher be well suited to undertake a participant observation study of the interactions between psychiatric nurses and their clients? Why or why not?

5. Read one of the following articles, and indicate how, if at all, you would augment the self-report data collected in this study with participant observation:

   • Cypress, B. S. (2010). The intensive care unit: Experiences of patients, families, and their nurses. *Dimensions of Critical Care Nursing, 29,* 94–101.
   • Gonzalez-Guarda, R., Oetega, J., Vasquez, E., & DeSantis, J. (2010). La *Mancha Negra:* Substance abuse, violence, and sexual risks among Hispanic males. *Western Journal of Nursing Research, 32,* 128–148.
   • Shigaki, C., Moore, C., Wakefield, B., Campbell, J., & LeMaster, J. (2010). Nurse partners in chronic illness care: patients' perceptions and their implications for nursing leadership. *Nursing Administration Quarterly, 34,* 130–140.

6. Read the introduction and method section of one of the following reports. Use the critiquing guidelines in Box 22.3 of the textbook (available as a Word document in the Toolkit ✪) to critique the data collection aspects of the study:

   • Kresheh, R., & Barclay, L. (2010). The lived experience of Jordanian women who received family support during labor. *MCN: The American Journal of Maternal/Child Nursing, 35,* 47–51.

- Meyer, M., & Champion, J. (2010). Protective factors for HIV infection among Mexican American men who have sex with men. *Journal of the Association of Nurses in AIDS Care, 21,* 53–62.
- Murphy, F., & Philpin, S. (2010). Early miscarriage as "matter out of place": An ethnographic study of nursing practice in a hospital gynaecological unit. *International Journal of Nursing Studies, 47,* 534–541.

■ C. Application Exercises

EXERCISE 1: STUDY IN APPENDIX B

Read the method section of the article by Cricco-Lizza ("Rooting for the breast") in Appendix B—paying special attention to the subsection labeled "Data Collection." Then answer the following questions:

Questions of Fact

a. Did the researcher collect any self-report data? If no, could self-reports have been used? If yes, what concepts were captured by self-report?
b. What specific types of qualitative self-report methods were used?
c. Were examples of questions included in the report?
d. Does the report provide information about how long interviews took, on average?
e. How were the self-report data recorded?
f. Did this study collect any data through observation? If no, could observation have been used? If yes, what concepts were captured through observation?
g. If there were observations, how were observational data recorded?
h. Were any other types of data collected in this study?
i. Who collected the data in this study?

Questions for Discussion

a. Comment on the adequacy of the researcher's description of her data collection methods.
b. Comment on the data collection approaches Cricco-Lizza used. Did she fully capture the concepts of interest in the best possible manner?
c. If examples of specific questions were included in the report, do they appear appropriate for collecting the desired information? If they were not included, does the absence of such examples undermine your ability to fully understand the quality of evidence the study yielded?
d. If the report describes how long the interviews were, do you feel the interviews were sufficiently long to obtain the desired information? If such information was missing, does its absence undermine your ability to fully understand the quality of evidence the study yielded?
e. Comment on the procedures used to collect and record data in this study. Were adequate steps taken to ensure the highest possible quality data?

EXERCISE 2: STUDY IN APPENDIX E

Read the method section of the article by Beck ("The arm") in Appendix E.
Then answer the following questions:

Questions of Fact

a. Did Beck collect any self-report data? If no, could self-reports have been used? If yes, what concepts were captured by self-report?
b. What specific types of qualitative self-report methods were used?
c. Were examples of questions included in the report?
d. Does the report provide information about how long interviews took, on average?
e. How were the self-report data recorded?
f. Did this study collect any data through observation? If no, could observation have been used? If yes, what concepts were captured through observation?
g. If there were observations, how were observational data recorded?
h. Who collected the data in this study?

Questions for Discussion

a. Comment on the adequacy of the researcher's description of her data collection methods.
b. Comment on the data collection approaches Beck used. Did she fully capture the concepts of interest in the best possible manner?
c. If examples of specific questions were included in the report, do they appear appropriate for collecting the desired information? If they were not included, does the absence of such examples undermine your ability to fully understand the quality of evidence the study yielded?
d. If the report describes how long the interviews were, do you feel the interviews were sufficiently long to obtain the desired information? If such information was missing, does its absence undermine your ability to fully understand the quality of evidence the study yielded?
e. Comment on the procedures used to collect and record data in this study. Were adequate steps taken to ensure the highest possible quality data?

■ D. The Toolkit

For Chapter 22, the Toolkit on the accompanying CD-ROM contains a Word file with the following:

- Guidelines for Critiquing Unstructured Data Collection Methods (Box 22.3 of the textbook)
- Example of a topic guide for a semistructured interview*
- Example of an agenda for a focus group session*

- Focus groups versus in-depth personal interviews: Guide to selecting a method*
- Example of a protocol for a windshield (community mapping) survey*
- Examples of types of information relevant in unstructured observation (from textbook)
- Example of an observation protocol for unstructured observation*
- Useful Websites for Chapter 22: Resources for Unstructured Data Collection

---

*These items do not appear in the textbook.

CHAPTER 23

Qualitative Data Analysis

■ A. Crossword Puzzle

Complete the crossword puzzle below, which uses terms and concepts presented in Chapter 23. (Puzzles may be removed for easier viewing.)

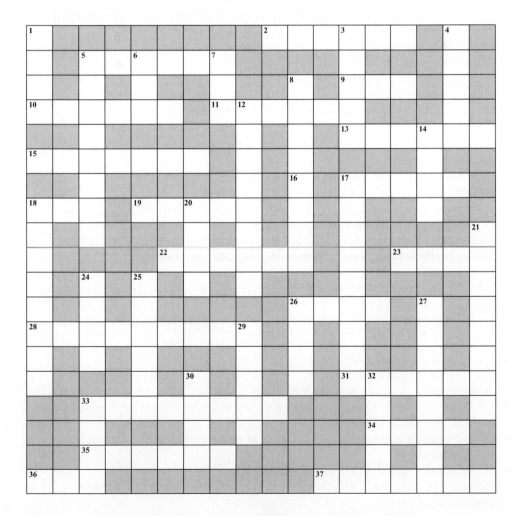

ACROSS

2. A sociogram can be used to map the flow of conversation between a _____ of a focus group and others in the group.
5. Phenomenological analysis involves the identification of essential _____.
9. In Glaser & Strauss' method, there are theoretical codes and _ _ _stantive codes.
10. In ethnographies, a broad unit of cultural knowledge
11. In the hierarchy of grounded theory codes, in vivo codes are _____ codes.
13. The hermeneutic _____ involves movement between parts and whole of a text being analyzed.
15. _ _ _ _ _ _ _i was a prominent analyst and writer in the Duquesne school of phenomenology.
16. In Diekelmann's approach, the discovery of a constitutive _____ forms the highest level of analysis.
18. In grounded theory, the developing categories of the substantive theory must _____ the data.
19. The phenomenologist _ _ _ _ _i did not espouse validating themes with peers or study participants.
22. The hermeneutic approach developed by _____ includes an analysis of exemplars.
23. Transcribed interviews are usually the main form of _____ in phenomenological analysis.
26. Timelines and _____ charts are devices that can be used to highlight time sequences in qualitative analysis.
28. The ability to "make meaning" from qualitative texts depends on researchers' _____ in and closeness to the data.
31. After a categorization system is developed, the main task involves _____ the data.
33. A Dutch phenomenologist who encouraged the use of artistic data sources
34. Sometimes qualitative _____ analysis is described as a content analysis.
35. Before analysis can begin, qualitative researchers have to develop a categorization _____.
36. All of a phenomenologist's transcribed interviews would comprise a qualitative data _____.
37. One of the two major schools of phenomenology (a Dutch school)

DOWN

1. A recurring _____ in a set of interviews can be the basis for an emerging theme.
3. One type of core variable in grounded theory is a _____ social process that evolves over time.
4. A type of coding in Strauss and Corbin's approach wherein the analyst links subcategories
5. A preliminary guide for sorting narrative data
6. When voice recognition software is used, oral transcriptionists still need to _ _ _t the text to correct errors.

7. In grounded theory, _ _ _ective coding focuses on the core variable.
8. A device sometimes used as part of an analytic strategy, especially by interpretive phenomenologists
12. Themes and conceptualizations are viewed as _____ in qualitative analysis.
14. In grounded theory, the _____ category is a central pattern that is relevant to participants.
17. The second level of analysis in Spradley's ethnographic method
18. Glaser originally proposed 18 _____ of theoretical codes to help grounded theorists conceptualize relationships.
20. The first stage of constant comparison involves _____ coding.
21. _____ cases are strong examples of ways of being in the world.
24. Grounded theorists document an idea in an analytic _____.
25. The nurse researcher who helped develop an alternative approach to grounded theory
26. In manual organization of qualitative data, excerpts are cut up and inserted into a conceptual _____.
27. In Van Manen's _____ approach, the analyst sees the text as a whole and tries to capture its meaning.
29. The field _____ of an ethnographer are an important source of data for analysis.
30. Van _____ was a phenomenologist from the Duquesne school.
32. The purpose of developing a categorization scheme is to impose _____ on the narrative information.
33. The amount of data collected in a typical qualitative study typically is _____.

■ B. Study Questions

1. Ask two people to describe their conception of preventive healthcare and what it means in their daily lives. Pool descriptions with those of other classmates, and develop a category scheme to organize responses.

2. If possible, listen to an audiotaped interview and transcribe a few minutes of it. Compare your transcription with that of another classmate, or with that of the professional transcriber.

3. What is wrong with the following statements?
   a. Hall conducted a grounded theory study about coping with a miscarriage in which she was able to identify four major themes.
   b. Lowe's ethnographic analysis of Haitian clinics involved gleaning related thematic material from French poetry.
   c. Allen's phenomenological study of the lived experience of Parkinson's disease focused on the domain of fatigue.
   d. Dodd's grounded theory study of widowhood yielded a taxonomy of coping strategies.
   e. In her ethnographic study of the culture of a nursing home, MacLean used a rural nursing home as a paradigm case.

4. A descriptive category scheme for coding interviews with recently divorced women follows:

**CODING SCHEME FOR STUDY
OF ADJUSTMENT TO DIVORCE**

---

1. Divorce-related issues
   a. Adjustment to divorce
   b. Divorce-induced problems
   c. Advantages of divorce

2. General psychological state
   a. Before divorce
   b. During divorce
   c. Current

3. Physical health
   a. Before divorce
   b. During divorce
   c. Current

4. Relationship with children
   a. General quality
   b. Communication
   c. Share activities
   d. Structure of relationship

5. Parenting
   a. Discipline and child-rearing
   b. Feelings about parenthood
   c. Feelings about single parenthood

6. Friendship/social participation
   a. Dating and marriage
   b. Friendships
   c. Social groups, leisure
   d. Social support

7. Employment/education
   a. Employment experiences
   b. Educational experiences
   c. Job and career goals
   d. Educational goals

8. Workload
   a. Coping with workload
   b. Schedule
   c. Child care arrangements

9. Finances

Read the following excerpt, taken from a real interview. Use the coding scheme to code the topics discussed in this excerpt.

> I think raising the children is so much easier without the father around. There isn't two people conflicting back and forth. You know, like . . . like you discipline them during the day. They do something wrong, you're not saying, "When daddy gets home, you're going to get a spanking." You know, you do that. The kid gets a spanking right then and there. But when two people live together, they have their ways of raising and you have your ways of raising the children and it's so hard for two people to raise children. It's so much easier for one person. The only reason a male would be around is financial-wise. But me and the kids are happier now, and we get along with each other better, cause like, there isn't this competitive thing. My husband always wanted all the attention around here.

5. Read the method and results sections of one of the following reports. Use the critiquing guidelines in Box 23.3 of the textbook (available as a Word document in the Toolkit ⊗) to critique the data analysis aspects of the study:

- Foli, K. (2010). Depression in adoptive parents: A model of understanding through grounded theory. *Western Journal of Nursing Research, 32,* 379–400.
- Juthberg, C., & Sundin, K. (2010). Registered nurses' and nurse assistants' lived experience of troubled conscience in their work in elderly care—a phenomenological hermeneutic study. *International Journal of Nursing Studies, 47,* 20–29.
- Werner, P., Goldstein, D., & Buchbinder, E. (2010). Subjective experience of family stigma as reported by children of Alzheimer's disease patients. *Qualitative Health Research, 20,* 159–169.

■ C. Application Exercises

EXERCISE 1: STUDY IN APPENDIX E

Read the "Data Analysis" and "Results" sections of the article by Beck ("The arm") in Appendix E. Then answer the following questions:

Questions of Fact

a. Did Beck organize her data manually or with the assistance of computer software? If the latter, what software was used?
b. Did Beck calculate any quasi-statistics?
c. Which phenomenological analytic approach was adopted in this study?
d. Did Beck prepare any analytic memos?
e. Did Beck describe the coding process? If so, what did she say?
f. How many themes emerged in Beck's analysis? What were they?
g. Did Beck provide supporting evidence for her themes, in the form of excerpts from the data?

Questions for Discussion

a. Discuss the thoroughness of Beck's description of her data analysis efforts. Did the report present adequate information about the steps taken to analyze the data?
b. Was there any evidence of "method slurring"—that is, did Beck apply any analytic procedures that are inappropriate for a phenomenological approach?
c. Discuss the effectiveness of Beck's presentation of results. Does the analysis seem sensible, thoughtful, and thorough? Was sufficient evidence provided to support the findings? Were data presented in a manner that allows you to be confident about Beck's conclusions?

EXERCISE 2: STUDY IN APPENDIX G

Read the "Data Analysis" and "Results" sections of the article by Rasmussen and colleagues ("Young women with type I diabetes") in Appendix G. Then answer the following questions:

Questions of Fact

a. Did the researchers audiotape and transcribe the interviews? If yes, who did the transcription? Did the report state how many pages of data comprised the data set?
b. Was constant comparison used in analyzing the data?
c. Did Rasmussen and colleagues create conceptual files? Was a computer used to analyze the data? If yes, what software was used?
d. Did the researchers calculate any quasi-statistics?
e. Which grounded theory analytic approach was adopted in this study?
f. Did the researchers prepare any analytic memos?
g. Did the authors describe the open coding process? If so, what did they say?
h. Did the authors describe the process of theoretical coding? If so, what did they say? Did they offer any examples of their theoretical codes?
i. How many categories emerged in the analysis? How many major categories were ultimately developed and refined? What were they?
j. What was the BSP? What does the BSP entail?
k. Did the report include a figure that represented the grounded theory?

Questions for Discussion

a. Discuss the thoroughness of Rasmussen and colleagues' description of their data analysis efforts. Did the report present adequate information about the coding of the data and the steps taken to analyze the data?
b. Was there any evidence of "method slurring"—that is, did Rasmussen and colleagues apply any analytic procedures that are inappropriate for a grounded theory approach?
c. Discuss the effectiveness of the researchers' presentation of results. Does the analysis seem sensible, thoughtful, and thorough?
d. Were data presented in a manner that allows you to be confident about the researchers' conclusions? Comment on the inclusion or noninclusion of figures that graphically represent the grounded theory.

■ D. The Toolkit

For Chapter 23, the Toolkit on the accompanying CD-ROM contains a Word file with the following:

- Guidelines for Critiquing Qualitative Analyses and Interpretations (Box 23.3 of the textbook)
- Example of a Memo from Beck's (2002) Study on Mothering Multiples*
- Example of a Codebook from Beck's (2005) Study of the Benefits of Participating in Internet Interviews*
- Example of Coding Hierarchy from Beck's (2002) Study on Mothering Multiples*
- Useful Websites for Chapter 23: Resources for Qualitative Analysis

---

*These items do not appear in the textbook.

Trustworthiness and Integrity in Qualitative Research

■ A. Crossword Puzzle

Complete the crossword puzzle below, which uses terms and concepts presented in Chapter 24. (Puzzles may be removed for easier viewing.)

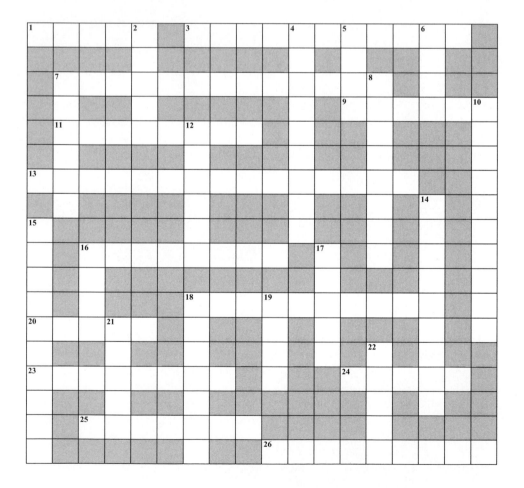

ACROSS

1. Confirmability can be addressed through a scrutiny of documents and procedures in an inquiry _____.
3. A key criterion for assessing quality in qualitative studies, in both frameworks described in the textbook
7. Use of multiple means of converging on the truth
9. _ _ _ _ _ _ ability refers to the stability of data over time and conditions, analogous to reliability.
11. _ _ _ _ _ _ _ _ ness is a secondary criterion in the Whittemore and colleagues framework, referring to the ability to follow researchers' decisions and interpretations.
13. Extent to which qualitative findings can be applied to other settings
16. Auditability can be enhanced by maintaining a log of each _____, that is, by documenting judgments and choices.
18. A secondary criterion in the Whittemore and colleagues framework, referring to interconnectedness
20. Collecting data in multiple sites is a form of _____ triangulation.
23. Credibility in qualitative inquiry has been described as analogous to _____ validity in quantitative inquiry.
24. _ _ _ _ ness involves the presentation of rich, artful descriptions that highlight salient themes in the data.
25. A(n) _____ audit involves a scrutiny of data and supporting documents by an external reviewer.
26. Persistent _____ refers to a focus on the aspects of a situation that are relevant to the phenomena being studied (abbr.).

DOWN

2. An audit _____ is a systematic collection and assembly of materials for an independent auditor.
4. A word used by some as an overarching goal for qualitative inquiry, in lieu of validity
5. A music player (brand name—unrelated to research!)
6. _____ triangulation involves collecting data about a phenomenon at multiple points.
7. With _____ triangulation, researchers use competing hypotheses or conceptualizations in their analysis and interpretation of data.
8. A process by which researchers revise their interpretations by including cases that appear to disconfirm earlier hypotheses is a(n) _____ case analysis.
10. Credibility can be enhanced through a thorough search for _____ing evidence.
12. One method of addressing credibility involves going back to participants to do member _____.
14. _ _ _ _ _ _ _ _ _ ity is a quality criterion indicating the extent to which the researchers fairly and faithfully show a range of different realities.

15. _ _ _ _ _ _ _ _ _ _ or triangulation is achieved by having 2+ researchers make key decisions and interpretations.

16. Interviewing patients *and* family members about a phenomenon is an example of _____ source triangulation.

17. Qualitative researchers strive for the _ _ _ _ _worthiness of their data and their methods.

18. _ _ _ _ _ _ _ity is a secondary criterion in the Whittemore et al. framework, reflecting challenges to traditional ways of thinking.

19. Lincoln and _____ proposed criteria for evaluating the trustworthiness of qualitative inquiries.

21. Researchers typically "_____" transcribed data by comparing transcriptions to recordings and making necessary corrections.

22. A term that is hotly debated in terms of appropriateness for evaluating quality in qualitative inquiry.

■ B. Study Questions

1. Suppose you were conducting a grounded theory study of couples' coming to terms with infertility. What might you do to incorporate various types of triangulation into your study?

2. In the previous chapter, one study question involved a class exercise to elicit descriptions of people's conceptions of preventive healthcare and what it means in their daily lives (Study question B.1 in Chapter 23). Describe efforts you could take to enhance the integrity of this inquiry.

3. What is your opinion about the value of member checking as a strategy to enhance credibility? Defend your position.

4. Read a research report in a recent issue of the journal *Qualitative Health Research*. Identify several examples of "thick description." Also, identify areas of the report in which you feel additional thick description would have enhanced the inquiry.

5. Read one of the following reports. Use the critiquing guidelines in Box 24.1 of the textbook (available as a Word document in the Toolkit ✪) to evaluate the integrity and quality of the study—augmented, as appropriate, by questions in Table 24.1 of the textbook:

   • Cruickshank, S., Adamson, E., Logan, J., & Brackenridge, K. (2010). Using syringe drivers in palliative care within a rural, community setting: Capturing the whole experience. *International Journal of Palliative Nursing, 16,* 126–132.

   • Gangenes, J. E. (2010). Adaptations to achieve physical activity in rural communities. *Western Journal of Nursing Research, 32,* 401–419.

   • Kong, E., Deatrick, J., & Evans, L. (2010). The experiences of Korean immigrant caregivers of non-English-speaking older relatives. *Qualitative Health Research, 20,* 319–329.

■ C. Application Exercises

EXERCISE 1: STUDY IN APPENDIX E

Read the report by Beck ("The Arm") in Appendix E. Then answer the following questions:

Questions of Fact

a. Did Beck devote a section of her report to describing quality-enhancement strategies? If so, what was it labeled? If not, where was information about such strategies located?
b. What types of triangulation, if any, were used in Beck's study?
c. Were any of the following methods used to enhance the credibility of the study and its data?

- Prolonged engagement and/or persistent observation
- Member checks
- Search for disconfirming evidence
- Researcher credibility
- Other methods

d. Describe what methods (if any) were used to enhance the following aspects of the study:

- Dependability
- Transferability
- Authenticity
- Explicitness

Questions for Discussion

a. Discuss the thoroughness with which Beck described her efforts to enhance and evaluate the quality and integrity of her study.
b. Discuss the extent to which Beck made efforts to enhance the transferability of her study findings.
c. How would you characterize the integrity and trustworthiness of this study, based on Beck's documentation?

EXERCISE 2: STUDY IN APPENDIX G

Read the report by Rasmussen and colleagues ("Young women with type I diabetes") in Appendix G. Then answer the following questions:

Questions of Fact

a. Did the researchers devote a section of their report to describing their quality-enhancement strategies? If so, what was it labeled? If not, where was information about such strategies located?

b. What types of triangulation, if any, were used in this study?
c. Were any of the following methods used to enhance the credibility of the study and its data?
   - Prolonged engagement and/or persistent observation
   - Peer review and debriefing
   - Member checks
   - Search for disconfirming evidence
   - Researcher credibility
d. Describe what methods (if any) were used to enhance the following aspects of the study:
   - Dependability
   - Confirmability
   - Transferability
   - Authenticity
   - Explicitness

Questions for Discussion

a. Discuss the thoroughness with which Rasmussen and colleagues described their efforts to enhance and evaluate the quality and integrity of her study.
b. In the section titled "Rigor and Credibility," the authors state that their strategies "were all very important, assuring credibility." Comment on this statement.
c. How would you characterize the integrity and trustworthiness of this study, based on the researchers' documentation?

■ D. The Toolkit

For Chapter 24, the Toolkit on the accompanying CD-ROM contains a Word file with the following:

- Guidelines for Evaluating Quality and Integrity in Qualitative Studies (Box 24.1 of the textbook)
- Questions for Self-Scrutiny during a Study: Whittemore et al.'s Primary Qualitative Validity Criteria (Table 24.1 of the textbook)
- Questions for Self-Scrutiny during a Study: Whittemore et al.'s Secondary Qualitative Validity Criteria (Table 24.1 of the textbook)
- Questions for Post Hoc Assessments of a Study: Whittemore et al.'s Primary Qualitative Validity Criteria (Table 24.1 of the textbook)
- Questions for Post Hoc Assessments of a Study: Whittemore et al.'s Secondary Qualitative Validity Criteria (Table 24.1 of the textbook)
- Useful Websites for Chapter 24: Resources for Qualitative Integrity

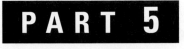

PART 5

Designing and Conducting Mixed Methods Studies to Generate Evidence for Nursing

CHAPTER 25

Overview of Mixed Methods Research

■ A. Crossword Puzzle

Complete the crossword puzzle below, which uses terms and concepts presented in Chapter 25. (Puzzles may be removed for easier viewing.)

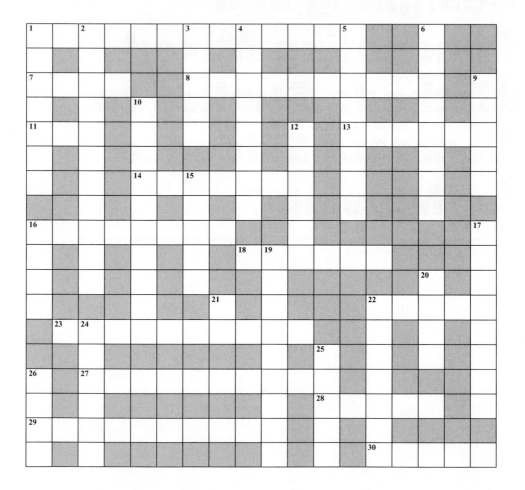

ACROSS

1. The purpose of the _____ design is to obtain different, but complementary, data about the central phenomenon under study.
7. Structured and unstructured _____ are analyzed in a mixed methods study.
8. The paradigmatic basis of mixed methods research is sometimes said to be _____.
11. In an explanatory or exploratory design, there is a time _____ between phases of the study.
13. Inference _ _ _ _ _ erability is the degree to which mixed methods conclusions can be applied in other contexts.
14. In mixed methods study, researchers sometimes _____ one type of data into a different type (e.g., qualitizing).
16. Researchers give equal _____ to the QUAL and QUAN strands in some mixed methods studies.
18. Mixed methods studies can involve both *intramethod* (e.g., structured and unstructured self-reports) and *intermethod* (e.g., biophysiologic measures and unstructured observation) approaches to _____ data collection methods.
22. In selecting a design, mixed methods researchers should have a basic grasp of the project's theoretical _____.
23. Mixed methods research is often used to develop and test a(n) _____.
27. Mixed methods designs that have multiple phases are called _____ designs.
28. In mixed method notation, the symbol used when one strand is completed prior to starting the other strand.
29. Quality criteria for evaluating *interpretive rigor* include interpretive and _ _ _ _ _ _ _ _ _ l consistency—that is, conceptual congruence.
30. A _ _ _ _ _ level relationship involves selecting samples from different levels of a hierarchy.

DOWN

1. Mixed methods researchers who have written extensive methodologic advice are _____ and Tashakkori.
2. Mixed methods research can only achieve its full potential for enhanced insights when _____ of the two types of data or results occurs.
3. The strand that has the dominant status is often symbolized in _____ case letters.
4. In a convergence model (QUAN + QUAL), data for the two strands are collected and analyzed in parallel and then the results of the two separate _____ are compared and contrasted.
5. Mixed methods designs are often portrayed using a _____ system developed by nurse researcher Janice Morse.
6. When one strand has higher priority than another strand in mixed methods research, it is said to have _____ status.

9. _ _ _ _ _ence quality is the overarching criterion for evaluating the quality of results and interpretations in mixed methods research.

10. In _____ designs, the two strands of data are collected simultaneously.

12. One tool to support mixed methods analyses is a meta-_____.

15. One of many sources of data in mixed methods studies could be field _____.

16. The _____ symbol is used to designate simultaneous collection of the two strands.

17. In a(n) _____ design, one type of data is used solely in a supportive capacity.

19. _____ sampling occurs when the same participants are in both strands of a mixed methods study.

20. To avoid _____, it is prudent to consider whether qualitative or quantitative data should be collected first.

21. An acronym for mixed methods research

22. Mixed methods designs can be represented in a visual _____.

24. In _____ sampling, participants in the qualitative strand are a subset of the participants in the quantitative strand.

25. Creswell and _____ Clark are two prominent mixed methods scholars.

26. A _____ inference is a conclusion generated by integrating inferences from both strands of a mixed methods study.

■ B. Study Questions

1. Read one of the following studies, in which quantitative data were gathered and analyzed to address a research question. What was the primary research question in this study? Write one or two related research questions that could be addressed with qualitative data to strengthen the study's inference quality or enhance its interpretability:

   - Benson, S., Hahn, S., Tan, S., Janssen, O., Schedlowski, M., & Eisenbruch, S. (2010). Maladaptive coping with illness in women with polycystic ovary syndrome. *Journal of Obstetric, Gynecologic & Neonatal Nursing, 39,* 37–45.
   - Kalisch, B., & Begeny, S. (2010). Preparation of nursing students for change and innovation. *Western Journal of Nursing Research, 32,* 157–167.
   - Rattray, J., Crocker, C., Jones, M., & Connaghan, J. (2010). Patients' perceptions of and emotional outcome after intensive care: results from a multicentre study. *Nursing in Critical Care, 15,* 86–93.

2. How would you design a mixed methods study to address the combined questions you developed for Exercise B.1? Draw a visual diagram of the design that you think would be especially well suited, and indicate the appropriate mixed methods notation.

3. Read one of the following studies, in which qualitative data were gathered and analyzed to address a research question. What was the primary research question in this study? Write one or two related research questions that could be addressed with quantitative data to strengthen the study's inference quality:

- Harris, R., Bennett, J., Davey, B., & Ross, F. (2010). Flexible working and the contribution of nurses in mid-life to the workforce: a qualitative study. *International Journal of Nursing Studies, 47,* 418–426.
- Noone, J., & Young, H. (2010). Rural mothers' experiences and perceptions of their role in pregnancy prevention for the adolescent daughters. *Journal of Obstetric, Gynecologic & Neonatal Nursing, 39,* 27–36.
- Oliffe, J., Bottorff, J., Johnson, J., Kelly, M., & LeBeau, K. (2010). Fathers: Locating smoking and masculinity in the postpartum. *Qualitative Health Research, 20,* 330–339.

4. How would you design a mixed methods study to address the combined questions you developed for Exercise B.3? Draw a visual diagram of the design that you think would be especially well suited, and indicate the appropriate mixed methods notation.

5. Below is a brief description of a mixed methods study, followed by a critique. Do you agree with this critique? Can you add other comments regarding the study design? Comment, for example, on the researcher's design and sampling strategies.

> **Fictitious Study.** Davis conducted a study designed to examine the emotional well-being of women who had a mastectomy. Davis wanted to develop an in-depth understanding of the emotional experiences of women as they recovered from their surgery, including the process by which they handled their fears, their concerns about their sexuality, their levels of anxiety and depression, their methods of coping, and their social supports.
>
> Davis's basic study design was a descriptive qualitative study. She gathered information from a sample of 26 women, primarily by means of in-depth interviews with the women on two occasions. The first interviews were scheduled within 1 month after the surgery. Follow-up interviews were conducted about 12 months later. Several women in the sample participated in a support group, and Davis attended and made observations at several meetings. Additionally, Davis decided to interview the "significant other" (usually the women's husbands) of most of the women, when it became clear that the women's emotional well-being was linked to the manner in which the significant other was reacting to the surgery.
>
> In addition to the rich, in-depth information she gathered, Davis wanted to be able to better interpret the emotional status of the women. Therefore, at both the original and follow-up interview with the women, she administered a psychological scale known as the Center for Epidemiological Studies Depression Scale (CES-D), a quantitative measure that has scores that can range from 0 to 60. This scale has been widely used in community populations and has cut-off scores designating when a person is at risk of clinical depression (i.e., a score of 16 and above).

Davis's qualitative analysis showed that the basic process underlying psychological recovery from the mastectomy was something she labeled "Gaining by Losing," a process that involved heightened self-awareness and self-respect after an initial period of despair and self-pity. The process also involved, for some, a strengthening of personal relationships with significant others, whereas for others, it resulted in the birth of awareness of fundamental deficiencies in their relationships. The quantitative findings confirmed that a very high percentage of women were at risk of being depressed at 1 month after the mastectomy, but at 12 months, the average level of depression was actually modestly lower than in the general population of women.

Critique. In her study, Davis embedded a quantitative measure into her fieldwork in an interesting manner. The bulk of data were qualitative—in-depth interviews and in-depth observations. However, she also opted to include a well-known measure of depression, which provided her with an important context for interpreting her data. A major advantage of using the CES-D is that this scale has known characteristics in the general population and, therefore, provided a built-in "comparison group."

Davis used a flexible design that allowed her to use her initial data to guide her inquiry. For example, she decided to conduct in-depth interviews with significant others when she learned their importance to the women's process of emotional recovery. Davis did do some advance planning, however, that provided loose guidance. For example, although her questioning undoubtedly evolved while in the field, she had the foresight to realize that to capture a process as it evolved, she would need to collect data longitudinally. She also made the up-front decision to use the CES-D to supplement the in-depth interviews.

In this study, the findings from the qualitative and quantitative portions of the study were complementary. Both portions of the study confirmed that the women initially had emotional "losses," but eventually they recovered and "gained" in terms of their emotional well-being and their self-awareness. This example illustrates how the validity of study findings can be enhanced by the blending of qualitative and quantitative data. If the qualitative data alone had been gathered, Davis might not have gotten a good handle on the degree to which the women had actually "recovered" (*vis à vis* women who had never had a mastectomy). Conversely, if she had collected only the CES-D data, she would have had no insights into the process by which the recovery occurred.

6. Read one of the following mixed methods studies. Use the critiquing guidelines in Box 25.1 of the textbook (available as a Word document in the Toolkit ✪) to critique the study:

   • Tluczek, A., Gabos, T., Ballenas, V., & Rutledge, R. (2010). When the cystic fibrosis label does not fit: A modified uncertainty theory. *Qualitative Health Research, 20,* 209–223.
   • Wilson, D. R. (2010). Stress management for adult survivors of childhood sexual abuse: A holistic inquiry. *Western Journal of Nursing Research, 32,* 103–127.

- Young, C., Armstrong, M., Roberts, A., Mello, I., & Angel, E. (2010). A triad of evidence for care of women with genital piercings. *Journal of the American Academy of Nurse Practitioners, 22*, 70–80.

■ C. Application Exercises

EXERCISE 1: STUDY IN APPENDIX B

Read the article by Cricco-Lizza ("Rooting for the breast") in Appendix B. Was this a mixed methods study? If yes, describe its design. If no, redesign the study in such a fashion that it would involve mixed methods. In your design, specify the following: (a) the new question(s) that would be addressed; (b) the specific design, using symbols to designate priority and sequence; (c) the sampling design that would be used; and (d) the additional data that would be collected.

EXERCISE 2: STUDY IN APPENDIX F

Read the article by Jurgens and colleagues ("Responding to heart failure symptoms") in Appendix F. Then answer the following questions:

Questions of Fact

a. Was this a mixed methods study? If yes, what was the purpose of the quantitative strand, and what was the purpose of the qualitative strand?
b. Which strand had priority in the study design?
c. Was the design sequential or concurrent?
d. Using the design names used in the textbook, what would the design be called?
e. How would the design be portrayed using the notation system described in the textbook? Did the researchers themselves use this notation?
f. What sampling design was used in this study?
g. Were any quantitative data qualitized? Were any qualitative data quantitized?
h. What did the report say about integrating the two strands?

Questions for Discussion

a. Evaluate the use of a mixed methods approach in this study. Did the approach yield richer or more useful information than would have been achieved with a single-strand study?
b. Discuss the researchers' choice of a specific research design and the sampling design. Would an alternative mixed methods design have been preferable? If so, why?
c. How would you characterize the way in which the researchers integrated the two strands? Do you think the integration maximized the benefits of having used a mixed methods approach?

▪ D. The Toolkit

For Chapter 25, the Toolkit on the accompanying CD-ROM contains a Word file with the following:

- Guidelines for Critiquing Mixed Methods Studies (Box 25.1 of the textbook)
- Examples of Integrative Mixed Methods Research Questions, by Type of Design*
- Useful Websites for Chapter 25: Resources for Mixed Methods Research

---

*This item does not appear in the textbook.

CHAPTER 26

Developing Complex Nursing Interventions Using Mixed Methods Research

■ A. Crossword Puzzle

Complete the crossword puzzle below, which uses terms and concepts presented in Chapter 26. (Puzzles may be removed for easier viewing.)

ACROSS

1. People who have an involvement with an intervention or with the group being treated are often called _ _ _ _ _ _ _ _ _ _rs.
7. It takes a considerable amount of time and _____ to develop, implement, and test an intervention.
8. A design decision concerns the intervention _____—the place where the intervention will be implemented.
11. One of many goals of early development work is to develop _____ strategies to keep participants in the study.
12. One of the many _____ of intervention research is that some people do not want to be randomized.
15. Before an intervention is created or tested, a lot of _ _ _ _ _ _ _ _ _ _nt work is needed (Phase I).
17. An ideal intervention addresses a pressing problem, and is efficacious, cost-effective, and _____.
18. In designing an intervention, consultation with _____ is especially useful if the existing evidence base is thin.
23. A major _____ in developing interventions concerns the fact that human beings are involved.
25. When an intervention is being tested, both proximal and _____ outcomes must be considered.
26. _ _ _ specific effects are the effects from factors other than those conceptualized as being driven by the intervention.
27. Patient _____ can often affect how acceptable an intervention is, and so it should be taken into account in designing the intervention.
28. One of the theories that has been found useful in designing health interventions is the Health _____ Model.
30. A literature _____ is one of the first steps in planning an intervention project.
31. The focus of the Phase IV work in the original MRC framework is usually on testing the _____ of the intervention in controlled settings.
32. A widely used framework for intervention development and testing was developed in this British organization (acronym).
34. An intervention that involves multiple components and that unfolds over a 10-week period would be considered a com_ _ _ _ intervention.

DOWN

2. The people who deliver the intervention are sometimes called intervention _____.
3. When it comes to intervention development, researchers must "_____" the problem the intervention is addressing.
4. The type of mixed methods design used in intervention research is often a(n) _____ design.
5. A(n) _____ theory is the basis for predicting how important outcomes can be achieved.

6. In Phase III of an intervention project, the design is often _ _ _ _ (qual).
9. Health intervention research often involves an interdisciplinary _____ of researchers.
10. A(n) _____ phase is almost always needed so that refinements to the intervention can be made and its acceptability can be assessed.
13. A key product of Phase II work is usually a lot of _____ learned.
14. A primary objective in Phase II is to assess the _____ of the intervention in a real-world setting.
16. During Phase I, exploratory and _____ research can pave the way for better understanding a problem and the target group.
19. A theory that has been found useful in designing health interventions is Theory of _____ Behavior.
20. In designing an intervention, a decision needs to be made about the potency and _____ (the "dose") of the treatment.
21. Intervention protocols can be subjected to content _ _ _ _ _ation by a panel of experts.
22. The _ _ _ _ _cal Research Council revised its widely used intervention framework in 2008.
24. Although often portrayed as a 4-phase process, intervention development and testing is rarely a(n) _____ process.
29. It is useful to have a _ _ _ _ _ work to guide the myriad tasks of intervention research.
33. A widely used symbol for a medical prescription

■ B. Study Questions

1. Read the 2009 pilot intervention study by Nolan and Lawrence ("A pilot study of a nursing intervention protocol to minimize maternal-infant separation after Cesarean birth." *Journal of Obstetric, Gynecologic, & Neonatal Nursing, 38,* 430–442). How might the pilot findings be used to refine procedures for a full RCT of the intervention?

2. Read one of the following pilot studies. What were the key "lessons learned"? To what extent are these lessons similar to and different from pilot lessons described in the textbook?
   • Beddoe, A., Lee, K., Weiss, S., Kennedy, H., & Yang, C. (2010). Effects of mindful yoga on sleep in pregnant women: A pilot study. *Biological Research for Nursing, 11,* 363–370.
   • Simpson, C., & Carter, P. (2010). Pilot study of a brief behavioral sleep inter vention for caregivers of individuals with dementia. *Research in Gerontological Nursing, 3,* 19–29.
   • Woodward, S., Norton, C., & Barribal, K. (2010). A pilot study of the effectiveness of reflexology in treating idiopathic constipation in women. *Complementary Therapies in Clinical Practice, 16,* 41–46.

3. Suppose you wanted to develop an educational intervention for women at risk of osteoporosis. Read the following review:

- Smith, C. A. (2010). A systematic review of health care professional-led education for patients with osteoporosis or those at high risk for the disease. *Orthopedic Nursing, 29,* 119–132.

  Then, make a list of the kind of questions you might want to address in further descriptive research with the patient population or key stakeholders before designing the intervention. (Alternatively, read a systematic review on a topic of interest to you and then proceed to list questions.)

4. Read one of the following studies. Use the relevant critiquing guidelines in Box 26.2 of the textbook (available as a Word document in the Toolkit ✖) to critique the study:

- Cowart, L., Biro, D. J., Wasserman, T., Stein, R., Reider, L., & Brown, B. (2010). Designing and pilot-testing a church-based community program to reduce obesity among African Americans. *ABNF Journal, 21,* 4–10.
- Hirani, S., Karmaliani, R., McFarlane, J., Asad, N., Madhani, F., Shehzad, S., & Ali, N. (2010). Development of an economic skill building intervention to promote women's safety and child development in Karachi, Pakistan. *Issues in Mental Health Nursing, 31,* 82–88.
- McGrath, B., & Ka'lili, T. (2010). Creating Project Talanoa: A culturally based community health program for U.S. Pacific Islander adolescents. *Public Health Nursing, 27,* 17–24.

■ C. Application Exercises

EXERCISE 1: STUDY IN APPENDIX A

Read the article by Kennedy and Chen ("Changes in childhood risk taking") in Appendix A. Then answer the following questions:

Questions of Fact

a. Could the intervention that was tested in this study be described as a complex intervention? If yes, along which dimensions is it complex?
b. Was there an intervention theory that guided the development of the intervention?
c. Did the researchers complete developmental research that facilitated the development of the intervention?
d. Was the intervention under scrutiny in this study pilot tested? If not, was this study itself a pilot test? If no to both questions, how did the researchers come to conclusions about the feasibility of the project?
e. Was a mixed methods approach used in the part of the study described in this article?

Questions for Discussion

a. Suppose that the study described here *was* the pilot test for the intervention. What changes, if any, would you make to the intervention or the study design, based on the study results?
b. What additional research questions could this study have addressed through the collection of qualitative data? What types of qualitative data would you recommend to address those questions?

EXERCISE 2: STUDY IN APPENDIX D

Read the article by Whittemore and colleagues ("Diabetes prevention program") in Appendix D. Then answer the following questions:

Questions of Fact

a. Could the intervention that was tested in this study be described as a complex intervention? If yes, along which dimensions is it complex?
b. Was there an intervention theory that guided the development of the intervention?
c. Did the researchers complete developmental research that facilitated the development of the intervention?
d. Was the intervention under scrutiny in this study pilot tested? If not, was this study itself a pilot test? If no to both questions, how did the researchers come to conclusions about the feasibility of the project?
e. Was this a mixed methods study? If yes, what was the purpose of the quantitative strand, and what was the purpose of the qualitative strand?
f. Which strand had priority in the study design?
g. Was the design sequential or concurrent?
h. How would the design be portrayed using the notation system described in the textbook? Did the researchers themselves use this notation?

Questions for Discussion

a. Comment on the complexity of the intervention in this project. Do you think it was *too* complex? Insufficiently complex? What might be some of the advantages and disadvantages of making it simpler?
b. Evaluate the use of a mixed methods approach in this study. Did the approach yield richer or more useful information than would have been achieved with a single-strand study?
c. What additional types of data (if any) might have been useful as a supplement to the data that the researchers gathered? Would such data collection change the mixed methods design?

■ D. The Toolkit

For Chapter 26, the Toolkit on the accompanying CD-ROM contains a Word file with the following:

- Guidelines for Critiquing Aspects of Intervention Projects (Box 26.2 of the textbook)
- Examples of Exploratory Research Questions for Designing an Evidence-Based Intervention*
- Examples of Questions for Expert Consultants and Team Brainstorming in Designing an Intervention*
- Useful Websites for Chapter 26: Resources for Intervention Research

---

*These items do not appear in the textbook.

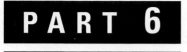

PART 6

Building an Evidence Base for Nursing Practice

Systematic Reviews of Research Evidence: Meta-Analysis, Metasynthesis, and Mixed Studies Review

■ A. Crossword Puzzle

Complete the crossword puzzle below, which uses terms and concepts presented in Chapter 27. (Puzzles may be removed for easier viewing.)

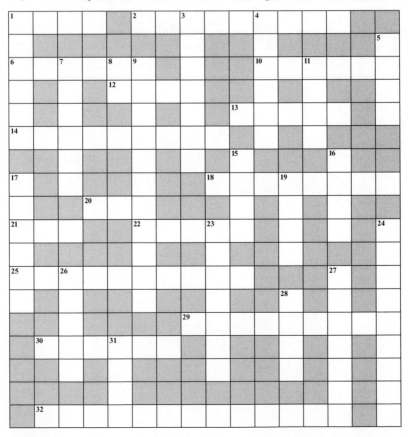

ACROSS

1. A(n) _____-safe number estimates the number of studies with nonsignificant results that would be needed to reverse the conclusion of a significant effect.
2. A(n) _____ effect size in a metasummary is the ratio of reports with a particular thematic finding, divided by all reports relating to a phenomenon.
6. The type of model used in meta-analysis that takes both within-study and between-study variability into account is called _____ effects.
10. One theory-building integration approach is _____ grounded theory.
12. Meta-_ _ _ _ession is a method of analyzing the effect of multiple clinical and method factors on variation in effect size.
13. Study quality can be examined in relation to effect size using either a component or _____ approach.
14. The _____ level ($5k + 10$) is the number against which a fail-safe number is compared.
18. In a meta-analysis, a(n) _____ analysis involves examining the extent to which effects differ for different types of studies, people, or intervention elements.
20. The numerator for computing a weighted average effect is the _____ of each primary study's ES times the weight for each study.
21. A common test of the null hypothesis for heterogeneity is the _____-squared test.
22. Analysts must choose a(n) _____ for the meta-analysis that addresses the issue of heterogeneity
25. Another name for the effect index d is standardized mean _____.
29. A concern in a systematic review is the _____ bias that stems from identifying only studies in journals and books (abbr.).
30. One way to address primary study quality is to do a(n) _ _ _ _ _ _ _ivity analysis that includes and then excludes studies of low quality.
32. A meta-analyst must make decisions about how to address the inevitable _____ of effects across studies.

DOWN

1. A(n) _____ plot is a graphic display of the effect size (including CIs) of each primary study.
3. A pre-analysis task in systematic reviews is to _____ information about study and sample characteristics from each primary study.
4. Each primary study in a meta-analysis must yield a quantitative estimate of the _____ of the independent variable on the dependent variable.
5. A funnel _____ is often used to detect publication biases.
7. One of the originators of a widely used approach to meta-synthesis (meta-ethnography)
8. One of several effect size indicators for dichotomous outcomes (acronym)

9. A(n) _____, which involves calculating manifest effect sizes, can lay the foundation for a metasynthesis.

11. Extraction and quality assessment should be done by more than one reviewer so that intercoder _ _ _ _ability can be assessed.

15. There is evidence of a bias against the _____ hypothesis in published studies.

16. An early question in a quantitative systematic review is whether it is justifiable to _____ results across studies statistically.

17. A coding manual should be developed for reviewers who will extract and _____ information from primary studies in the systematic review.

19. The body of unpublished studies is sometimes referred to as _____ literature.

23. In a meta-analysis, researchers may decide to _____ primary studies whose reports are written in certain languages (e.g., those not in English).

24. A(n) _____ effect size is the ratio of the number of themes represented in one report, divided by all relevant themes relating to a phenomenon across all reports.

26. In a(n) _____ effects model, it is assumed that one true effect size underlies all study results.

27. _____ appraisal is undertaken in most systematic reviews, although approaches to using the information vary.

28. In a meta-ethnography, a critical step involves a _ _ _ _ -of-argument synthesis.

31. The index *d* provides an estimate of effect _____ for comparing means.

▪ B. Study Questions

1. Read one of the following meta-analysis reports:
   - Conn, V., Valentine, J., & Cooper, H. (2002). Interventions to increase physical activity among aging adults: A meta-analysis. *Annals of Behavioral Medicine, 24*, 190–200.
   - Fetzer, S. J. (2002). Reducing venipuncture and intravenous insertion pain with eutectic mixture of local anesthetic. *Nursing Research, 51*, 119–124.
   - Floyd, J., Medler, S., Ager, J., & Janisse, J. (2000). Age-related changes in initiation and maintenance of sleep: a meta-analysis. *Research in Nursing & Health, 23*, 106–117.
   - Hill-Westmoreland, E. E., Soeken, K., & Spellbring, A. M. (2002). A meta-analysis of fall prevention programs for the elderly: How effective are they? *Nursing Research, 51*, 1–8.

   Then, search the literature for related quantitative primary studies published *after* this meta-analysis. Are new study results consistent with the conclusions drawn in the meta-analytic report? Are there enough new studies to warrant a new meta-analysis?

2. Read one of the following metasynthesis reports:
   - Goodman, J. H. (2005). Becoming an involved father of an infant. *Journal of Obstetric, Gynecologic, & Neonatal Nursing, 34*, 190–200.
   - Lefler, L., & Bondy, L. (2004). Women's delay in seeking treatment with myocardial infarction: A meta-synthesis. *Journal of Cardiovascular Nursing, 19*, 251–268.
   - Nelson, A. M. (2002). A metasynthesis: Mothering other-than-normal children. *Qualitative Health Research, 12*, 515–530.

   Then, search the literature for related qualitative primary studies published *after* this metasynthesis. Are new study results consistent with the conclusions drawn in the metasynthesis report? Are there enough new studies to warrant a new metasynthesis?

3. Read the following report, which involved a systematic review without a meta-analysis. Did the authors adequately justify their decision not to conduct a meta-analysis?
   - Lee, O., & Johnson, L. (2005). A systematic review for effective management of central venous catheters and catheter sites in acute care paediatric patients. *Worldviews on Evidence-Based Nursing, 2*, 4–13.

4. Read one of the following reports, and use the critiquing guidelines in Box 27.1 (available as a Word document in the accompanying Toolkit ✪) to evaluate the integration.
   - Choi, S., Rankin, S., Stewart, A., & Oka, R. (2008). Effects of acculturation on smoking behavior in Asian Americans: A meta-analysis. *Journal of Cardiovascular Nursing, 23*, 67–73.
   - Conn, V., Hafdahl, A., Brown, S., & Brown, L. (2008). Meta-analysis of patient education interventions to increase physical activity among chronically ill adults. *Patient Education and Counseling, 70*, 57–172.
   - Hammer, K., Mogensen, O., & Hall, E. (2010). The meaning of hope in nursing research: A meta-synthesis. *Scandinavian Journal of Caring Science, 24*, 200–212.
   - Lo, S., Chang, C., Hu, W., Hayter, M., & Chang, Y. (2009). The effectiveness of silver-releasing dressings in the management of non-healing chronic wounds: a meta-analysis. *Journal of Clinical Nursing, 18*, 716–728.
   - Reid, B., Sinclair, M., Barr, O., Dobbs, F., & Crealey, G. (2009). A meta-synthesis of pregnant women's decision-making processes with regard to antenatal screening for Down syndrome. *Social Science & Medicine, 69*, 1561–1573.

5. Identify a topic of interest and explore whether it might be possible to undertake a mixed studies synthesis on the topic. Alternatively, investigate whether a mixed studies synthesis might be feasible for systematic reviews cited in Exercise B.4.

■ C. Application Exercises

EXERCISE 1: STUDY IN APPENDIX K

Read the article by Han and colleagues ("Interventions to promote mammography") in Appendix K. Then answer the following questions:

Questions of Fact

a. What was the stated purposed of this review?

b. How many bibliographic databases were searched? Was there an effort to identify and locate "grey literature"?

c. Were non-English language primary study reports excluded from the review? What other exclusion criteria were in place?

d. How many initial citations were obtained? How many citations were reviewed in depth? How many primary studies were included in the analysis?

e. If a primary study was an RCT that examined the effect of an intervention on breast self-examination, would it have been included in the review?

f. Did the researchers develop quality assessment scores for each study in the dataset? If yes, how many study elements were appraised? What was the highest possible quality score? What was the average quality score for the studies used in the meta-analysis? How many people scored the studies for quality? Was inter-rater agreement assessed?

g. Did the researchers set a threshold for study quality as part of their inclusion criteria? If yes, what was it? Were any studies excluded because of a low quality rating?

h. What effect size measure was used in the analysis? What were the effect sizes weighted by?

i. Was a fixed effects or random effects model used? Did the researchers perform any tests for heterogeneity?

j. How many subjects were there in total, in all studies combined?

k. What was the overall (pooled) effect size? What does this mean?

l. Were any subgroup analyses performed? What were the characteristics used to form subgroups of studies?

m. Answer the following questions regarding information in Table 2:

- How many studies had individually directed interventions?
- Among the intervention types, which had the largest effect size? Which had the smallest? How many of the different types had *significant* effects?
- In which type of setting were the interventions found to be most effective?
- For which ethnic group were intervention effects significantly positive?
- Did quality of the study play a big role in the size of the intervention effect?

n. Was a meta-regression performed?

o. Did the researchers do any sensitivity analyses based on study quality or sample size?

p. Did this meta-analysis address the issue of publication bias?

Questions for Discussion

a. Was the size of the sample (studies and subjects) sufficiently large to draw conclusions about the overall effect of screening-promotion interventions and about subgroup effects?
b. What other subgroups might have been interesting to examine (assume there was sufficient information in the original studies)?
c. Did the researchers draw reasonable conclusions about the quality, quantity, and consistency of evidence?
d. How would you assess the overall rigor of this meta-analysis? What would you recommend to improve the quality of this systematic review?
e. Were the authors' recommendations consistent with their findings?

EXERCISE 2: STUDY IN APPENDIX L

Read the article by Xu ("Strangers in strange lands") in Appendix L. Then answer the following questions:

Questions of Fact

a. What was the stated purpose of this metasynthesis? What was the central phenomenon and how was it defined?
b. Which bibliographic databases were searched? What key words were used? Was there an effort to identify and locate "grey literature"? In addition to electronic database searches, what did Xu do to locate relevant studies?
c. What was Xu's position in the debate regarding integration across research traditions?
d. How many primary studies were included in the integration? Were the primary studies described?
e. Were primary studies appraised for quality? Were any studies excluded because of poor quality?
f. Were the data in the primary studies derived from interviews, observations, or both?
g. What approach was used to conduct this metasynthesis? Was the analytic process described?
h. Was a metasummary performed?
i. How many study participants were there in all of the studies combined?
j. How many shared themes were identified in this metasynthesis? What were those themes?
k. Was Xu's analysis supported through the inclusion of raw data from the primary studies?
l. Did the report discuss the metasynthesis findings? Did Xu present possible implications?

Questions for Discussion

a. Was the size of the sample (studies and subjects) sufficiently large to conduct a meaningful metasynthesis? Did the diversity of the sample (in terms of participant characteristics, timing of data collection, or research tradition) enhance the study or weaken it?

b. Did the analysis and integration appear reasonable and thorough?

c. Were primary studies adequately described?

d. Did Xu draw reasonable conclusions about the quality and consistency of evidence?

e. How would you assess the overall rigor of this metasynthesis? What would you recommend to improve its quality?

f. Based on this metasynthesis, what is the evidence regarding the experiences of immigrant Asian nurses working in western countries? What are the implications for nursing practice, nursing administration, or healthcare policy?

▪ D. The Toolkit

For Chapter 27, the Toolkit on the accompanying CD-ROM contains a Word file with the following:

- Guidelines for Critiquing Systematic Reviews (Box 27.1 of the textbook)
- Example of a Data Extraction Form for a Meta-Analysis*
- Template for Flow Diagram for Inclusion of Primary Studies (as recommended in PRISMA)*
- Selected Formulas for Calculating a Standardized Mean Difference Effect Size (d)*
- Template for a Table Summarizing Characteristics of Studies Included in a Meta-Analysis or Systematic Review*
- Template for a Summary Table for a Metasynthesis*
- Template for a Table Summarizing Meta-Findings in a Metasummary*
- Useful Websites for Chapter 27: Resources for Systematic Reviews

----

*These items do not appear in the textbook.

CHAPTER 28

Disseminating Evidence: Reporting Research Findings

■ A. Crossword Puzzle

Complete the crossword puzzle below, which uses terms and concepts presented in Chapter 28. (Puzzles may be removed for easier viewing.)

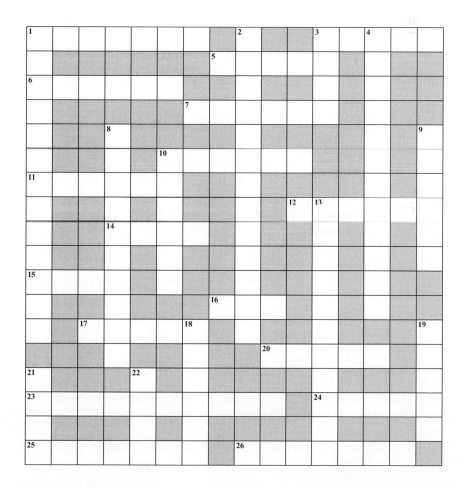

ACROSS

1. The guidelines now used by many medical and health journals for reporting randomized controlled trials (RCTs)
3. Some schools permit students to prepare a(n) _____-format thesis that incorporates reports ready to submit for publication.
5. All reports should have a succinct, descriptive _____ that provides guidance to prospective readers.
6. Most scholarly journals have a policy of blind peer _____ of submitted manuscripts.
7. Many journals require authors to sign a copyright tr _ _ _ _ _ _ form prior to publication.
10. In qualitative reports, key _____ are often used as subheadings of the results section.
11. At professional conferences, research results can often be communicated visually in a(n) _____ session.
12. A journal's _____ factor is the ratio between citations to a journal and recent citable items published.
14. The traditional method of communicating research results at a conference is a(n) _____ presentation to an audience of attendees.
15. Acronym for one of the top ranking journals listed in the nursing subset of the *Journal Citation Reports*
16. STROBE guidelines are to _____ experimental studies what the CONSORT guidelines are to RCTs.
17. The _____ author of a report is usually the lead author.
20. The traditional organization for quantitative reports is the _____ format.
23. _ _ _ _ _ _ _ _ _ _ ments give credit to individuals or institutions that contributed to the study.
24. Presentations at conferences are enhanced through effective visual materials such as _____ Point slides.
25. Cover _____ to journal editors typically provide assurances that the manuscript has not been submitted elsewhere.
26. Quantitative reports are more likely to be written in the _____ voice than qualitative reports.

DOWN

1. The _____ author is the author with whom journal editors communicate during the review stage of the publication process.
2. The final phase of a research project, involving communication of results
3. Manuscripts submitted to a journal are usually subjected to _____ review by several experts in the field.
4. An important communication outlet for research findings is a(n) _____ at a professional conference.

8. _____ credit on a report should be based on a person's having made a substantial contribution to the study, and to the writing and review of the paper.
9. Decisions about acceptance or rejection of a manuscript are usually communicated by a journal's _____.
10. The "T" in CONSORT stands for _____.
13. Papers or documents that are not (yet) published
18. Most quantitative reports include statistical _____ to summarize results efficiently.
19. The type of letter sent to journal editors to ascertain their interest in a manuscript
21. Associations sponsoring a conference usually issue a(n) "_____ for Abstracts" months before the conference.
22. The acronym for the reporting guidelines for meta-analyses of non-RCT primary studies is M _ _ _ _.

■ B. Study Questions

1. The following sentences or titles have stylistic flaws. Suggest ways in which the sentences could be improved.
   a. ICU nurses experience more stress than nurses on a general ward ($t = 2.5$, $df = 148$, $p < .05$).
   b. "A Study Investigating the Effect of Primary Care Nursing on the Emotional Well-Being of Patients in a Cardiac Care Unit."
   c. The nonsignificant results demonstrate that there is no relationship between diet and hyperkinesis.
   d. It has, therefore, been proved that people have a more negative body image if the age of onset of obesity is before age 20 years.
   e. The positive, significant relationship indicates that occupational stress causes sleep disturbances.

2. Suppose that you were the author of a research article with the titles indicated below. For each, name two different journals to which your article could be submitted for publication. At least one of the journals should be a specialty journal.
   a. "Parental attachment to children with Down's syndrome."
   b. "Sexual functioning among the elderly: The lived experience of noninstitutionalized men and women in their 70s."
   c. "Comparison of therapists' and clients' expectations regarding psychiatric therapy."
   d. "The effects of fetal monitoring on selected birth outcomes."
   e. "Effectiveness of alternative methods of relieving pressure sores."

3. Read one of the following reports, and use the critiquing guidelines in Box 28.2 (available as a Word document in the accompanying Toolkit ✪) to evaluate the presentation of the report.

- Beeber, L., Holditch-Davis, D., Perreira, K., Schwartz, T., Lewis, V., Blanchard, H., Canuso, R., & Goldman, B. D. (2010). Short-term in-home intervention reduces depressive symptoms in early Head Start Latina mothers of infants and toddlers. *Research in Nursing & Health, 33,* 60–76.
- Hu, J., Wallace, D., & Tesh, A. (2010). Physical activity, obesity, nutritional health and quality of life in low-income Hispanic adults with diabetes. *Journal of Community Health Nursing, 27,* 70–83.
- Woods-Giscombé, C. (2010). Superwoman schema: African American women's views on stress, strength, and health. *Qualitative Health Research, 20,* 668–683.
- Wu, H., Chi, T., Chen, L., Wang, L., & Jin, Y. (2010). Occupational stress among hospital nurses: cross-sectional survey. *Journal of Advanced Nursing, 66,* 627–634.

■ C. Application Exercises

STUDIES IN APPENDICES A–L

Answer the following questions with regard to the 12 research reports included in appendices in this *Resource Manual:*

Questions of Fact

a. Were any articles published in journals that do not have an impact factor rating?
b. Which articles in the appendices were published in journals that had an impact factor greater than 1.00 in 2009?
c. Which, if any, of the articles in the appendices deviated from a traditional IMRAD format?
d. In articles that had multiple authors, were the authors listed alphabetically?
e. Which, if any, of the reports used first-person narratives to describe aspects of the study methods or results?

Questions for Discussion

a. Comment on the extent to which the abstracts for the studies in the appendices adequately captured key concepts and the population of interest.
b. Which report title had the greatest appeal to you—that is, which one most intrigued you and made you want to read the study?
c. Select one or two reports and comment on how effectively the authors used figure and tables to enhance or streamline communication.

▪ D. The Toolkit

For Chapter 28, the Toolkit on the accompanying CD-ROM contains a Word file with the following:

- Guidelines for Preparing Statistical Tables (Box 28.1 of textbook)
- Guidelines for Critiquing the Presentation of a Research Report (Box 28.2 of textbook)
- CONSORT 2010 Checklist of Information to Include when Reporting a Randomized Trial*
- Template for the CONSORT 2010 Flow Diagram*
- Useful Websites for Chapter 28: Resources for Writing and Disseminating Research

---

*These items do not appear in the textbook.

CHAPTER 29

Writing Proposals to Generate Evidence

■ A. Crossword Puzzle

Complete the crossword puzzle below, which uses terms and concepts presented in Chapter 29. (Puzzles may be removed for easier viewing.)

ACROSS

3. In applications to NIH, the study purpose is described in the section called _____ Aims.
5. The costs of a project over and above specific project-related costs
8. Specific project-related costs
9. The funding mechanism that gives researchers considerable discretion in what to study and how best to study it
10. A mechanism for soliciting grant application using broad guidelines about the type of projects of interest (acronym)
12. In the United States and most countries, the entity that funds most research (abbr.)
13. A type of NIH award for institutions that have not historically received much NIH funding is an R15 or _____ grant (acronym).
15. Applications to NIH typically go through _____ rounds of review.
16. A frequent criticism by peer reviewers of grant applications to NIH is insufficient _____ work.
17. The form used for NIH grant submissions is the _ _ 424.
18. It is prudent to consider whether there is a current "hot _____" that will make a grant application more appealing to reviewers.
19. The R03, or _____ Grant Program, is mainly for pilot or feasibility studies (backwards).
20. Indirect costs, or _____, are institutional costs associated with doing research (e.g., for space, administrators, etc.).
21. Acronym for an NIH award program, and often associated with the name "Ruth Kirschstein"
22. Grant applications are reviewed by a(n) _____ and secondary reviewer prior to the meeting date, whose preliminary scores affect whether an application will be formally scored.

DOWN

1. In the NIH scoring system, the score signifying "exceptional"
2. The set of skills needed to secure funding for a research project
3. The informal name for an NIH peer review group (two words)
4. The funding mechanism for a specific study that a government or entity wants to have done
6. The formal name for a peer review panel for NIH (acronym)
7. Writing proposals is time-consuming, so a good strategy is to _____ early!
11. Scored grant applications to NIH are given a(n) _____ score that reflects average ratings of merit, multiplied by 10.
14. _____ budgets, paid in blocks of $25,000, are appropriate for most NIH applications requesting $250,000 or less per year of direct costs.

15. NIH F-series awards are for _____ fellowships.
17. Each applicant to NIH is sent a(n) _____ sheet that includes reviewers' comments.

■ B. Study Questions

1. Chapter 29 of the text described four major sections or subsections of NIH grant applications (Specific Aims, Research Strategy: Significance, Research Strategy: Innovation, and Research Strategy: Approach). In which section would the following statements ordinarily be found?

   a. Study participants, who will include young adults who have been treated for a drug overdose, will initially be recruited through the emergency room of a local hospital. Network sampling will then be used to contact a broader population of those with an overdose experience.

   b. It is hypothesized that paraplegics who receive pool therapy will perform better on tests of muscle strength than those who receive other types of exercise.

   c. Two members of the research team have recently completed an in-depth longitudinal study of the coping mechanisms of parents with a Down syndrome infant.

   d The major threat to the internal validity of the proposed study is selection bias, which will be dealt with through the careful selection of comparison subjects and through statistical adjustment of preexisting differences.

   e. Prior studies have found that people undergoing cancer treatment experience a complex array of disease- and treatment-related symptoms.

   f. The proposed research will have the potential of restructuring the delivery of healthcare in rural areas.

2. Go to the RePORT database (*http://projectreporter.nih.gov/*) and find an NINR-funded grant nearing completion, on a topic that interests you. Write to the Principal Investigator (PI) to inquire about any conference presentations or published papers that have resulted from the grant.

■ C. Application Exercises

EXERCISE 1: APPENDIX M

Appendix L contains a successful grant application, "Older adults' response to health care practitioner pain communication." This application was submitted by Dr. Deborah Dillon McDonald to NINR for funding under a program announcement PA-03-152, "Biobehavioral Pain Research." Before reviewing Dr. McDonald's grant application and the associated materials in Appendix L, scan the program announcement (available at (*http://grants.nih.gov/grants/guide/pa-files/pa-03-152.html*) and answer the following questions:

a. Did this PA fund projects through the R01 mechanism only?
b. When did this program announcement expire for R01 applications?
c. How many institutes within NIH, besides NINR, participated in this program announcement?
d. Would this funding mechanism be appropriate for funding research on the effectiveness of pain treatments and interventions?
e. Would this funding mechanism be appropriate for funding basic research on affective responses to pain?

EXERCISE 2: APPENDIX M

Read through the grant application forms and research proposal submitted by Dr. McDonald in Appendix L. (Note that this application was submitted on form PHS398, the form that was used before the SF424 electronic filing form became mandated. Also, the scoring of applications at that time was different, with scores ranging from 100 for the highest possible score to 500 for the lowest possible score.) Then answer the following questions:

Questions of Fact

a. What were the total *direct* costs requested for the entire research project for all project years? What are the *total* requested funds, for both direct and indirect costs?
b. What were the proposed time frames for the study?
c. How many people were listed as key personnel for the proposed study? How much of the PI's time was proposed for this project?
d. Did the research plan section of the grant application conform to the page restrictions for this PA?
e. In what section of the application did McDonald present her hypothesis? Is this placement consistent with guidelines?
f. In what section did McDonald describe her own prior research relating to pain communication? How many relevant prior studies had she undertaken?
g. McDonald divided her "Research Design and Methods" section into several subsections. What were they?
h. What type of research design did McDonald propose?
i. What sample size did McDonald propose? Was the proposed sample size based on a power analysis?
j. According to the proposal, who would be blinded in this study?
k. Did the application stipulate that a stipend would be given to subjects? If yes, what incentive would be offered?
l. In the analysis plan, were any multivariate analyses proposed? If so, what type of analysis would be undertaken?

Questions for Discussion

a. Before reading any of the reviewers' comments, critique McDonald's proposed design, sampling plan, data collection, and data analysis strategies. Then compare your comments with the reviewers' comments about the proposed methods.
b. What do you think the weakest aspect of the proposed project is?

EXERCISE 3: APPENDIX M

Appendix L also includes the summary sheet for McDonald's grant application, together with McDonald's response to reviewers' concerns. Read through these materials and then answer the following questions.

a. The application number indicates the NIH funding mechanism for the proposed project. What was the funding mechanism?
b. Which study section reviewed the grant application? On what date did the study section meet?
c. What was this grant application's priority score? (Note that this application was scored under an earlier system; in that system, scores under 200 were competitive.)
d. What was the primary concern of the study section—that is, what part was deemed "unacceptable" and required McDonald to elaborate on proposed methods?

▪ D. The Toolkit

For Chapter 29, the Toolkit on the accompanying CD-ROM contains a Word file with the following:

- Checklist for a Quantitative Grant Application*
- Selected NIH Grant Application Forms (Not Fillable—for Review Purposes Only)*
- Useful Websites for Chapter 29: Resources for Proposal Writing and Grantsmanship

---

*These items do not appear in the textbook.

CHANGES IN CHILDHOOD RISK TAKING AND SAFETY BEHAVIOR AFTER A PEER GROUP MEDIA INTERVENTION

Christine Kennedy • Jyu-Lin Chen

EDITOR'S NOTE

Materials documenting the review process for this article are posted at http://www.nursing-research-editor.com

▶ **Background:** Risk taking is a significant health-compromising behavior among children that often is portrayed unrealistically in the media as consequence-free. Physical risk taking can lead to injury, and injury is a leading cause of hospitalization and death during childhood.

▶ **Objective:** The aim of this study was to examine the effectiveness of a 4-week program for school-age children in reducing risk-taking behaviors and increasing safety behaviors.

▶ **Methods:** A two-group, experimental, repeated-measures design was used to compare 122 White and Latino children randomly assigned to an intervention group or a wait-list group at baseline and at 1, 3, and 6 months after intervention. Children received a behaviorally based intervention delivered in four 2-hour segments conducted over consecutive weeks. The thematic concept of each week (choices, media, personal risk taking, and peer group risk taking) moved from the general to the specific, focusing on knowledge and awareness, the acquisition of new skills and behaviors, and the supportive practice and application of skills.

▶ **Results:** Participants increased their safety behaviors ($p = .006$), but risk-taking behaviors remained unchanged. Families in the intervention group increased their consistent use of media rules ($p = .022$), but decreases in media alternatives suggest difficulty in taking up other habits and activities. Coping effectiveness was predictive of safety behaviors ($p = .005$) at 6 months, and coping effectiveness plus television watching was predictive of risk taking ($p = .03$).

▶ **Conclusions:** Findings from this study suggest that interventions that influence children's media experiences help enhance safety behaviors and that strategies to aid parents in finding media alternatives are relevant to explore.

▶ **Key Words:** children · risk taking · safety behaviors · television

Risk taking is a significant behavior that compromises health, and an expansive literature that describes the rapidly deteriorating and interrelated nature of health risk behaviors in American youth has emerged. Physical risk taking can lead to injury, and injury is a leading cause of hospitalization during childhood. Speltz, Gonzales, Sulzbacher, and Quan (1990) found that children with two injuries or more scored significantly higher on risk taking ($M = 33.7$), using a primary-care–based tool, the Injury Behavior Checklist (IBC),

2009

than did children with no ($M = 22$) or one ($M = 24$) injury. Kennedy replicated those results, finding that the IBC was predictive of the injury outcome in both White (Kennedy & Lipsitt, 1998) and Latino (Kennedy & Rodriguez, 1999) children. Unintentional injury is the leading cause of death for children more than 1 year of age; more children die from injuries than from all diseases combined.

Injury is a phenomenon that is underrepresented in nursing research, which is surprising given the focus on health promotion in the field (Sommers, 2006). This lack of research on injury is especially critical given that rates for counseling about injury prevention remain low and have not changed in the past two decades in primary care except in two specific areas (poison control and bike helmet use). However, research based on the national Injury Control and Risk Survey and earlier studies has shown that counseling by healthcare providers about injury prevention promotes safer behaviors (Chen, Kresnow, Simon, & Dellinger, 2007).

Health science researchers have established that children's media consumption affects their health behaviors and is one of the factors that influence risk taking in children. Risk taking is portrayed in the media as consequence-free, and outcomes are rarely depicted realistically. Harmful outcomes are depicted in only 3% of prime-time television shows. If these shows were realistic, viewers would see 15 injuries per hour in adult shows, 24 injuries per hour during Saturday morning shows, and 46 injuries per hour in afternoon children's shows. Potts, Doppler, and Hernandez (1994) experimentally manipulated children's exposure to television cartoons that depicted high- or low-risk behaviors and demonstrated that the children who saw the high-risk content reported a greater willingness to take risks. Potts and Swisher (1998) demonstrated that exposure to safety education videos decreased a child's willingness to take physical risks. Children are aware of their risk-taking behavior, and their intentions to take risk closely align with how they behave in risk situations (Morrongiello, 2004; Potts, Martinez, & Dedmon, 1995).

> Risk taking is portrayed in the media as consequence-free, and outcomes are rarely depicted realistically.

Kennedy (2000a) found that preschool-age children who often take physical risks watch more television and have parents with little media knowledge and few family media rules who provide little media monitoring. Gender, acculturation, and ethnicity influenced both the types of shows viewed and the amount of viewing time among White and Latino children and the rates of risk taking and injuries (Kennedy, 2000a, 2000b). Young school-age children report television as a *friend* and look upon it not only as entertainment but more importantly as a source of information, educating them on how to act in the world of grown-ups—a world that, developmentally, they are anxious to join and fit into (Kennedy, Strzempko, Danford, & Kools, 2002). Some work suggests that television viewing is chosen by children as a coping strategy, albeit a strategy that they view as not very effective (Chen & Kennedy, 2005). Children also report that at least 50% of their viewing time is by default, in that they watch television to spend time with their parents who are themselves watching television (Kennedy, 2000b; Kennedy et al., 2002). Despite parents' avowed beliefs that they regulate their child's exposure to negative media influences and encourage only positive shows, a serious gap exists between this belief and the actual viewing of television by children (Kennedy, 2000a).

Few researchers have documented how other healthier choices can be developed in school-age children. In general, the body of research tends to be focused on teenagers and the remediation of poor choices once such choices have been established. Recent work focused on identifying assets within the teenage years suggests that identifying the antecedents to these positive behaviors would be appropriate for health interventionists. Children's health beliefs, perceptions, and practices such as risk-taking behaviors are stable by 9 to 11 years of age;

therefore, efforts to influence these behaviors should be made with younger school-age children. Most interventions to reduce television viewing are prescriptive, and even successful approaches to reducing daily television viewing time leave one to wonder whether the behavior can be maintained. It seems justifiable to enhance children's understanding of the skewed media portrayal and to do so via a self-choice and self-care model.

Risk taking by children is influenced by a variety of persons (child, parent, and teachers), environmental factors (neighborhood and culture), and social factors (peers and media). Given the adverse health consequences of media consumption by children and the developmental trajectory of negative health behaviors, the socialization of children's health behaviors remains surprisingly underexplored by nursing.

One model that includes socialization of health behaviors is Cox's Interaction Model of Client Health Behavior (IMCHB). This conceptual model is grounded in a multidisci-plinary perspective on the dynamic interplay between clients, the health professional's inter-action with the child and family, and health outcomes (Figure 1; Carter & Kulbok, 1995; Farrand & Cox, 1993). The model suggests that changes in children's health behaviors by healthcare interventions occur via a change in the child's cognitive appraisal (i.e., their health perception) and that intrinsic motiva-tion and affective response (i.e., perceived self-competency) exert their influence on the child's cognitive appraisal. Farrand and Cox (1993) reported a fairly strong confirmation of the model's proposed linkages, identifying gender-specific determinants of children's health behaviors. They reported that the cen-tral role of cognitive appraisal/health percep-tion is to mediate the effects of affective responses (perceived competency) and motiva-tion on the outcome of health behaviors. Although the published model does not address coping specifically, our earlier work supported investigating it because children reported television watching as one of their

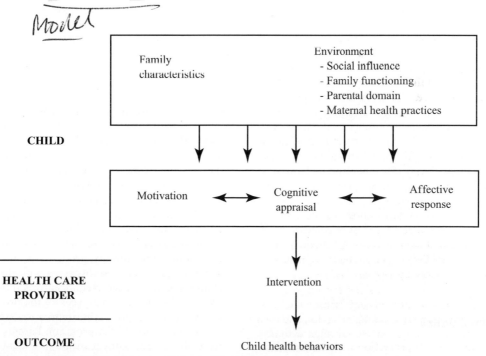

Model

Figure 1. Child health behaviors and intervention model.

most frequent, but ineffective, coping strategies (Chen & Kennedy, 2005).

The primary aim of this prospective, randomized, 4-year longitudinal study was to test a peer group intervention aimed at decreasing physical risk-taking behaviors by influencing children's media behaviors, understanding, and choices. Guided by the IMCHB, factors that were examined included the child's motivation, health perceptions, and self-competencies. Children's coping strategies; parents' safety, media practices, and beliefs; and family functioning also were explored.

■ Methods

A two-group, experimental, longitudinal design was used to compare children who were randomly assigned to the intervention group ($n = 57$) or to a wait-list control group ($n = 65$) at four times: baseline and 1, 3, and 6 months after the intervention.

PARTICIPANTS

Sixteen sites provided a total of 34 groups with an average of four children in a group. Of the 145 parents and children who were approached to participate, 11 declined because of time or activity conflicts and another 12 did not meet eligibility requirements. A total of 122 children (ages 8 and 9 years) and their mothers participated in the study (58 White and 64 Latino); the randomly assigned sample included 58 girls (47.5%) and 64 boys (52.5%). The groups were balanced in distribution by gender and ethnicity. No attrition or loss of participants was noted during the study. All children and parents completed the baseline assessment and the three follow-up assessments.

PROCEDURES

Human subject protection was approved by the University of California, San Francisco,

Committee on Human Research. Upon approval, participants were solicited from community sources and after-school programs in Northern California. Eight-year-old children and their parents were eligible for enrollment if they met the following criteria: (a) the adult and child self-identified their ethnicity as either Latino or White; (b) the child was in good health, defined as free of an acute or life-threatening disease and able to attend to activities of daily living such as going to school; (c) parents, in addition to speaking either English, Spanish, or both, were able to read in one of the two languages in order to fill out questionnaires written at a fourth- to sixth-grade level; and (d) parent and child participants resided in the same household.

After written consent was obtained from a parent, White and Latino families were assigned randomly to an intervention group or a control (wait-list) group using a random numbers table. Intervention groups received a 4-week program and completed measures at baseline (before the intervention) and 1, 3, and 6 months after the intervention. The wait-list control groups completed the same measures at the same time intervals. After the 6-month data collection, the control group also received the intervention. All children's data were self-reported and obtained at each child care site by using an interactive game on a laptop with software designed for the study (Kennedy, Charlesworth, & Chen, 2003). Each child logged on with a password-protected ID number, their data were encrypted, and the data were uploaded and transferred to SPSS files. Parents used traditional pen-and-paper questionnaires in their preferred language and returned the completed forms by mail.

Verbal assent was obtained from all children, and confidentiality, group rules, and general guidelines were discussed with the children. Children received incentives (books and small surprises) each week of the program and a $20 gift certificate to a toy store upon completion of the program. Parents were given a $20 gift certificate to a local food market.

INTERVENTION

The intervention program was designed for small groups of four to six children, facilitated by a research team nurse or health counselor. Four interventionists were trained by the primary investigator and project director in a group workshop model and utilized a standardized procedural manual for each of the sessions. The project director routinely monitored the delivery of sessions through random direct observation visits, and all interventionists participated in training refresher sessions every 6 months. Details of the behavioral basis of the program, process evaluation, and treatment fidelity are reported elsewhere (Kennedy & Floriani, 2008).

The program comprised four content segments, conducted during consecutive weekly sessions. The thematic concept of each week moved from the general to the specific, focused on knowledge and awareness, the acquisition of new skills and behaviors, and the supportive practice and application of the skills. Essential to learning and internalizing the information presented, each week of the program allowed for repetition and practice within the group and at home. Although parents did not participate directly in the program, they did receive weekly information packets containing media and health concepts similar to the content the children received that week. The concept of each program segment was reviewed further during the following week, in relation to the activities children had practiced at home and as an introduction for the related successive concept.

MEASURES

Five age-appropriate instruments designed for children and five instruments for parents that had literacy levels established at lower-grade-school readability were used (Table 1).

Affective. The Self-Perception Profile (SPP) is a 36-item questionnaire used for assessing self-perceptions of competencies in children in third grade and older (Table 1).

Child's Health Behaviors. The reported overall health behaviors of the child were measured with a 36-item Likert scale called How Often Do You? Stember, Swanson-Kaufman, Goodwin, Rogers, and Mathews (1984) reported that content and concurrent validity was demonstrated sufficiently by this instrument (Table 1).

Cognitive. The Child's Health Self-Concept Scale is used to measure children's cognitive appraisal (perception) of health (Hester, 1984). This 45-item scale takes approximately 15 minutes for the child to complete. Based on a diverse sample of 940 children, the authors originally created four subscales (Table 1), but because further analysis suggested that a single attribute is being measured, only a total score is reported.

Coping. The Schoolager's Coping Strategies Inventory is a 26-item self-report instrument used to measure the type, frequency, and effectiveness of coping strategies used by children (Ryan-Wenger, 1990). Each child identifies a stressor and then scores each coping strategy for frequency of use and for degree of helpfulness (Table 1).

Family Characteristics. Demographics were collected with a 31-item parent questionnaire for educational, financial, and social descriptive data. A 12-item Short Acculturation Scale (Marin, Sabogal, Marin, Oter-Sabogal, & Perez-Stable, 1987) was used to measure the acculturation level of Latino families. The Acculturation Scale has demonstrated good psychometric properties in both its English and Spanish versions (Table 1).

Family Functioning. The Family Assessment Device (FAD) has six specific subscales (Epstein, Baldwin, & Bishop, 1983) and a 12-item general functioning subscale that has been used as a global assessment of general health of the family (Table 1). Several studies have reported the concurrent validity of the FAD as ranging from 0.48 to 0.53 and reliabilities

Table 1. Instruments Used to Assess Children and Their Families

Instrument	Assessment	Subscales	Score range	Psychometric properties
Self-Perception Profile	Affect in children 8 to 12 years old	Scholastic competence Athletic competence Social acceptance Physical appearance Behavioral conduct Global self-worth	Likert scale, 1 (low) to 4 (high)	Internal consistency reliability α: .80 to .85 for scholastic competence, .80 to .86 for athletic competence, .75 to .80 for social acceptance, .76 to .82 for physical appearance, .71 to .77 for behavioral conduct, and .78 to .84 for global self-worth
How Often Do You?	Child's health behaviors	Safety Junk food Activity Nutrition Hygiene Assertiveness	1 (low frequency) to 4 (high frequency)	Cronbach's α = .86−.91
Child's Health Self-Concept Scale	Children's perception of their health	Psychosocial issues Physical health Values Energy and healthiness	Summative rating scale from 1 (negative health self-concept) to 4 (positive health self-concept)	Moderate stability High internal consistency reliability (.82) Evidence of content validity
Schoolager's Coping Strategies Inventory	Coping in children aged 8 to 12 years	Frequency of use of coping strategy Effectiveness of coping strategy	0 (low) to 3 (high)	Construct validity Internal consistency (r = .79) Test–retest reliability (r = .73−.82) Cronbach's α reliability coefficients: .84 for frequency subscale, .85 for effectiveness subscale

Short Acculturation Scale	Acculturation of Latino families	Validity criteria: respondents' generation, length of residence in the United States, and age on arrival in the United States	Average of scores on Likert scale from 1 to 5: scores ≤2.99, low; scores >2.99, high	Correlated with respondents' generation ($r = .69$), length of residence in the United States ($r = .76$), and age on arrival in the United States ($r = .72$)
Family Assessment Device	Family functioning	Problem solving / Communication / Roles / Affective responsiveness / Affective involvement / Behavior control / General functioning	Likert scale, 1 ("strongly agree") to 4 ("strongly disagree") Higher scores indicate poorer function	Cronbach's α: .73 for problem solving, .72 for communication, .70 for roles, .69 for affective responsiveness, .64 for affective involvement, .52 for behavior control, and .82 for general functioning
Media Quotient	Family media habits and beliefs	Media use / Monitoring / Consistency / Media effects / Media knowledge / Alternative activities	Likert scale: "always" (1) to "never" (5)	Reliability coefficients: media use, $\alpha = .75$; monitoring, $\alpha = .89$; consistency, $\alpha = .73$; media effects, $\alpha = .63$; media knowledge, $\alpha = .25$; and alternative activities, $\alpha = .66$ Test–retest correlations: media use, $r = .96$; monitoring, $r = .82$; consistency, $r = .89$; media effects, $r = .84$; media knowledge, $r = .81$; alternative activities, $r = .82$
Health Self-Determinism Index–Children	Motivation of children	Self-determinism in health behavior / Competency in health matters / Internal–external cue responsiveness / Self-determinism in health judgment	1 (maximum extrinsic orientation) to 4 (maximum intrinsic orientation)	Internal consistency (Cronbach's α) of .78 2-week test–retest correlation for total tool of .83

(continued)

Table 1. *(Continued)*

Instrument	Assessment	Subscales	Score range	Psychometric properties
Injury Behavior Checklist	Parents report on frequency of children's risk-taking behaviors in past 6 months	24 items describing risk-taking behaviors	0 = "not at all" 1 = "very seldom, has happened once to twice" 2 = "sometimes, about once a month" 3 = "pretty often, about once a week" 4 = "very often, more than once a week" Total sum for all 24 items, 0 to 96	Internal consistency of .84–.92 1-month test–retest correlation of .81 Specificity adequate
Framingham Safety Survey	Parents describe home-based safety practices	19 questions on injury prevention and safety behaviors	1 (low) to 3 (high) safety for each response, with a total score from 19 to 57. Higher scores reflect greater safety behaviors	Internal reliability (Cronbach's α) External reliability Validity

from .69 to .86 (Kabakoff, Miller, Bishop, Epstein, & Keitner, 1990; Miller, Ryan, Keitner, Bishop, & Epstein, 2000).

Family Media. The Media Quotient was used to measure family media habits and beliefs about the effects of media (Gentile & Walsh, 2002). The reliability coefficients and test–retest correlations for the six indices of the Media Quotient are listed in Table 1. Gentile and Walsh (2002) reported that the low reliability coefficient for the Media Knowledge index was expected because of the wide range of topics measured by this index (it was a heterogeneous index, whereas other indices were homogeneous). Across all items, the mean test–retest correlation is .75. The mean test–retest correlation for the six indices is .85. Validity was supported by the negative correlations between children's television viewing and each of the indices.

Motivation. The Health Self-Determinism Index–Children (HSDI-C) is composed of 32 forced-choice Likert-format items divided over four subscales (Cox, 1985). Children were asked to decide which kind of *kid* is most like themselves and then are asked whether this is *only sort of true* or *really true* for them (Table 1).

Risk Taking. The IBC is a reporting measure for parents that contains 24 items describing various specific risk-taking behaviors and minor injurious mishaps for children up to age 9 years (Table 1). The IBC score is predictive of subsequent injuries; reported mean scores range from 18 to 33 in diverse populations (Bass & Mehta, 1980; Bernardo, 1996; Kennedy & Rodriguez, 1999; Potts et al., 1995, 1997).

Safety Behaviors. The American Academy of Pediatrics Framingham Safety Survey (FSS) for ages 5 to 9 years is a 19-question parent report on home-based safety practices used to gather information so that caregivers in primary care clinical settings can provide counseling about injury prevention and safety behaviors (Table 1). The FSS also is referred to as The Injury

Prevention Program Safety Survey. Five developmentally age-specific versions of the FSS are available in both English and Spanish. Psychometric properties (Table 1) reported for the younger FSS support acceptable internal and external reliability and validity for parent report (Mason, Christoffel, & Sinacore, 2007).

DATA ANALYSIS

Descriptive statistics were examined initially for demographic characteristics and all major study variables. The intervention and control groups were compared by using t tests to check for any major dissimilarity between the study groups at baseline. Partial correlation coefficients, controlling for gender, weight status, ethnicity, and group membership (intervention vs. control), were computed to examine variables related to risk taking and safety behaviors. Stepwise regressions were used to examine factors from the baseline data that contributed to children's safety and risk-taking behaviors. Examined was whether the rate of change in children in the intervention group was different than the rate among children in the control group by fitting linear mixed-effects models that include functions of time and group effects to the repeated child data. Analyses were performed with SPSS 15.0, and mixed modeling was performed by using SAS version 8.

▪ Results

Approximately 86% of White and 22% of Latina mothers had completed a high school education. Four percent of White families and 38% of Latino families had annual incomes less than $20,000, whereas 82% of White families and 8% of Latino families had annual incomes greater than $40,000. Significantly more Latino mothers (77%) than White mothers (66%) were married ($\chi^2 = 13.05$, $p = .023$). Most of the Latino mothers (93%) were highly acculturated; 40% were U.S. natives. The 60% who were born elsewhere had resided in the United States for more than 10 years.

Total scores on risk taking were significantly higher in boys (14.6) than in girls (11.0; $t = 2.23$, $p < .02$) and in normal-weight children (15.0) than in overweight children (10.0; $t = 2.59$, $p < .01$). Mean scores for the major child model variables did not differ significantly between the children in the two groups at baseline (Table 2).

Partial correlation coefficients were used to examine correlations between family variables and children's behaviors, and regression models were computed to explore factors contributing to children's risk-taking and safety behaviors at baseline. When gender, ethnicity, weight, and group membership were controlled for, it was found that increased television viewing time was related to less use of safety behaviors ($r = -.34$, $p = .009$) and to less use of positive media ($r = -.32$, $p = .012$). Higher risk taking in children was related significantly to parents' belief that media do not affect children ($r = -.27$, $p = .036$). Higher amounts of television watching also correlated with the child having a negative health self-concept ($r = -.54$, $p < .001$).

Stepwise regression models were computed to examine factors contributing to children's safety and risk-taking behaviors. The children's age and ethnicity were first, followed by seven subscales of the FAD (problem solving, communication, roles, affective involvement, affective responsiveness, behavior control, and general functioning), six indices from the Media Quotient (alternatives, consistency, effects, knowledge, monitoring, and media use), and total hours of television viewing. At baseline, five variables contributed to lower safety behaviors (adjusted $R^2 = .37$, $F = 9.93$, $p < .0001$): poorer problem solving in the family ($sr^2 = .25$), unhealthy (high) affective involvement in the family ($sr^2 = .08$), high use of alternative media in families ($sr^2 = .08$), high television viewing times among children ($sr^2 = .06$), and high use of positive media in the family ($sr^2 = .07$). Four variables were significant in predicting children's risk-taking behaviors (adjusted $R^2 = .21$, $F = 6.70$, $p < .0001$): being White ($sr^2 = .16$), being a boy ($sr^2 = .03$), poor affective responsiveness in the family ($sr^2 = .10$), and better media con-

sistency (consistent use of media rules) in the family ($sr^2 = .08$; Table 3).

No significant differences were found between groups in children's affect (SPP), cognition and health perceptions (CHSCS), coping strategies, motivation (HSDI-C), or general health behaviors (How Often Do You?) during the 6-month period (Table 2). Children evidenced significant decreases in self-determined health judgment (HSDI-C subscale) over time ($F = 3.09$, $p = .03$), but no interaction was found between groups and time ($F = 1.9$, $p = .13$). Children, on average, watched 18 hours of television weekly. Television watching in the intervention group had decreased to 17 hours weekly by 6 months after the intervention, although this difference was not statistically significant ($t = -1.90$, $p = .07$). In the hierarchical mixed model, the intervention group significantly increased their safety behaviors ($F = 4.37$, $p = .006$). No difference was found in risk taking over time or between groups ($F = 0.23$, $p = .87$; Table 4). At the 6-month follow-up, families in the intervention group reported two additional changes: an increase in the consistent use of media rules ($t = -0.241$, $p = .022$) but a decrease in use of alternative activities ($t = 2.21$, $p = .032$). To explore these results further, a regression analysis was run on children's baseline variables as predictors of safety and risk-taking behaviors at 6 months after the intervention. More effective coping by the child at baseline was predictive of higher use of safety behaviors 6 months later (adjusted $R^2 = .13$, $F = 8.69$, $p = .005$). Higher television watching time and less effective coping at baseline were predictive of higher risk-taking behaviors at 6 months after the intervention (adjusted $R^2 = .21$, $F = 4.78$, $p = .034$).

■ Discussion

THEORETICAL MODEL

These findings raise issues about the need for further refinement and testing of the IMCHB

Table 2. Child Variables (Means and SD)

Variable	Intervention				Control			
	T1	T2	T3	T4	T1	T2	T3	T4
Framingham Safety Survey	41.41 (0.68)	43.95 (0.74)	44.70 (0.70)	45.09 (0.66)	43.48 (0.68)	44.19 (0.89)	43.87 (0.76)	44.09 (0.79)
Injury Behavior Checklist	13.62 (1.10)	14.20 (1.29)	11.91 (1.19)	11.31 (1.14)	12.50 (1.11)	12.13 (1.51)	12.93 (1.30)	11.58 (1.35)
Health Self-Determinism Index–Children								
Behavior	35.94 (6.31)	37.33 (7.10)	37.27 (6.16)	37.09 (6.87)	36.51 (6.05)	37.12 (6.68)	36.85 (5.63)	36.16 (8.96)
Internal–External cue	14.15 (4.27)	14.06 (4.20)	13.27 (3.75)	13.54 (6.87)	13.37 (3.97)	14.38 (4.00)	14.33 (4.28)	14.00 (4.27)
Competence	15.70 (4.07)	14.90 (5.01)	14.75 (4.04)	13.92 (4.20)	15.37 (3.97)	14.20 (3.90)	14.21 (4.06)	14.91 (4.41)
Judgment	7.31 (2.43)	7.21 (2.84)	6.72 (2.66)	6.06 (2.37)	6.92 (2.67)	6.65 (2.80)	6.47 (2.76)	7.03 (2.9)
Self-Perception Profile								
Scholastic competence	17.75 (4.22)	18.63 (3.59)	18.61 (4.09)	18.45 (4.08)	17.61 (3.64)	18.12 (3.64)	18.31 (3.42)	17.46 (4.48)
Social acceptance	16.48 (4.03)	16.61 (4.57)	17.43 (4.63)	16.90 (4.89)	16.50 (3.10)	16.79 (3.59)	16.97 (3.53)	17.16 (3.97)
Athletic competence	17.06 (3.81)	16.73 (4.16)	17.31 (3.71)	17.43 (4.28)	16.71 (3.51)	16.38 (3.97)	16.21 (4.33)	16.27 (4.00)
Physical appearance	18.91 (3.87)	19.12 (4.24)	19.00 (3.85)	19.19 (4.27)	17.98 (4.33)	18.23 (3.89)	18.41 (3.77)	18.03 (4.4)
Behavioral conduct	18.25 (2.95)	19.47 (3.26)	19.27 (3.28)	18.34 (3.92)	18.25 (3.46)	18.84 (3.16)	19.04 (3.18)	18.84 (3.88)
Global self-worth	19.52 (4.11)	19.08 (3.73)	19.29 (3.60)	19.55 (3.85)	18.99 (3.00)	19.32 (3.77)	19.75 (3.71)	18.97 (3.75)
Child's Health Self-Concept Scale	133.12 (15.02)	134.34 (17.48)	136.67 (17.55)	136.21 (17.15)	133.45 (14.86)	136.52 (14.44)	135.45 (15.28)	133.68 (14.66)
How Often Do You?	114.81 (10.04)	113.35 (11.94)	115.92 (10.72)	116.10 (10.29)	111.87 (11.43)	114.00 (11.29)	113.19 (10.86)	114.94 (11.58)
Schoolager's Coping Strategies Inventory								
Frequency	38.30 (10.39)	37.84 (10.59)	38.81 (8.30)	37.45 (10.30)	37.21 (10.74)	36.91 (8.61)	35.68 (8.80)	38.31 (9.41)
Effectiveness	44.68 (10.46)	42.97 (10.06)	45.46 (9.24)	42.10 (9.90)	45.42 (11.71)	42.64 (8.53)	42.99 (8.75)	44.39 (9.52)

Note. T1 is baseline, T2 is 1 month after baseline, T3 is 3 months after baseline, and T4 is 6 months after baseline.

Table 3. Stepwise Multiple Regression Summary Table

Source	Adjusted R^2	β	sr^2	df	F	p
Low safety behaviors						
Overall	.37			5, 70	9.93	.0001
Poorer problem solving		−.457	.25	5, 70	23.37	.0001
High affective involvement		.230	.08	5, 70	5.90	.018
Better media use		−.250	.07	5, 70	4.96	.029
High use of alternative media		−.283	.08	5, 70	6.22	.015
High television viewing time		−.199	.06	5, 70	4.31	.041
High risk taking						
Overall	.21			4, 83	6.70	.0001
White		−.470	.16	4, 83	15.24	.0001
Boy		−.170	.03	4, 83	2.97	.05
Poorer affective response		.378	.10	4, 83	9.70	.003
Better media consistency		.265	.08	4, 83	7.21	.009

Table 4. General Mixed Model Summary Table

Variables	−2 Log Likelihood	Group $F(p)$	Time $F(p)$	Group × Time $F(p)$
Framingham Safety Survey	1,327.3	0.01 (.908)	9.17 (.001)	4.37 (.0062)
Injury Behavior Checklist	1,948.6	0.017 (.6827)	0.50 (.6684)	0.23 (.8742)
HSDI-C behavior	516.6	0.11 (.7421)	0.38 (.7697)	0.23 (.8744)
HSDI-C competence	596.6	0.000 (.9884)	1.22 (.3078)	0.70 (.5532)
HSDI-C internal/external	658.7	0.33 (.5644)	1.50 (.2201)	1.60 (.1926)
HSDI-C judgment	661.2	0.08 (.7839)	3.09 (.0314)	1.90 (.1340)
SPP athletic competence	576.1	0.96 (.3304)	1.03 (.3836)	0.66 (.5783)
SPP behavioral conduct	553.3	0.09 (.7664)	1.40 (.2442)	0.72 (.5414)
SPP physical appearance	590.9	1.93 (.1673)	0.39 (.7625)	0.47 (.7071)
SPP scholastic competence	581.4	0.77 (.3812)	0.96 (.4162)	0.66 (.5809)
SPP social acceptance	568.9	0.01 (.9258)	0.25 (.8617)	0.16 (.9219)
SPP global self-worth	563.3	0.34 (.5588)	0.57 (.6340)	0.56 (.6441)
Child's Health Self-Concept	90.3	0.03 (.8533)	0.64 (.5936)	0.66 (.5776)
How Often Do You?	2,527.9	0.33 (.5671)	1.53 (.2108)	1.37 (.2537)

Note. HSDI-C = Health Self-Determinism Index–Children; SPP = Self-Perception Profile.

in pediatric nursing research. As suggested by Carter and Kulbok (1995), it is possible that cognitive appraisal (a) should not be captured only as "perceived health status," (b) needs further development as a construct, and (c) may not be sensitive to developmental change over time. Morrongiello and Mark (2008) reported that by targeting specific risk-taking cognitions, in contrast to general perceived health cognitions, they could reduce children's risk-taking intentions by using an induced-hypocrisy intervention. Regarding the second point, in construct validity testing, the CHSCS did not discriminate into its original five sub-scales, suggesting little support for the construct validity of the subscales and leaving unknown the construct validity of it as a measure of a single attribute. Our study is the first to use a longitudinal and repeated-measures design in children; thus, from a developmental perspective, we believe that the third point also has merit.

In both groups, self-determined health judgment decreased significantly in the 6 months after the intervention, reflecting movement from an intrinsic to extrinsic orientation. This result is in contrast to the results originally reported by Cox, Cowell, Marion, and Miller (1990), who found a linear trend from extrinsic to intrinsic motivation with increasing age. Those values, however, were based on cohort studies and not on longitudinal changes with the same study population, and they reflect a much wider age range (third–seventh grade). Cox et al. noted that the 1-year test–retest α values decreased and suggested that the measure might be capturing state versus trait behavior. Further psychometric property testing should address whether the HSDI-C is stable for midrange periods such as 6 months if it is to be used fruitfully in future short-term longitudinal studies.

A child's coping effectiveness was predictive of both safety and risk-taking behaviors 6 months later. This finding suggests that coping strategies should continue to be investigated as a relevant facet of children's health intervention work, especially given reports that training in coping skills enhances behav-

> As expected, boys scored higher than girls scored on risk taking.

ioral interventions in diverse areas such as pediatric diabetes (Grey, Boland, Davidson, Li, & Tamborlane, 2000) and weight reduction (Berry, Savoye, Melkus, & Grey, 2007).

MEDIA

At 18 hours a week, the total television watching time of the children in this sample is less than the national average of 21 hours a week but is still not at the American Academy of Pediatrics' recommendation of 2 hours or less a day (14 hours weekly). Higher risk taking in children was significantly related to parents' belief that media do not affect children, and yet large amounts of television watching did correlate significantly with children reporting a more negative perception self-concept of their own health. Greater television viewing time was also related to less use of safety behaviors in households.

At the 6-month follow-up, families in the intervention group reported a significant increase in the consistent use of media rules but a decrease in use of alternative activities. These findings suggest that families still need help in creating and maintaining lifestyles that enhance activity choices other than watching television. Future studies attempting to address media use in the parent–child dyad or (even more challenging) the family as a whole will be critical.

RISK TAKING AND SAFETY

As expected, boys scored higher than girls did on risk taking. This finding is in concert with the robust gender differences reported in the injury literature. As in most other studies, we have operationalized risk taking as a physical activity, which might also account for the significantly lower rates of risk taking in overweight children compared with children of normal weight in the study. Green (1997) found that physical risk taking is an important factor in the creation of boys' social identity. Results of a recent ethnographic study suggest that girls are risk takers when social domains are included and that children's risk engagement and risk taking are a balancing act between risk willingness and self-care within the context of social relationships, emotional excitement, and connections and activities with other children (Christensen & Mikkelsen, 2008). Possibly, the intervention was not motivating enough to lower risk-taking behavior because it did not attend to the social identity and perceptions of other peers in the group. A second potential explanation is that the lack of change might reflect a "floor effect," where reduction of risk taking is less likely in a group that is already low in risk taking. A third arises from a recent report by Morrongiello, Lassenby-Lessard, and Matheis (2007), who used IBC scores reported by the child rather than the parent. They found that school-age children routinely engage in greater risk taking than their parents would have them do and that parents often were not told about minor injuries or risk-taking behaviors. This suggests potential underreporting of risk taking by parents of school-age children.

Intervention families showed a significant increase in safety behaviors, and this effect was sustained for the 6 months. The intervention activities of the children that were practiced at home and, possibly, the parental materials that were sent home influenced modifications in the home environment, as measured by the safety behaviors. Given the baseline predictors of safety behaviors, we suggest that the intervention engaged mothers' affective-based perspectives and enhanced maternal problem solving. Decisions by mothers to engage in safety practices are driven by affect rather than knowledge, that is, by changes in perception of their specific child's characteristics that they believe make their child vulnerable (Morrongiello & Kiriakou, 2004). Our finding that poor affective involvement is related to low safety behaviors among mothers supports this interpretation. Perhaps, the safety behaviors meas-

ured in the FSS tap those behaviors that the mothers could effectively change. Kronenfeld, Reiser, Glik, Alatorre, and Jackson (1997), reported direct effects and greater use of safety behaviors in mothers who had high stress levels and high coping skills (affect variables) and only an indirect effect for cognitive variables in increasing the use of safety behaviors.

Despite these limitations, the intervention increased use of safety behaviors and thus affected one part of the injury equation. Future research with high risk-taking populations and approaches that enhance the social/emotional milieu are necessary for further refinement of interventions. If some physical risk taking is a necessary social developmental experience in the context of peer play and risk engagement, then the very low rates of physical risk taking among overweight children suggest additional psychological issues that intervention programs to reduce sedentary activity and increase physical activity will have to address for health promotion.

In conclusion, Sommers (2006) suggests that four strategies are needed for nurses to build injury science: identification of individuals at risk, development of models to explain the association between risk taking and injury, development and testing of interventions to prevent and control injury, and refinement of interventions that are culturally relevant. The results of this study contribute to these goals to foster a child and family approach for nurses practicing in primary care and community settings.

Christine Kennedy, PhD, RN, FAAN, is Professor; and Jyu-Lin Chen, PhD, RN, is Assistant Professor, Department of Family Health Care, School of Nursing, University of California, San Francisco.

Accepted for publication March 20, 2009.
This study was funded by the National Institute of Nursing Research, National Institutes of Health (RO1 NR04680).
Thank you to Annemarie Charlesworth-Suring MA, project director, and Ms. Emma Passalacqua, BA, staff coordinator, of the Kids TV study.

Corresponding author: Christine Kennedy, PhD, RN, FAAN, School of Nursing, University of California, San Francisco, Box 0606, 2 Koret Avenue, San Francisco, CA 94143 (e-mail: Christine.Kennedy@ ucsf.edu).

REFERENCES

Bass, J. L., & Mehta, K. A. (1980). Developmentally-oriented safety surveys: Reported parental and adolescent practices. *Clinical Pediatrics, 19*(5), 350–356.

Bernardo, L. M. (1996). Parent-reported injury-associated behaviors and life events among injured, ill, and well preschool children. *Journal of Pediatric Nursing, 11*(2), 100–110.

Berry, D., Savoye, M., Melkus, G., & Grey, M. (2007). An intervention for multiethnic obese parents and overweight children. *Applied Nursing Research, 20*(2), 63–71.

Carter, K. F., & Kulbok, P. A. (1995). Evaluation of the Interaction Model of Client Health Behavior through the first decade of research. *Advances in Nursing Science, 18*(1), 62–73.

Chen, J., Kresnow, M. J., Simon, T. R., & Dellinger, A. (2007). Injury-prevention counseling and behavior among US children: Results from the second Injury Control and Risk Survey. *Pediatrics, 119*(4), e958–e965.

Chen, J. L., & Kennedy, C. (2005). Cultural variations in children's coping behaviour, TV viewing time, and family functioning. *International Nursing Review, 52*(3), 186–195.

Christensen, P., & Mikkelsen, M. R. (2008). Jumping off and being careful: Children's strategies of risk management in everyday life. *Sociology of Health & Illness, 30*(1), 112–130.

Cox, C. L. (1985). The Health Self-Determinism Index. *Nursing Research, 34*(3), 177–183.

Cox, C. L., Cowell, J. M., Marion, L. N., & Miller, E. H. (1990). The Health Self-Determinism Index for Children. *Research in Nursing & Health, 13*(4), 237–246.

Epstein, N., Baldwin, L., & Bishop, S. (1983). The McMaster Family Assessment Device. *Journal of Marital and Family Therapy, 9*(2), 171–180.

Farrand, L., & Cox, C. L. (1993). Determinants of positive health behaviors in middle childhood. *Nursing Research, 42*(4), 208–213.

Gentile, D. A., & Walsh, D. A. (2002). A normative study of family media habits. *Journal of Applied Developmental Psychology, 23*(2), 157–178.

Green, J. (1997). Risk and the construction of social identity: Children's talk about accidents. *Sociology of Health & Illness, 19*(4), 457–479.

Grey, M., Boland, E., Davidson, M., Li, J., & Tamborlane, W. V. (2000). Coping skills training for youth with diabetes mellitus has long-lasting effects on metabolic control and quality of life. *Journal of Pediatrics, 137*(1), 107–113.

Hester, N. O. (1984). Child's Health Self-Concept Scale: Its development and psychometric properties. *Advances in Nursing Science, 7*(1), 45–55.

Kabakoff, R., Miller, I., Bishop, D., Epstein, N., & Keitner, G. (1990). A psychometric study of the McMaster Family Assessment Device in psychiatric, medical, and nonclinical samples. *Journal of Family Psychology, 3*(4), 431–439.

Kennedy, C. M. (2000a). Television and young Hispanic children's health behaviors. *Pediatric Nursing, 26*(3), 283–294.

Kennedy, C. M. (2000b). Examining television as an influence on children's health behaviors. *Journal of Pediatric Nursing, 15*(5), 272–281.

Kennedy, C. M., Charlesworth, A., & Chen, J. L. (2003). Interactive data collection: Benefits of integrating new media into pediatric research. *Computers, Informatics, Nursing, 21*(3), 120–127.

Kennedy, C. M., & Floriani, V. (2008). Translating research on healthy lifestyles for children: Meeting the needs of diverse populations. *Nursing Clinics of North America, 43*(3), 397–417.

Kennedy, C. M., & Lipsitt, L. P. (1998). Risk-taking in preschool children. *Journal of Pediatric Nursing, 13*(2), 77–84.

Kennedy, C. M., & Rodriguez, D. A. (1999). Risk taking in young Hispanic children. *Journal of Pediatric Health Care, 13*(3 Pt. 1), 126–135.

Kennedy, C. M., Strzempko, F., Danford, C., & Kools, S. (2002). Children's perceptions of TV and health behavior effects. *Journal of Nursing Scholarship, 34*(3), 289–294.

Kronenfeld, J. J., Reiser, M., Glik, D. C., Alatorre, C., & Jackson, K. (1997). Safety behaviors of mothers of young children: Impact of cognitive, stress and background factors. *Health, 1*(2), 205–225.

Marin, G., Sabogal, F., Marin, B. V., Oter-Sabogal, R., & Perez-Stable, E. J. (1987). Development of a short acculturation scale for Hispanics. *Hispanic Journal of Behavioral Sciences, 9*(2), 183–205.

Mason, M., Christoffel, K. K., & Sinacore, J. (2007). Reliability and validity of The Injury Prevention Project Home Safety Survey. *Archives of Pediatrics & Adolescent Medicine, 161*(8), 759–765.

Miller, I. W., Ryan, C. E., Keitner, G. I., Bishop, D. S., & Epstein, N. B. (2000). The McMaster Approach to Families: Theory, assessment, treatment and research. *Journal of Family Therapy, 22*(2), 168–189.

Morrongiello, B. A. (2004). Do children's intentions to risk take relate to actual risk taking? *Injury Prevention, 10*(1), 62–64.

Morrongiello, B. A., & Kiriakou, S. (2004). Mothers' home-safety practices for preventing six types of childhood injuries: What do they do, and why? *Journal of Pediatric Psychology, 29*(4), 285–297.

Morrongiello, B. A., Lassenby-Lessard, J., & Matheis, S. (2007). Understanding children's injury-risk behaviors: The independent contributions of cognitions and emotions. *Journal of Pediatric Psychology, 32*(8), 926–937.

Morrongiello, B. A., & Mark, L. (2008). "Practice what you preach": Induced hypocrisy as an intervention strategy to reduce children's intentions to risk take on playgrounds. *Journal of Pediatric Psychology, 33*(10), 1117–1128. doi:10.1093/jpepsy/ jsn011. Advance Access.

Potts, R., Doppler, M., & Hernandez, M. (1994). Effects of television content on physical risk-taking in children. *Journal of Experimental Child Psychology, 58*(3), 321–331.

Potts, R., Martinez, I. G., & Dedmon, A. (1995). Childhood risk taking and injury: Self-report and informant measures. *Journal of Pediatric Psychology, 20*(1), 5–12.

Potts, R., Martinez, I. G., Dedmon, A., Schwarz, L., DiLillo, D., & Swisher, L. (1997). Brief report: Cross-validation of the Injury Behavior Checklist in a school-age sample. *Journal of Pediatric Psychology, 22*(4), 533–540.

Potts, R., & Swisher, L. (1998). Effects of televised safety models on children's risk taking and hazard identification. *Journal of Pediatric Psychology, 23*(3), 157–163.

Ryan-Wenger, N. M. (1990). Development and psychometric properties of the Schoolagers' Coping Strategies Inventory. *Nursing Research, 39*(6), 344–349.

Sommers, M. S. (2006). Injury as a global phenomenon of concern in nursing science. *Journal of Nursing Scholarship, 38*(4), 314–320.

Speltz, M. L., Gonzales, N., Sulzbacher, S., & Quan, L. (1990). Assessment of injury risk in young children: A preliminary study of the Injury Behavior Checklist. *Journal of Pediatric Psychology, 15*(3), 373–383.

Stember, M., Swanson-Kaufman, K., Goodwin, L., Rogers, S., & Mathews, S. (1984). *How often do you?* Denver, CO: University of Colorado Health Services Center.

ROOTING FOR THE BREAST: BREASTFEEDING PROMOTION IN THE NICU

Roberta Cricco-Lizza, PhD, MPH, RN

ABSTRACT

▶ **Purpose:** This study explored the structure and process of breastfeeding promotion in the NICU.

▶ **Methods:** An ethnographic approach was used with the techniques of participant observation, interviewing , and artifact assessment. This 14-month study took place in a level IV NICU in Northeastern US children's hospital. General informants consisted of 114 purposively selected NICU nurses. From this group, 18 nurses served as key informants. There was an average of 13 interactions with each key informant and 3.5 for each general informant. Audiotaped interviews, feeding artifacts, and observational notes were gathered for descriptions of breastfeeding promotion. Data were coded and analyzed for recurring patterns. NUD*IST-aided data management and analysis.

▶ **Findings:** There were three main findings: (1) organizational and human resources were developed to create a web of support to promote breastfeeding in the NICU; (2) variations in breastfeeding knowledge and experience within the nursing staff, marketing practices of formula companies, and insufficient support from other health professionals served as sources of inconsistent breastfeeding messages; and (3) promotion of breastfeeding in this NICU is evolving over time from a current breast milk feeding focus to the goal for a future breastfeeding process orientation.

▶ **Clinical Implications:** NICU nurses should advocate for organizational and human resources to promote breastfeeding in the unit. To decrease inconsistent messages, staff development should be expanded to all professionals, and formula marketing practices should be curtailed.

▶ **Keywords:** breastfeeding · NICU · nurses · promotion.

This study explored the structure and process of breastfeeding promotion in the neonatal intensive care unit (NICU). Mother's milk is particularly important for the health of premature and high-risk infants (American Academy of Pediatrics, 2005; Ip et al., 2007). Ingestion of breast milk in the NICU by low birth weight infants has been linked to beneficial health outcomes and enhanced cognitive development (Vohr et al., 2006). Breast milk provides protection against infections, sepsis, necrotizing enterocolitis, and retinopathy of prematurity (Furman, Taylor, Minich, & Hack, 2003; Hylander, Strobino, Pezzullo, & Dhannireddy, 2001; Schanler, Lau, Hurst, & Smith, 2005). The American Academy of Pediatrics recommends direct breastfeeding and/or use of mother's own pumped milk for high-risk infants; however, these reported rates are low for NICU babies (Espy & Senn, 2003). In addition to maternal and neonatal issues, staff and hospital factors also influence NICU breastfeeding rates (Lessen & Crivelli- Kovach, 2007; Merewood, Philipp, Chawla, & Cimo, 2003).

Maternity practices in the United States are often not evidence based and have been shown to impede breastfeeding (Centers for Disease

Control and Prevention, 2008; DiGirolamo, Grummer-Strawn, & Fein, 2001). The World Health Organization (WHO) and the United Nations Children's Fund (UNICEF) (1992) launched the Baby-Friendly Hospital Initiative (BFHI) to protect, promote, and support breastfeeding in birth environments. The recommended practices in this Initiative have been linked to improved breastfeeding rates, but they generally pertain to routine births in hospitals and birthing centers (Kramer et al., 2001). Mothers of high-risk infants face unique challenges to the initiation and continuation of breastfeeding (Meier, 2001; Spatz, 2006). Hospitals must address these challenges to prepare the NICU staff to support breastfeeding families. However, mothers have reported problems with hospital routines and inadequate support for breastfeeding from nurses and physicians in the NICU (Cricco-Lizza, 2006). Hospitals with NICU breastfeeding promotion programs have positively influenced breastfeeding rates (Dall'Oglio et al., 2007; do Nascimento & Issler, 2005).

More research is needed about effective ways to promote breastfeeding in the NICU. Structures and processes in an organization can advance or can hamper the implementation of health promotion strategies, and much can be gained by exploring the context of everyday practices (Yano, 2008). This report is part of a larger qualitative study of NICU nurses and infant feeding. In a previous publication from this study, nurses' personal contexts of infant feeding outside of the NICU were examined. The nurses identified a formula feeding norm during their own childhoods and described limited exposure to breastfeeding in nursing school (Cricco-Lizza, 2009). The current article examines the structures and processes that were developed to promote breastfeeding in the NICU.

▪ Methods

An ethnographic approach was used with the techniques of participant observation,

interviewing, and artifact analysis. By combining these three techniques, multiple sources of information were obtained for a comprehensive view of breastfeeding promotion in the NICU. The sample consisted of 114 nurses who were considered "general informants," purposefully selected to provide a wide angle view of breastfeeding promotion, and 18 "key informants" chosen from that group who were followed more intensively for an in-depth view. Both key and general informants were selected for maximal variety of infant feeding and NICU clinical experiences. The 14-month study was conducted in a level IV NICU in a freestanding children's hospital in the Northeastern United States. This study was approved by the Human Subjects' Committees and study information was provided to the nurses through the intranet, staff meetings, and individual encounters in the NICU. Nurses who served as key informants for the study signed informed consent before formal interviews.

SAMPLE

From 250 nurses employed in this NICU, 114 served as the general informants; 96 of these were White, 9 African American, 8 Asian, and 1 Hispanic. Only one was a male. About 30% of the general informants had taken a hospital breastfeeding course developed before this study was initiated. The age of the 18 key informants ranged from 22 to 51 (mean = 33). Of these, 17 were female; 16 were White and 2 were African American. Two had diplomas in nursing, 1 had an associate degree, 14 had a BSN, and 1 had a master's degree. The key informants were almost evenly divided among all four expertise levels of the clinical ladder, from novices to clinical experts. About half of these key informants had taken the hospital breastfeeding course and almost one-fourth were on the breastfeeding committee.

DATA COLLECTION

Participant Observation. Unobtrusive observations focused on the nurses' behaviors during interactions with babies, families, nurses, and other healthcare professionals throughout everyday NICU activities. Included in these observations were feedings and routine care, shift reports, breastfeeding committee meetings, nutrition meetings, psychosocial rounds, and nurse-run breastfeeding support groups for parents. There were 128 observation sessions, which took place for 1 to 2 hours during varying days and times of the week. The investigator introduced herself as a nurse researcher who was interested in learning about NICU nurses' perspectives about infant feeding. The researcher role evolved from observation to informal interviews over time. The nurses were asked about breastfeeding promotion within the context of everyday nursing care in the NICU. The general informants were observed/informally interviewed an average of 3.5 times each (range 1–24) over the study period. All observational data and informal interview data were documented immediately after each session.

Artifact Analysis. Documents can serve as a resource for investigating social meaning and practice (Miller & Alvarado, 2005). Breastfeeding standards of care, teaching plans, and policies and procedures were purposefully gathered and reviewed early in the study. These documents provided insight into officially recognized standards of care for infant feeding in this NICU. They also served as a springboard for lines of inquiry that were further developed during observations and interviews. In addition, parent education materials, posters on the unit, and signs placed at the bedside provided other sources of data about breastfeeding promotion in this NICU.

Nurses who had taken the breastfeeding course said that it helped them feel "comfortable," "competent" and "prepared" to teach breastfeeding to families.

Formal Interviewing. Each of the 18 key informants engaged in a formal, 1-hour, tape-recorded interview in a private room near the NICU. Open-ended interview questions probed nursing perspectives about breastfeeding promotion in the NICU. In addition to the formal interview, they were also informally interviewed and/or observed a total of 3 to 43 times each (mean of 13.1) over the entire study. The formal interviews were transcribed verbatim and the transcriptions and tapes were reviewed for accuracy.

DATA ANALYSIS AND VERIFICATION

The data from formal and informal interviews, observations, NICU artifacts, and ongoing memos were analyzed concurrently with data collection. QSR NUD*IST was used to facilitate data management, retrieval, and analysis. The data were examined line-by-line in an iterative fashion and codes were inductively derived for meaning. These codes were restructured into categories and then analyzed for patterns. Ongoing contact with general and key informants facilitated pattern identification and verification. The findings were continuously verified through triangulation of interviewing, participant observation, and artifact assessment and this helped to decrease bias. A peer-review group of pre- and post-doctoral nurse researchers also provided oral and written critique throughout the course of the study.

■ Findings

ORGANIZATIONAL AND HUMAN RESOURCES WERE DEVELOPED TO CREATE A WEB OF SUPPORT TO PROMOTE BREASTFEEDING IN THE NICU

Organizational Resources. There was consistent evidence that organizational resources had been developed in the NICU to encourage breastfeeding. A general informant described how multidisciplinary NICU representatives had reviewed the state of the science on breastfeeding. She said that they used these findings to conceptualize *"a continuum from informed decision making, pump access with establishment and maintenance of milk supply, breast milk feeding, skin-to-skin care, nonnutritive sucking, transition to breast, to preparation for discharge."*

A review of unit documents demonstrated that breastfeeding standards of care and policies and procedures clearly communicated unit-approved statements supporting the use of human milk and breastfeeding in the NICU. Breastfeeding teaching plans and educational materials were observed to be readily available on the unit and examination of the content showed that these documents focused on the specific needs of families with high-risk infants. The general and key informants referred to these documents and discussed how they were used during interactions with parents. One nurse said, *"We try to give them information. We have booklets, printouts, whatever about breastfeeding."* Another stated, *"We present them with breastfeeding information as soon as they come in the door."* The admission packet for parents described breastfeeding as a *"wonderful"* decision for the health of the baby.

Discussion with general and key informants revealed an understanding of the breast milk management system in this NICU. These breast milk handling procedures were generally followed by the nurses, although discussion between the nurses and mothers about milk supply was sometimes overlooked, and occasionally this information did not get transmitted in shift reports. Observations in the unit showed that pump rooms were easily accessible and used by NICU mothers. These spaces had high visibility and accessibility in a central location. Rolling breast pumps were also on hand for bedside pumping and a rental station was available to support breast pumping away from the NICU. Observations also revealed that current literature about medications and breast milk was on reserve in the NICU. All of these structures and

processes provided a foundation to promote breastfeeding.

Interviews of general and key informants demonstrated that these organizational resources were initiated by the NICU lactation and nursing professionals in this NICU, and further developed through the combined actions of the NICU breastfeeding committee members. NICU nurses, along with the lactation staff, served on this committee and they met on a monthly basis to discuss any ongoing issues related to breastfeeding on the unit. Observations demonstrated that the nurses who served on this committee were the leaders in all phases of breastfeeding promotion on the unit. Specific activities observed during this study included conference planning, quality improvement studies, World Breastfeeding Week events, and skin-to-skin care promotion. These activities had ripple effects throughout the unit. For example, one key informant stated, *"We had posters all around for World Breastfeeding Week, and a mother read... about all the benefits... and said, 'you know because of that I'm breastfeeding my baby.'"* Observations also demonstrated that there was an increase in mothers asking about doing skin-to-skin care after the breastfeeding committee members placed skin-to-skin posters in the NICU.

Efforts were also expended beyond the NICU to strengthen intra- and extra-hospital support for breastfeeding promotion. The breastfeeding committee successfully lobbied the hospital foundation to remove a public display panel within the hospital corridors that promoted bottle feeding. This committee also designated annual awards to staff nurses who were most active in breastfeeding promotion. Furthermore, the committee members conducted an annual breastfeeding conference and they were observed sharing the latest research-based feeding practices with NICU nurses from the varied hospitals in this perinatal catchment area. In addition, they used conference gatherings as opportunities to encourage staff nurses to become politically active in support of statewide breastfeeding legislation.

Human Resources. Staff development factors were also important for breastfeeding promotion in the unit. The NICU had lactation consultants and a nursing clinical specialist who provided weekday support for mothers who wanted to breastfeed their NICU babies. Bedside staff nurse support was important for initial referral and continuing assistance of these mothers. All nurses in the NICU were required to complete a Web-based module about the handling, storage, and management of breast milk. General and key informants also talked about the additional 16-hour breastfeeding course that had been developed before this study took place, and had been offered over the past few years at this hospital. They said that this course included information about breastfeeding benefits, anatomy and physiology of lactation, and specific NICU issues of pumping, lacto-engineering, skin-to-skin care, transition to the breast, test weights, and concerns related to the transfer of viruses and drugs. They stated that they also received clinical experience with assessment of positioning, latch, and breastfeeding. The nurses who completed this course identified that they learned important information for their NICU nursing practice. Some nurses said: *"A lot of the things were new to me"* and *"It was excellent, very informative."* Other nurses said that this course helped them feel *"comfortable," "competent,"* and *"prepared"* to teach breastfeeding to families. One new graduate nurse stated, *"I don't hesitate to . . . help the baby latch on . . . try different holds . . . try different techniques."* There was also evidence that the benefits of this course extended to personal experiences outside of the NICU setting. For example, one nurse said that this course was the biggest influence on her decision to breastfeed her own child. She stated, *"From working here and becoming educated [and] knowing all the benefits it has for the baby and for the mom . . . I just thought that it would be a good thing to do."*

The nurses who completed this breastfeeding course were expected to act as bedside breastfeeding supporters and some of them served on the breastfeeding committee or helped to coordinate the parents' breastfeeding support group. Observations in the NICU demonstrated that the nurses who had taken this course were very positive about breastfeeding promotion. In varied situations these nurses were observed encouraging mothers who had low supplies and educating them about steps to take to increase yield. In one particular situation on the night shift, a new graduate nurse worked closely supporting and teaching new parents how to assess intake. She said that she felt pleased with her ability to facilitate their infant feeding. Another nurse was heard telling parents *"We want to help you"* when the mother was discouraged with pumping.

VARIATIONS IN BREASTFEEDING KNOWLEDGE AND EXPERIENCE WITHIN THE NURSING STAFF, MARKETING PRACTICES OF FORMULA COMPANIES AND INSUFFICIENT SUPPORT FROM OTHER HEALTH PROFESSIONALS SERVED AS SOURCES OF INCONSISTENT MESSAGES FOR BREASTFEEDING

Breastfeeding Knowledge and Experience of the NICU Nurses. There were considerable variations in the breastfeeding knowledge and experience of the NICU nurses. The 16-hour breastfeeding course was a requirement for all orientees, but for the rest of the NICU staff, it was optional. One of the key informants said, *"There's no requirement"* for existing NICU staff members to take the breastfeeding classes. During the study there were about 45 nurses out of 250 who had completed these classes and all had been paid for their time in class. Another key informant stated that nurses who had not taken this course were *"not practicing based on evidence right now; they are practicing based on their beliefs."* The NICU nurses freely spoke about their education for infant feeding and whether or not they had taken the breastfeeding course. One of the NICU nurses who had chosen not to take the course stated, *"I feel like for me if there's certain stuff I need to know, I'd rather know how to give a kid a* bolus and do different stuff like that than breastfeed. I'd rather grab somebody else you know, a resource nurse or lactation consultant." Another nurse voiced similar reasons why she had decided not to take the breastfeeding course. She asserted, "If you give me a list of 10 different things to pursue interest-wise, breastfeeding would be somewhere towards the bottom. It's not something that I have ever gone out of my way to get involved in." She said, "If I have to go to an in-service I will, but I don't go out of my way to pursue [breastfeeding] conferences."

The nurses who had not completed the breastfeeding course were generally more detached from breastfeeding promotion activities. Observations throughout the study demonstrated that these nurses were more likely to miss opportunities for breast-feeding promotion during the work day. Nurses who had not taken this course some-times treated breast milk and formula as equivalent or did not promote direct breast-feeding to pumping mothers. For example, a mother who was committed to breastfeeding expressed concern to her nurse over her baby's difficulty eating. She asked the nurse what the goal was for her child. This nurse said that she had to take a certain amount of "p.o. feeds" or the rest would be given by tube. When the mother asked the meaning of the term "p.o. feeds," the nurse replied, "all of the feeds by bottle." This general informant seemed unaware that she had dismissed breastfeeding.

Formula Company Marketing. The marketing practices of formula companies also presented challenges for breastfeeding promotion. The nurses frequently identified formula companies when they talked about infant feeding information that was perceived as educational. One key informant said, "Formula reps come in and do a little lunch and do a little slideshow." Many of the informants said that they attended these formula company-sponsored in-services and they talked confidently about the messages learned there. One nurse said that she was

told that a certain formula "is better for eye and brain development." Another nurse stated that a particular formula company publishes "a calendar every year with kids that have been on some of their different formulas, very specialized formulas, just to show you. . . how these kids have progressed [and] grown." She said, "They help them because they have these special formulas available." One other nurse also went to these in-services and said that it helped in, "finding . . . what formulas [were] most like breast milk and really helped the baby with digestion." Another nurse stated that the formula companies have an annual conference and the "topics are nonformula related so you can get a big audience of nurses to go, but in between the speakers it's almost commercial breaks for the product." She said that they offer "good topics and it's really reasonable and you get really good food. . . and you get contact hours for certification." This nurse declared that the formula companies were "trying to push the science of 'this is such a superior product' and that may catch the nurses." One of the nurses who supported breastfeeding also sarcastically referred to "the cutest lunch bags" that the formula representative was giving to the staff.

Insufficient Support from other Healthcare Professionals. Other challenges for breastfeeding promotion included the varied feeding approaches of other professionals. Some of the nurses did not feel that the physicians promoted breastfeeding. One key informant said, "The doctors here are more totally focused on the disease process, getting the baby better. . . getting the baby out of here. I don't think I've EVER heard. . . a doctor here question the mom about how she was planning to feed the baby. I think they're too busy. And it's just the LAST thing on their list of priorities."

Observations at the bedside established that the lactation staff and nurses were the most likely to promote breastfeeding with the parents. Nurses' interactions with mothers and members of other disciplines were frequently observed. The physicians rarely mentioned breastfeeding. The speech/infant feeding therapists focused on bottle feeding and in one case, one of them made deprecating comments to the nurse and parents about the pumping advice of the lactation staff. Infant feeding instructions posted at the bedside by these therapists consistently described procedures for the use of pacifiers and bottles.

Promotion of Breastfeeding in This NICU Is Evolving Over Time From a Current Breast Milk Feeding Focus To the Goal for a Future Breastfeeding Process Orientation

The general and key informants identified that there had been significant changes in breastfeeding promotion in the NICU over the past 5 years. The NICU had not documented rates of breastfeeding or breast milk feeding prior to instituting their efforts to promote breastfeeding. However, one key informant repeated a common refrain when she said, *"We really have grown."* Another nurse described her individual growth and the changes that had occurred in the unit since she took the breastfeeding course. She said: *"I feel since I started here we have come a long way as far [as] educating nurses and I think people are a lot more comfortable now, educating families and mothers about breastfeeding. Although I was a new nurse and really hadn't been exposed that much to breastfeeding, I didn't know much about it. You know it was a little uncomfortable for me . . . because people asked me questions and I didn't know what to tell them or how to help them. But now that we've been educated, I think that it's a lot easier."*

There was general acknowledgement that support for breastfeeding still varied in the NICU. One nurse said, *"I think that more* [nurses] *are understanding the importance of breast milk but I don't think that 100% of them are."* This nurse felt that some nurses' *"lack of information"* and *"lack of awareness of its importance"* interfered with breastfeed-

> "I feel since I started here we have come a long way as far [as] educating nurses and I think people are a lot more comfortable now, educating families and mothers about breastfeeding."

ing promotion. Another nurse said, *"I would say some nurses do a better job at trying to steer them* [mothers] *towards breastfeeding or pumping than other nurses."*

There were variations in the breastfeeding measures currently collected by the staff on the unit. During the study, monthly rates for percent of NICU babies ever receiving any human milk varied from 53% to 95% with an average of 71%. The nurses did not gather measures about any differences in the percentage of feeds of breast milk consumed or rates of transition to actual breastfeeding. In general, the nurses were more oriented to breast milk feeding than actual breastfeeding. Frequently, the nurses mentioned the scientific advantages of breast milk when they engaged in breastfeeding promotion. During the parents' breastfeeding support meetings, the nurses often used cards that listed varying science-based statements about the properties of breast milk. Likewise one of the breastfeeding promotion signs on the unit was worded, *"Breast milk is more than nutrition. It is protection."* The focus was usually on breast milk as a scientific product rather than breastfeeding as human process between mother and baby.

Interviews and observations demonstrated that breast milk feeding was more widespread than actual breastfeeding. Overall one of the key informants said, *"We've come a long way here. More* [babies] *receive breast milk at this point than ever in our past."* Another key informant further clarified this. She said, *"We are trying to work on the notion that baby can go to breast for the first oral feed. It doesn't need to be the bottle. That's a hard notion."* Other nurses concurred that it was the *"transition to the breast"* that was the area most in need of improvement. During observations some of the nurses could be seen handing a defrosted bottle of breast milk to a mother instead of helping her to breastfeed. When one key informant was asked about this practice, she stated, *"It does get overlooked sometimes definitely . . . I know that plenty of time we feed the kid the bottle."* Another key informant spoke for many when she attributed this practice to: *"Doctors and nurses being uncomfortable with the breastfeeding, extra work for the nurses, getting the test weight scale, and making sure that the screens are up and appropriate. And just, you know, it IS a lot of extra work."*

There was also evidence that attempts to make the NICU more breastfeeding supportive occasionally took its toll on the staff. One general informant who was a member of the breastfeeding committee said that it was discouraging because one nurse helps with breastfeeding and the next one does not. A key informant described the continuing struggle to promote breastfeeding in the NICU. She said: *"But the difficult thing is trying to change culture and practice in this unit. It's very difficult . . . For instance with breastfeeding, we've made such headway in the last couple of years, but sometimes we have to stop and look back and say we are making headway because on a daily basis, at times, it doesn't feel that way because you are constantly struggling or you feel like that somebody is always trying to undo something that you've done."*

Nevertheless, the breastfeeding committee members remained committed to breastfeeding promotion and to changing the NICU culture to support high-risk families with this process. One of them reflected a common sentiment when she stated: *"I think we send the message that it's important . . . That we've made such a change in our culture and it's not 100% across the board, but there are enough of us that we are making a change happen. And* [it is one] *that moms really value."* These nurses had a long term view of the change process in the NICU and decided to work together over time to overcome the hurdles. Another breastfeeding committee member said: *"It's really up to us. It's not fair if we*

> "It is really up to us. It's not fair if we don't provide the adequate education and . . . give the parents the proper information to make an informed decision . . . and WE CAN, as NICU nurses, we can get there. "

don't provide the adequate education and be able to give the parents the proper information to make an informed decision. . . . And WE CAN, as NICU nurses, we can get there."

■ Discussion/Clinical Nursing Implications

The BFHI has provided clear guidelines to promote breastfeeding in birth settings; however, high-risk infants require special care to safeguard their need for breastfeeding. These infants face distinctive challenges related to their compromised physical states and their separation from their mothers, and many questions exist about how NICUs can support these vulnerable families. This study used an ethnographic approach to examine the organizational and human resource support for breastfeeding promotion in the NICU and detailed the multifaceted elements that should be considered in a high-risk setting.

The staff in this particular NICU had limited experience and exposure to breastfeeding during their formative years and in their nursing school education (Cricco-Lizza, 2009). This greatly increased the demand on the institution to develop resources to meet the needs for breastfeeding promotion. Leaders in lactation and nursing spearheaded the changes that initiated this still evolving process. They started a breastfeeding committee that actively involved the staff nurses in this evidence-based change process. As a group they developed systems of support and material resources for pumping and breast milk management, and constructed wide ranging policy, procedure, and teaching materials as staff resources. This infrastructural support was highly visible for the staff and parents and clearly communicated the value of breastfeeding within the daily activities of the unit. The group also took these changes outside of the NICU into the hospital itself, the multiple hospitals in this perinatal catchment area and on to legislators in this state. In such a manner they built a multifaceted web of support. This web could be further enhanced by efforts to gather more detailed data about breast milk and breastfeeding rates. These rates could guide breastfeeding promotion efforts within the unit.

Development of human resources met with mixed success. The breastfeeding course was specifically geared for breastfeeding promotion in an acute care setting. The staff members who completed this 2-day session served as extensions of the lactation staff and as bedside sources of breastfeeding expertise. Siddell, Marinelli, Froman, and Burke (2003) demonstrated that a breastfeeding educational intervention significantly increased NICU nurses' breastfeeding knowledge and altered some attitudes about breastfeeding. The findings of this ethnographic study support this and showed that these nurses not only served as leaders on the unit, but some also took this knowledge back into their personal lives outside of the NICU. Jones, Shapiro, and Roshon (2007) determined that an organized team of experts coupled with training and continued troubleshooting could affect culture change in an acute care setting. During the time of the study, about 45 NICU nurses had fulfilled the course requirements to serve as these bedside supporters. These nurses promoted breastfeeding and acted as change agents in this NICU. Those nurses who did not take the course maintained a more detached stance in breastfeeding activities. In the demanding setting of the NICU, nurses without the breastfeeding training missed opportunities to promote and support breastfeeding. This uneven knowledge and skill with breastfeeding could serve as a source of inconsistent messages for families. This finding suggests that the time is right to implement the breastfeeding course for the entire staff.

Breastfeeding training for all staff members is a requirement for birth hospitals for BFHI and is probably even more important for the vulnerable babies in non-birth hospital NICUs.

Nurses were also exposed to formula marketing messages in educational forums for NICU staff. Many of these nurses had not attended the breastfeeding course and identified these formula programs as sources for infant feeding education. Bernaix (2000) found that knowledge about breastfeeding was predictive of maternal child nurses' supportive behaviors for breastfeeding, and emphasized the need for accurate knowledge. The NICU nurses in this current study repeated some of the non-evidence-based formula company claims, and some accepted small gifts and lunches from the sales representatives. The American Academy of Pediatrics (2005) has identified formula marketing as an obstacle to breastfeeding. This study suggests that direct infant formula marketing to professionals by formula representatives also compromises clear messages about breastfeeding promotion in the NICU. Sponsored educational offerings, gifts, and meals can create conflicts of interest and serve as threats to professional integrity (Erlen, 2008; Hagen, Pijl-Zieber, Souveny, & Lacroix, 2008; Stokamer, 2003).

Clinical Implications

NICU nurses should:

- Develop organizational and human resources for breastfeeding promotion
- Provide breastfeeding education for all NICU staff
- Encourage multidisciplinary representation for breastfeeding committees and projects
- Limit formula marketing practices in the NICU to avoid inconsistent feeding messages
- Utilize in-house experts to provide staff education about infant feeding
- Gather specific breastfeeding and breast milk feeding rates to guide promotion efforts

The nurses also perceived a lack of support for breastfeeding from other NICU healthcare professionals. The study findings demonstrated that there were inconsistent recommendations from health professionals in this NICU. Mothers have previously reported conflicting breastfeeding advice from professionals (McInnes & Chambers, 2008). do Nascimento and Issler (2005) found that a trained interdisciplinary team provided consistent information and attained a 94.6% rate for breast milk consumption at discharge from a Brazilian NICU. Multidisciplinary commitment is crucial for successful implementation of evidence-based practice in critical care units (Weinert & Mann, 2008).

This study also indicated that inconsistent messages can contribute to decreased morale and frustration for the nurses who do promote breastfeeding. The findings revealed that breastfeeding promotion in the NICU was not without its difficulties and that implementation occurred over time. Nevertheless, infrastructural and human resource development set the foundation for breastfeeding promotion and helped to buffer some of the inconsistent messages generated by formula marketing and the lack of breastfeeding education among some nurses and health professionals. To ensure that messages are clear and consistent, education about breastfeeding should be required for all staff members who interact with NICU parents. In addition, NICUs should reconsider whether outside corporations should be allowed access to the unit to market their products to the hospital staff. NICU babies should receive care based on scientific evidence that is not conflicting with commercial interests. Feeding education could be easily provided by experts in nutrition from within the NICU.

This article focused on structure and processes of breastfeeding promotion. Future manuscripts will shed further light on the nurses' infant feeding beliefs and experiences and how these get expressed in the everyday demands of nursing in the NICU setting.

ACKNOWLEDGMENTS

The author acknowledges funding from the National Institute of Nursing Research/National Institutes of Health Grant to the University of Pennsylvania School of Nursing, Research on Vulnerable Women, Children and Families (T32-NR-07100) and the Xi Chapter of Sigma Theta Tau International Honor Society of Nursing. The author also thanks Drs. Janet Deatrick, Sandra Founds, Diane Spatz, and Frances Ward for support during this study.

Roberta Cricco-Lizza, PhD, MPH, RN, is associated with Center for Health Disparities Research, University of Pennsylvania School of Nursing, Philadelphia, PA. She can be reached via e-mail at rcricco@nursing.upenn.edu
The author has disclosed that there are no financial relationships related to this article.

REFERENCES

American Academy of Pediatrics. (2005). Breastfeeding and the use of human milk. *Pediatrics, 115,* 496–506.

Bernaix, L. W. (2000). Nurses' attitudes, subjective norms, and behavioral intentions toward support of breastfeeding mothers. *Journal of Human Lactation, 16,* 201–209.

Centers for Disease Control and Prevention. (2008). Breastfeeding-related maternity practices at hospitals and birth centers—United States, 2007. *Morbidity and Mortality Weekly Review, 57,* 521–525.

Cricco-Lizza, R. (2006). Black non-Hispanic mothers' perceptions about the promotion of infant feeding methods by nurses and physicians. *Journal of Obstetric, Gynecologic and Neonatal Nursing, 35,* 173–180.

Cricco-Lizza, R. (2009). Formative infant feeding experiences and education of NICU nurses. *MCN The American Journal of Maternal Child Nursing.*

Dall'Oglio, I., Salvatori, G., Bonci, E., Nantini, B., D'Agostino, G., & Dotta, A. (2007). Breastfeeding promotion in neonatal intensive care unit: Impact of a new program toward a BFHI for high-risk infants. *Acta Paediatric 96,* 1626–1631.

DiGirolamo, A. M., Grummer-Strawn, L. M., & Fein, S. (2001). Maternity care practices: Implications for breastfeeding. *Birth, 28,* 94–100.

do Nascimento, M. B., & Issler, H. (2005). Breastfeeding the premature infant: Experience of a baby-friendly hospital in Brazil. *Journal of Human Lactation, 21,* 47–52.

Erlen, J. A. (2008). Conflict of interest: Nurses at risk! *Orthopedic Nursing, 27,* 135–139.

Espy, K. A., & Senn, T. E. (2003). Incidence and correlates of breast milk feeding in hospitalized preterm infants. *Social Science and Medicine, 57,* 1421–1428.

Furman, L., Taylor, G., Minich, N., & Hack, M. (2003). The effect of maternal milk on neonatal morbidity of very low-birth-weight infants. *Archives of Pediatrics Adolescent Medicine, 157,* 66–71.

Hagen, B., Pijl-Zieber, E. M., Souveny, K., & Lacroix, A. (2008). Let's do lunch? The ethics of accepting gifts from the pharmaceutical industry. *Canadian Nurse, 104,* (4), 30–35.

Hylander, M. A., Strobino, D., Pezzullo, J. C., & Dhanireddy, R. (2001). Association of human milk feedings in retinopathy of prematurity among very low birth weight infants. *Journal of Perinatology, 21,* 356–362.

Ip, S., Chung, M., Raman, G., Magula, N., DeVine, D., Trikalinos, T., et al. (2007). *Breastfeeding and maternal and infant health outcomes in developed countries* (Evidence Report/Technology Assessment No. 153). AHRQ Publication No. 07-E007. Rockville, MD: Agency for Healthcare Research and Quality.

Jones, A. E., Shapiro, N. I., & Roshon, M. (2007). Implementing early goal-directed therapy in the emergency setting: The challenges and experiences of translating research innovations into clinical reality in academic and community settings. *Academic Emergency Medicine, 14,* 1072–1078.

Kramer, M. S., Chalmers, B., Hodnett, E. D., Sevkovskaya, Z., Dzikovick, I., Shapiro, S., et al. (2001). Promotion of breastfeeding intervention trial (PROBIT): A randomized trial in the Republic of Belarus. *Journal of the American Medical Association, 285,* 413–420.

Lessen, R., & Crivelli-Kovach, A. (2007). Prediction of initiation and duration of breastfeeding for neonates admitted to the neonatal intensive care unit. *Journal of Perinatal Nursing, 21,* 256–266.

McInnes, R. J., & Chambers, J. A. (2008). Supporting breastfeeding mothers: Qualitative synthesis. *Journal of Advanced Nursing, 62,* 407–427.

Meier, P. P. (2001). Breastfeeding in the special care nursery: Prematures and infants with medical problems. *Pediatric Clinics of North America, 48* (2), 425–442.

Merewood, A., Philipp, B. L., Chawla, N., & Cimo, S. (2003). The baby-friendly hospital initiative increases breastfeeding rates in a US neonatal intensive care unit. *Journal of Human Lactation, 19,* 166–171.

Miller, F. A., & Alvarado, K. (2005). Incorporating documents into qualitative nursing research. *Journal of Nursing Scholarship, 37,* 348–353.

Schanler, R. J., Lau, C., Hurst, N. M., & Smith, E. O. (2005). Randomized trial of donor human milk versus preterm formula as substitutes for mothers' own milk in the feeding of extremely premature infants. *Pediatrics, 116,* 400–406.

Siddell, E., Marinelli, K., Froman, R. D., & Burke, G. (2003). Evaluation of an educational intervention on breastfeeding for NICU nurses. *Journal of Human Lactation, 19,* 293–302.

Spatz, D. L. (2006). State of the science: Use of human milk and breastfeeding for vulnerable infants. *Journal of Perinatal and Neonatal Nursing, 20,* 51–55.

Stokamer, C. L. (2003). Pharmaceutical gift giving: Analysis of an ethical dilemma. *Journal of Nursing Administration, 33,* 48–51.

Vohr, B. W., Poindexter, B. B., Dusick, A. M., McKinley, L. T., Wright, L. L., Langer, J. C., et al. (2006). Beneficial effects of breast milk in the neonatal intensive care unit on the developmental outcome of extremely low birth weight infants at 18 months of age. *Pediatrics, 118*(1), pp. e115–e123. Retrieved June 1, 2009, from http://pediatrics.aappublications.org/cgi/content/full/118/1/e115

Weinert, C. R., & Mann, H. J. (2008). The science of implementation: Changing the practice of critical care. *Current Opinion in Critical Care, 14,* 460–465.

World Health Organization and United Nations Children's Fund. (1992). Baby Friendly Hospital Initiative. Geneva: WHO/UNICEF.

Yano, E. (2008). The role of organizational research in implementing evidence- based practice: QUERI series. *Implementation Science, 3,* 29. Retrieved June 1, 2009, from http://www.pubmedcentral.nih.gov/articlerender.fcgi?tool=pubmed&pubmedid=18510749

A NURSE-FACILITATED DEPRESSION SCREENING PROGRAM IN AN ARMY PRIMARY CARE CLINIC

An Evidence-Based Project

Edward E. Yackel • Madelyn S. McKennan • Adrianna Fox-Deise

▶ **Background:** Depression, sometimes with suicidal manifestations, is a medical condition commonly seen in primary care clinics. Routine screening for depression and suicidal ideation is recommended of all adult patients in the primary care setting because it offers depressed patients a greater chance of recovery and response to treatment, yet such screening often is overlooked or omitted.

▶ **Objective:** The purpose of this study was to develop, to implement, and to test the efficacy of a systematic depression screening process to increase the identification of depression in family members of active duty soldiers older than 18 years at a military family practice clinic located on an Army infantry post in the Pacific.

▶ **Methods:** The Iowa Model of Evidence-Based Practice to Promote Quality Care was used to develop a practice guideline incorporating a decision algorithm for nurses to screen for depression. A pilot project to institute this change in practice was conducted, and outcomes were measured.

▶ **Results:** Before implementation, approximately 100 patients were diagnosed with depression in each of the 3 months preceding the practice change. Approximately 130 patients a month were assigned a 311.0 Code 3 months after the practice change, and 140 patients per month received screenings and were assigned the correct International Classification of Diseases, Ninth Revision Code 311.0 at 1 year. The improved screening and coding for depression and suicidality added approximately 3 minutes to the patient screening process. The education of staff in the process of screening for depression and correct coding coupled with monitoring and staff feedback improved compliance with the identification and the documentation of patients with depression. Nurses were more likely than primary care providers to agree strongly that screening for depression enhances quality of care.

▶ **Discussion:** Data gathered during this project support the integration of military and civilian nurse-facilitated screening for depression in the military primary care setting. The decision algorithm should be adapted and tested in other primary care environments.

▶ **Key Words:** decision algorithm · depression screening · evidence-based practice · military primary care clinic

Reprinted with permission from *Nursing Research*, 2009; 59(1S):S58–S65. Copyright © 2012 Wolters Kluwer Health I Lippincott Williams & Wilkins.

Mental illness ranks first among morbidities that cause disability in the United States, Canada, and Western Europe, with the associated healthcare cost in the United States estimated at $150 billion in 2003 (Centers for Disease Control and Prevention [CDC], 2003). A psychometric comparison of military and civilian populations in primary care settings revealed no statistical difference in the prevalence of mood disorders (Jackson, O'Malley, & Kroenke, 1999). However, Waldrep, Cozza, and Chun (2004) found that the deployment of a spouse or parent can challenge the ability of a military family member to cope with a preexisting medical or mental health illness. These authors recommended that clinicians identify those family members who require additional services and suggested actions that might mitigate the impact of deployment on the family unit.

Depression is a common medical condition seen frequently in primary care clinics. Patients with depression who present to primary care clinics have a greater chance of responding to treatment and recovery if primary care providers screen for depression using a short self-administered questionnaire as part of a comprehensive disease management program (DMP). The role of nurses in the process of screening for depression has yet to be delineated, so this evidence-based practice (EBP) project was designed to develop, to implement, and to evaluate a standardized nursing procedure to improve the screening of family members for depression at a military family practice clinic located on a U.S. Army infantry post in Hawaii. This EBP project was based on the Veterans Administration/ Department of Defense Behavioral Health Clinical Practice Guideline (VA/DoD BHCPG, 2002) for screening and treatment of depression as the DMP to guide practice change.

The absence in this clinic of a systematic method to screen family members of deployed soldiers for depression and the inability to estimate rates of depression in this clinical population were the problem-focused triggers for this project. National standards and guidelines that

call for the screening of all adults for depression in primary care settings, such as the VA/DoD BHCPG (2002) and the recommendations and rationale published by the U.S. Preventive Services Task Force (USPSTF, 2002), were the knowledge-focused triggers that guided practice change in this primary care clinic.

A multidisciplinary panel of stakeholders—advanced practice registered nurses (APRNs), physicians, certified nurse assistants (CNAs), registered nurses (RNs), psychologist, and clinic administrators—formed the EBP team. This team was led by a change champion (an APRN) and an opinion leader (a physician). The change champion was an expert clinician who had positive working relationships with other healthcare professionals and who was passionate and committed about screening for depression in primary care. Similarly, the opinion leader was viewed as an important and respected source of influence among his peer group, demonstrated technical competence, and excelled as a teacher and mentor on the subject of depression. The EBP team met to review both problem- and knowledge-focused triggers and determined that screening for depression was a priority for the organization. The EBP project received enthusiastic support throughout the organization and at the highest levels of nursing leadership.

Because of the relevance to the outpatient setting in taking into account clinical decision making, the clinician, and organizational perspectives (Titler et al., 2001), the Iowa Model of Evidence-Based Practice to Promote Quality Care (see the Titler and Moore editorial in this supplement) was chosen to guide an EBP improvement systematically in a military primary practice clinic.

LITERATURE REVIEW

The published medical and nursing literature was reviewed to identify studies evaluating the efficacy of screening for depression in primary care and methodological approaches to such screening. The MEDLINE, the Cochrane, and the Cumulative Index to Nursing and Allied Health Literature databases were searched for English-language articles using eight subject headings (primary care, clinical practice guidelines, mental health, depression instruments, depression screening, suicide screening, military healthcare, and deployment). In addition, bibliographies of the articles obtained were searched for relevant articles to generate additional references. Editorials were rejected, as were articles with data targeting pediatric populations exclusively. Two guidelines (graded as Level I), 3 Level I articles, 17 Level II articles, and 10 Level III articles were critiqued using USPSTF criteria by two APRNs, a physician, and a nurse researcher for inclusion in a literature synthesis. Level I articles included evidence obtained from at least one randomized controlled trial. Level II articles included evidence from well-designed controlled trials without randomization (classified as Level II-1), evidence from cohort or case–control analytic studies (Level II-2), and evidence from multiple time series with or without intervention (Level II-3). Level III articles included opinions of respected authorities that were based on clinical experience or descriptive studies and case reports (Harris et al., 2001). The literature synthesis (Table 1) facilitated the categorization of articles into three focus areas: (a) prevalence of depression in primary care populations; (b) depression management programs and evaluation of suicidal risk; and (c) depression screening instruments and their use in primary care settings.

Prevalence of Depression. Depression is a common medical condition associated with high direct and indirect healthcare costs (Badamgarav et al., 2003; Valenstein, Vijan, Zeber, Boehm, & Buttar, 2001). Dickey and Blumberg (2002) analyzed data from the 1999 National Health Interview Survey and found that 6.3% or 12.5 million noninstitutionalized U.S. adults suffer from major depression. The prevalence of major depression in primary care settings is 5% to 9% among adults, with half of these unrecognized and untreated

(Hirschfeld et al., 1997; Hunter, Hunter, West, Kinder, & Carroll, 2002; Simon & VonKorff, 1995). Depressive illness in primary care is less severe than in mental health settings; thus, the short-term prognosis, the chance of recovery, and the response to treatment are greater in primary care settings (Dickey & Blumberg, 2002; Pignone et al., 2002; Simon & VonKorff, 1995).

Within the next 20 years, depression is projected to be the second highest cause of disability in the world and to have a lifetime prevalence of 15% to 25% (Badamgarav et al., 2003). Depression has been shown to increase the morbidity and mortality associated with other chronic diseases, such as diabetes and cardiovascular disorders (Hunter et al., 2002; Pignone et al., 2002). Furthermore, family members of patients with depression have increased physical morbidity and psychopathology (Sobieraj, Williams, Marley, & Ryan, 1998). A majority of adult patients with mental health concerns such as depression will seek and receive care in primary care settings (Dickey & Blumberg, 2002; Pignone et al., 2002).

The lifetime suicide risk for all patients diagnosed with major depressive disorder has been estimated as 3.5% (Blair-West, Mellsop, & Eyeson-Annan, 1997). Harris and Barraclough (1997) found a 12- to 20-fold risk for suicide associated with depressive disorder using the general population for comparison. Suicide is the second-leading cause of death among those aged 25 to 34 years, accounting for 12.9% of all deaths annually (CDC, 2007). Luoma, Martin, and Pearson (2002) reviewed 40 studies examining rates of contact with primary care providers before suicide and found that approximately 45% of patients who committed suicide had contact with a primary care provider within 1 month of taking their lives, suggesting that screening for risk of suicide in patients with depression is important in primary care settings. Although the literature supports the efficacy of DMPs that include screening for depression, the USPSTF (2004) found insufficient evidence to recommend for or against screening for risk of suicide by

Table 1. Selected Literature Synthesis

Focus Area	Journal or Source	Year	Description	Level of Evidence
Prevalence of depression	General Hospital Psychiatry	1995	Literature review	Literature synthesis
	JAMA	2006	Population-based descriptive study	Level II-3
	Military Medicine	1999	Psychometric comparison: military vs. civilian	Level II-3
	Archives of Family Medicine	1995	Epidemiological study with 1-year follow-up	Level II-2
	Journal of the American Board Family Practice	2005	Descriptive study	Level III
	Military Medicine	2002	Comparative study: PHQ vs. progress notes	Level II-3
	Iraq War Clinicians Guide	2004	Opinion by respected authority	Level III
	American Journal of Psychiatry	2003	Meta-analysis	Level I
	National Mental Health Information Center	1999	Survey report	Level III
	JAMA	1997	Consensus statement	Level III
Depression management programs and evaluation of suicide risk	Annals of Internal Medicine	2002	Systematic literature review	Guideline/ Level I
	General Hospital Psychiatry	1992	Abstract	Level III
	American Journal of Psychiatry	2002	Meta-analysis of descriptive studies/ reports	Level III
	Journal of General Internal Medicine	1996	Structured interviews, comparison of three studies	Level II-1
	Annals of Family Medicine	2005	Randomized controlled trial	Level I
	British Journal of Psychiatry	1997	Meta-analysis	Level II-1
	Centers for Disease Control and Prevention	2007	Report/literature review	Level III

(continued)

Table 1. *(Continued)*

Focus Area	Journal or Source	Year	Description	Level of Evidence
Depression screening instruments	American Journal of Managed Care	2004	Psychometric comparison of one-item depression screen versus PHQ	Level II-3
	Journal of General Internal Medicine	1997	Comparing validity of PHQ-2 to validity of other known measures	Level II-2
	Medical Care	2003	Survey, nonrandomized	Level II-2
	Psychotherapy and Psychosomatics	2004	Descriptive comparison of three questionnaires	Level II-3
	Journal of General Internal Medicine	2001	PHQ-9 compared with other measures/nonrandomized	Level II-2
	Department of Veterans Affairs	2000	Clinical practice guideline	Guideline/level I
	JAMA	1999	Criterion standard study: PRIME MD	Level I
	American Journal of Obstetrics and Gynecology	2000	Validity study of PHQ in obstetrician-gynecologist patients	Level II-2

Note. Level I articles included evidence obtained from at least one randomized controlled trial. Level II articles included evidence from well-designed controlled trials without randomization (classified as Level II-1), evidence from cohort or case–control analytic studies (Level II-2), and evidence from multiple time series with or without intervention (Level II-3). Level III articles included opinions of respected authorities that were based on clinical experience or descriptive studies and case reports (Harris et al., 2001).

primary care clinicians. Focusing on the detection and care of patients with depression who are at higher risk for self-harm and improving the ability of primary care providers to identify and to treat those at risk for suicide are suggested strategies for suicide prevention efforts (Luoma et al., 2002; Schulberg et al., 2005).

DEPRESSION SCREENING INSTRUMENTS

A variety of self-administered questionnaires are available for assessing the severity of depression and risk of suicide in primary care. The Patient Health Questionnaire depression module (PHQ-9) and a two-item version of the PHQ depression module, the PHQ-2, provide primary care providers with valid and reliable measures to assess patients with depression in busy primary care settings (Kroenke, Spitzer, & Williams, 2001, 2003). The PHQ-9 is the self-administered depression module of the Primary Care Evaluation of Mental Disorders (a diagnostic instrument for common mental disorders designed for primary care providers to assess the cognitive and physical symptoms of depressive disorders; Hunter et al., 2002). Kroenke et al. (2001) examined the validity of the PHQ-9 by analyzing data from 6,000 patients aged 18 years or older who had completed the PHQ-9 in eight primary care clinics and seven obstetrics-gynecology clinics. Recent data show that the PHQ-9 has a sensitivity of 88% and a specificity of 88% for major depression, with excellent internal reliability ($\alpha = .89$) and validity in measuring the severity of depression (Corson, Gerrity, & Dobscha, 2004; Kroenke et al., 2001). Lowe et al. (2004) compared the criterion validity of the PHQ-9 for diagnosing depressive episodes with two other well-established instruments and concluded that the PHQ-9 demonstrated a diagnostic advantage and had superior criterion validity when compared with the other instruments. The last item of the PHQ-9 assesses patients for suicidal risk, which is one of the diagnostic criteria for depressive disorders. Feeling suicidal predicts plans to attempt suicide with 83% sensitivity, 98% specificity, and 30% positive predictive value when asked as a single self-report item (Olfson, Weissman, Leon, Sheehan, & Farber, 1996). Corson et al. (2004) reported that use of the PHQ-9 death or suicide item identified one third (7%) of patients in a VA primary care clinic with active suicidal ideation who would not have been treated otherwise.

Shorter screening tests with questions about depressed mood and anhedonia (inability to have pleasurable feelings) appear to detect a majority of depressed patients (Pignone et al., 2002). The PHQ-2 is a self-administered questionnaire used to ascertain the frequency of depressed mood and anhedonia over the past 2 weeks. Kroenke et al. (2003) established the criterion validity of the PHQ-2 by comparing its operating characteristics with an interview by an independent mental health provider and reported a sensitivity of 83% and a specificity of 92%. Corson et al. and Kroenke et al. reported 97% sensitivity and 91% specificity for depression when using the PHQ-2 to screen for this disorder in a VA primary care setting. Thus, the literature provides strong evidence for the validity of the PHQ-2 as a brief screening measure that facilitates the diagnosis of major depression. However, it is recognized as an initial step in a DMP that requires further assessment and implementation to care for

patients with major depression (Corson et al., 2004; Kroenke et al., 2003; USPSTF, 2002).

The VA/DoD BHCPG (2002) for screening and treatment of depression is an example of a DMP that includes screening for depression and suicide. The guideline is designed for use by providers who care for patients with depression in military primary care clinics. The VA/DoD BHCPG DMP describes (a) the screening and recognition of depression and suicidal ideation; (b) the assessment of physical and mental status; (c) the diagnostic criteria and assessment of risk factors; (d) a treatment plan that includes suggestions for managing medications, counseling, and referral criteria; (e) patient and family education; and (f) the monitoring and documentation of follow-up. The VA/DoD BHCPG is designed for the primary care setting and describes the role of primary care providers, but it does not explicate the role of nursing staff in implementing the process.

Evidence has been found that screening improves the identification of depressed patients and that effective follow-up and treatment of depressed adults decrease clinical morbidity in primary care settings (USPSTF, 2002). Evidence-based guidelines, patient education, collaborative and multidisciplinary care, and monitoring are used in DMPs to provide comprehensive care for patients with chronic diseases such as depression (Badamgarav et al., 2003). The DMPs that include screening for depression are more effective than the programs that are focused on depression screening alone (Bijl, van Marwijk, de Haan, van Tilburg, & Beekman, 2004; Pignone et al., 2002). Badamgarav et al. (2003) systematically reviewed the published medical literature evaluating the effectiveness of DMPs for chronic conditions such as depression and found that disease management improves the detection and care of patients with depression. Similarly, a systematic review and a meta-analysis of randomized controlled trials of DMPs for depression concluded that the costs of depression programs are within the cost range of other public health improvements and that enhanced quality of care is possible (Neumeyer-Gromen, Lampert, Stark, & Kallischnigg, 2004). Primary care providers play a vital role in DMPs to improve the detection and care of patients with depression. Notably absent from the literature are descriptors of nursing processes that facilitate screening for depression and the role that nurses play in the DMPs. The purpose of this EBP project was to implement and to evaluate the change process methodology involved in screening family members of military active duty soldiers for depression.

SETTING

The setting for this EBP project was a military family practice clinic with an enrollment of 14,322 family members and approximately 175 daily patient visits. Before implementation of the project, only female family members were screened routinely for depression (at well-woman visits), and nurses did not participate in screening for depression. This process resulted in 100 cases of depression being captured a month. Family members of military active duty soldiers older than 18 years who could read, write, and communicate in English were screened. Patient care was documented in a hard-copy medical record or in the military's electronic medical record, the Armed Forces Health Longitudinal Technology Application (AHLTA). The selection of the screening process for the EBP project was based on the VA/DoD BHCPG for screening and treatment of depression and similar patient populations studied by other investigators (Kroenke et al., 2003; Olfson et al., 1996). All military family members have open access to mental health services. Patients who require inpatient psychiatric care are referred by their primary care provider or mental health provider to a regional military medical center.

IMPLEMENTATION: DECISION ALGORITHM

Two questions from the PHQ-2 ("During the past month, have you often been bothered by

feeling down, depressed or hopeless?" and "During the past month, have you often been bothered by little interest or pleasure in doing things?") and one question from the PHQ-9 ("Do you have thoughts that you would be better off dead or hurting yourself in some way?") were selected for use in the project. The decision algorithm for nurses (Figure 1) integrates the PHQ-2 and the PHQ-9 questions as steps in the depression screening process. The first step of the depression screening process prompts nursing staff to ask the PHQ-2 questions in an effort to determine the presence of depressed mood or anhedonia. A negative response to the PHQ-2 questions concludes the depression screening process, and the primary care provider addresses the patient's primary complaint. The second step of the screening process directs nurses to ask the PHQ-9 question (suicidal ideation) when a positive response is given to either of the PHQ-2 questions. A patient who denies suicidal ideation is given a depression handout listing behavioral health support services, locations of clinics, and contact numbers. Subsequently, the patient is offered a follow-up appointment in 1 or 2 weeks with the primary care provider to discuss assessment and treatment of depression. The patient's appointment continues after the nurse reports the results of the depression screening to the primary care provider. A patient who responds positively to the PHQ-9 (*red flag*) question is referred immediately to a mental health professional for further evaluation. Documentation of the depression screening process is completed by nurses in the AHLTA system. Primary care providers are encouraged to use the VA/DoD BHCPG to assess and to treat patients with depression.

PILOTING THE CHANGE

Creating an environment for a practice change to occur is an important element in the EBP process; therefore, a pilot project was undertaken to identify barriers in implementing the decision algorithm. A physician, a CNA, and two RNs (a nurse researcher and a research

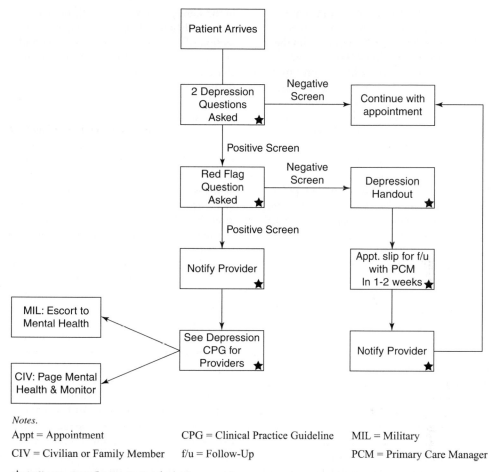

Notes.

Appt = Appointment	CPG = Clinical Practice Guideline	MIL = Military
CIV = Civilian or Family Member	f/u = Follow-Up	PCM = Primary Care Manager

★ indicates steps for nurses to take in the screening process

Figure 1. A decision algorithm for nurses.

assistant) from the EBP team were selected to model the change in clinical practice over a 3-day period. The experienced nurse researcher instructed the CNA on depression, depression screening, and integration of the EBP decision algorithm into existing screening practices by providing verbal education and written materials. The CNA was required to verbalize and to demonstrate the use of the decision algorithm before starting the pilot. All patients meeting the inclusion criteria were screened for depression using the decision algorithm. The experienced nurse researcher and research assistant observed screening practices during

the pilot to evaluate the process and outcomes and to make recommendations aimed at improving the process.

INSTITUTING THE CHANGE IN PRACTICE

Feedback from all participants in the pilot project was used to formulate six recommendations aimed at minimizing barriers in implementing the decision algorithm and in instituting the change in practice: (a) integrate the PHQ-2 and the PHQ-9 depression screening questions into both the hard-copy medical record and the AHLTA system to add continuity during unscheduled computer downtime; (b) educate staff (providers and nurses) on the decision algorithm and the documentation process for both hard-copy and electronic medical records; (c) provide depression awareness education by a mental health professional to increase the nursing staff's comfort when asking questions about depression; (d) post the decision algorithm at the nursing team center to foster recognition and comprehension; (e) display depression posters prominently in patient care areas to sensitize the patient population to this common mental health condition; and (f) educate providers (physicians, APRNs, and physician assistants) on the need to document and use the International Classification of Diseases, Ninth Revision (ICD-9) Code 311.0 (depressive disorder, not otherwise specified) consistently to simplify data retrieval from military medical databases. Forty staff members (RNs, LPNs, CNAs, APRNs, PAs, and MDs) were educated in using the decision algorithm and the documentation process for both the hard-copy and the electronic medical record by the family practice clinic head nurse (EBP team member). A psychologist provided depression education to 17 nurses (RN, LPN, or CNA). This included the definition of depression, how to approach asking questions on depression, and role playing the depression screening process. Thirteen of the family practice clinic providers (100%) were educated by the opinion leader on the use of Code 311.0 to document the diagnosis of depression. Depression posters were displayed in patient care areas, the decision algorithm was displayed at the nursing team center, and the PHQ-2 and the PHQ-9 questions were integrated into the hard-copy and the AHLTA medical record.

■ Results

OUTCOME MEASURES

Four measures were used to assess the success of implementing the EBP decision algorithm

in the family practice clinic: (a) number of patients diagnosed with depression; (b) satisfaction of providers and nurses; (c) compliance in documentation (measured via random chart audits); and (d) time–motion evaluation of the patient screening process. Data collection began 3 months after implementation of the decision algorithm by the RN researcher.

An assessment of the numbers of patients diagnosed with depression was based on data gathered from a military medical database to establish the number of family members diagnosed with depression in the family practice clinic using the ICD-9 Code 311.0 before and after the practice change. With nurses administering the depression screening to all adult patients (not just females) and providers using Code 311.0 to identify those with depression, approximately 130 patients a month were assigned a Code 311.0 3 months into the practice change and 140 patients a month at 1 year after the practice change (Figure 2). A possible correlation between deployment of soldiers to Iraq and increase in the number of family members presenting for treatment of depression was not examined.

The satisfaction of providers and nursing staff was measured at 3 and 12 months after the change in practice using one question answered on a 4-point Likert scale: ``Implementing depression screening enhances the quality of care in the family practice clinic.'' Participants rated their level of agreement from 1 (*strongly disagree*) to 4 (*strongly agree*). Three months after implementation, 64% of the nurses and 45% of the providers strongly agreed that screening for depression enhanced the quality of care in the clinic. At 1 year after the implementation of the decision algorithm, 95% of nurses and 54% of providers strongly agreed that screening for depression enhanced the quality of care.

The nurse researcher evaluated staff compliance in documenting the process of screening for depression using a standardized audit form to review systematically selected (every fourth record from 11 providers) electronic medical records. Thirty records that met selection criteria were audited at 3 months, and

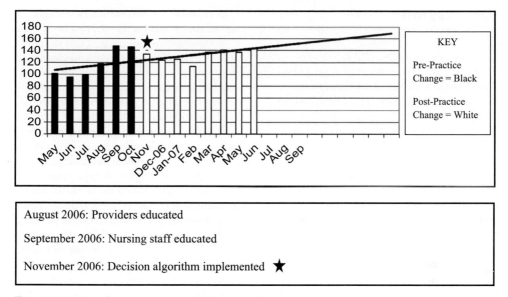

August 2006: Providers educated

September 2006: Nursing staff educated

November 2006: Decision algorithm implemented ★

Figure 2. Number of depression cases before and after practice change.

30 different records were audited at 6 months after the practice change was implemented. The number of records to audit was determined on the basis of patient visits per day and the rate of major depression in primary care (5–9%) obtained from the literature review. Three months into the practice change, 26 (87%) of 30 reviewed charts showed evidence of documentation for depression screening; 7 (27%) of 26 charts verified that patients screened for depression were positive for depressed mood or anhedonia without suicidal ideation. Six months after the practice change, evidence of documentation for depression screening was shown in 29 (97%) of the 30 charts, and patients who were screened for depression were positive for depressed mood or anhedonia without suicidal ideation in 10 (33%) charts. The nurse researcher was unable to determine the compliance of nursing staff in documenting notification of a mental health provider, given that no cases of suicidal ideation were identified in the audited charts. An important facet of compliance with documentation throughout the institutionalization of the decision algorithm was continual education and feedback to both providers and nurses on requirements.

Time–motion data were collected for the length of time it took to screen patients. The screening process included greeting the patient, obtaining weight and vital signs, escorting the patient into an examination room, reviewing demographic data, reviewing the screening questions on depression and suicide, and entering data into the AHLTA system. Variability among the nurses in the process for screening patients during the first month of the project initially resulted in a time variance of 11 minutes, with a range of 5 to 30 minutes for each screening. The clinic head nurse standardized the screening process by asking the nurses to enter data into the AHLTA in the examination rooms instead of returning to the team center. This resulted in a mean time reduction of 4 minutes, 58 seconds after the practice change. The mean time added per patient encounter after the practice change was 2 minutes, 53 seconds.

■ Discussion

Data gathered during the EBP project support the relevance of a nurse-facilitated program to screen for depression in a primary care setting. The VA/DoD BHCPG is designed for primary care and describes the role of primary care providers in the DMP but it does not describe the role of nurses in the depression screening process. The decision algorithm was a valuable tool defining the steps to be followed by nurses when screening patients for depression. More important, incorporating nurses into the depression screening process accomplished the first step of the VA/DoD BHCPG in a multidisciplinary effort consistent with recommendations found in the literature.

Nurses can be instrumental in depression screening in the primary care setting, leading to appropriate referral for further care. The prevalence, the morbidity, and the mortality associated with depression necessitate that nurses be involved integrally in this process as part of the healthcare team. In this pilot project, one provider, a CNA, and two RNs identified barriers in implementing the decision algorithm into the business practices of the family practice clinic. Although procedural barriers to the implementation of the decision algorithm were addressed, incorporating the process of screening for depression into existing screening practices was not clearly defined. The wide range seen in screening times during the first month of the project was most likely related to procedural differences in whether nursing staff entered vital signs and questionnaire data into the electronic medical record (the AHLTA) during or after seeing the patient. Standardization of the time of data entry improved screening times. A mandatory program for reconciling medications was implemented during the EBP project and may have affected the outcome of the time–motion study because the effects of implementing both screening for depression and medication reconciliation might have been measured.

A majority of staff members strongly agreed that screening for depression is a quality component of clinical practice, despite both providers and nurses acknowledging an increased workload because of the EBP project. The decision algorithm was designed to allow primary care providers the option of implementing the VA/DoD BHCPG upon notification of screening results by nurses. The hope was that if the nursing staff followed the procedural steps outlined in the decision algorithm, the need for providers to intercede in the process of screening for depression would be mitigated. However, clinical assessment of the presenting illness and trends in patients' healthcare utilization may have affected how providers responded to the screening results. Some providers were not comfortable with the process of screening for depression, which may have played a role also in how they responded to patients who reported anhedonia or depressed mood. Conversely, nurses who were comfortable with screening for depression were more likely to respond that such screening enhanced the quality of patient care. The difference between nurse and provider levels of comfort may have been the result of the difference in the educational offerings presented to each group. Nurses were offered depression awareness training and repeated education on the decision algorithm and documentation requirements, whereas providers were educated only on the management of depression in primary care and implementation of the decision algorithm. Standardization of educational offerings for all members of the healthcare team is recommended to provide consistent information and continuity of care and to foster trust in the depression screening process.

Both providers and nurses considered depression screening beneficial to family members of deployed soldiers. One year after the practice change, 10 providers were asked to reflect on how many patients had a positive screening for suicidal ideation that required immediate referral to a behavioral health specialist. These providers estimated that approximately 36 patients reported suicidal ideation who would not otherwise have been detected.

Although no data were obtained on the relationship between the deployment of soldiers and reports of depression and suicidal ideation by family members, further study on the relationship between these variables is recommended.

IMPLICATIONS FOR PRACTICE AND RESEARCH

The integration of a nurse-facilitated depression screening program into the business practices of a busy military family practice clinic was viewed by providers, nursing staff, and nursing leadership as a quality component of clinical practice that benefited the population served. The Iowa Model of Evidence-Based Practice to Promote Quality Care (Titler et al., 2001) and the decision algorithm for nurses were essential tools in implementing practice change and appear to have great utility in the primary care setting. The use of an EBP model provides a systematic method for nurses to evaluate critically, to define, and to implement changes in practice. The decision algorithm for nurses was a valuable tool in the depression screening process and should be tested in other primary care settings. In addition, further study is warranted to determine whether having nurses screen for depression influences the practice patterns of primary care providers when implementing a DMP such as the VA/DoD BHCPG.

Edward E. Yackel, MSN, RN, FNP-BC, is Lieutenant Colonel, U.S. Army Nurse Corps, McDonald Army Health Center, Fort Eustis, Virginia.
Madelyn S. McKennan, MSN, RN, FNP-BC, is Lieutenant Colonel, U.S. Army Nurse Corps, Schofield Barracks Army Health Clinic, Honolulu, Hawaii.
Adrianna Fox-Deise, RN, FNP, is Instructor, School of Nursing and Dental Hygiene, University of Hawaii at Manoa.

Accepted for publication September 30, 2009.
This project was funded by an award from the TriService Nursing Research Program, grant no. N03-P18. The Uniformed Services University of the Health Sciences (USUHS), 4301 Jones Bridge Rd., Bethesda, MD 20814-4799, is the awarding and administering office.
This project was sponsored by the TriService Nursing Research Program, Uniformed Services University of the Health Sciences; however, the information or content and conclusions do not necessarily represent the official position or policy of, nor should any official endorsement be inferred by, the TriService Nursing Research Program, Uniformed Services University of the Health Sciences, the Department of Defense, or the U.S. Government.
The following people contributed to the study: Nathan DeWeese, MD; Ms. Renee Latimer, RN, MPH; Mrs. Charlotte Grant, NA; Mr. Wesley Grant, NA; Richard Schobitz, PhD; and Mr. Adrian Santos, RN, BSN.
The authors thank LTC Debra Mark and LTC Mary Hardy, who were responsible for implementation of the Evidence-Based Practice Training Program at Tripler Army Medical Center, and CAPT Patricia Kelley, without whom we could not have conducted this project.
The views and opinions expressed in this article are solely those of the authors and do not reflect the policy or position of the Department of the Army, the Department of Defense, or the U.S. Government.
Corresponding author: Edward E. Yackel, MSN, RN, FNP-BC, U.S. Army Nurse Corps, McDonald Army Health Center, Fort Eustis, VA 23604 (e-mail: Ed.yackel@us.army.mil).

REFERENCES

Badamgarav, E., Weingarten, S. R., Henning, J. M., Knight, K., Hasselblad, V., Gano, A. Jr., et al. (2003). Effectiveness of disease management programs in depression: A systematic review. *American Journal of Psychiatry, 160*(12), 2080–2090.

Bijl, D., van Marwijk, H. W., de Haan, M., van Tilburg, W., & Beekman, A. J. (2004). Effectiveness of disease management programmes for recognition, diagnosis and treatment of depression in primary care. *European Journal of General Practice, 10*(1), 6–12.

Blair-West, G. W., Mellsop, G. W., & Eyeson-Annan, M. L. (1997). Down-rating lifetime suicide risk in major depression. *Acta Psychiatrica Scandinavica, 95*(3), 259–263.

Centers for Disease Control and Prevention. (2003). *Healthy people 2010: Progress review focus area 18.* Retrieved July 5, 2006, from http://www.cdc.gov/nchs/about/otheract/hpdata2010/focusareas/fa18-mentalhealth.htm

Centers for Disease Control and Prevention. (2007). *Suicide: Facts at a glance.* Retrieved July 22, 2007, from http://www.cdc.gov/injury

Corson, K., Gerrity, M. S., & Dobscha, S. K. (2004). Screening for depression and suicidality in a VA primary care setting: 2 items are better than 1 item. *American Journal of Managed Care, 10*(11 Pt. 2), 839–845.

Dickey, W. C., & Blumberg, S. J. (2002). *Prevalence of mental disorders and contact with mental health professionals among adults in the United States, National Health Interview Survey, 1999.* Retrieved July 5, 2006, from http://mentalhealth.samhsa. gov/publications/allpubs/SMA04-3938/Chapter08.asp

Harris, E. C., & Barraclough, B. (1997). Suicide as an outcome for mental disorders. A meta-analysis. *British Journal of Psychiatry, 170,* 205–228.

Harris, R. P., Helfan, M., Woolf, S. H., Lohr, K. N., Mulrow, C. D., Teutsch, S. M., et al. (2001). Current methods of the US Preventive Services Task Force: A review of the process. *American Journal of Preventive Medicine, 20*(Suppl. 3), 21–35.

Hirschfeld, R. M., Keller, M. B., Panico, S., Arons, B. S., Barlow, D., Davidoff, F., et al. (1997). The National Depressive and Manic- Depressive Association consensus statement on the undertreatment of depression. *JAMA, 277*(4), 333–340.

Hunter, C. L., Hunter, C. M., West, E. T., Kinder, M. H., & Carroll, D. W. (2002). Recognition of depressive disorders by primary care providers in a military *medical setting. Military Medicine, 167*(4), 308–311.

Jackson, J. L., O'Malley, P. G., & Kroenke, K. (1999). A psychometric comparison of military and civilian medical practices. *Military Medicine, 164*(2), 112–115.

Kroenke, K., Spitzer, R. L., & Williams, J. B. (2001). The PHQ-9: Validity of a brief depression severity measure. *Journal of General Internal Medicine, 16*(9), 606–613.

Kroenke, K., Spitzer, R. L., & Williams, J. B. (2003). The Patient Health Questionnaire-2: Validity of a two-item depression screener. *Medical Care, 41*(11), 1284–1292.

Lowe, B., Grafe, K., Zipfel, S., Witte, S., Loerch, B., & Herzog, W. (2004). Diagnosing ICD-10 depressive episodes: Superior criterion validity of the Patient Health Questionnaire. *Psychotherapy and Psychosomatics, 73*(6), 386–390.

Luoma, J. B., Martin, C. E., & Pearson, J. L. (2002). Contact with mental health and primary care providers before suicide: A review of the evidence. *American Journal of Psychiatry, 159*(6), 909–916.

Neumeyer-Gromen, A., Lampert, T., Stark, K., & Kallischnigg, G. (2004). Disease management programs for depression: A systematic review and meta-analysis of randomized controlled trials. *Medical Care, 42*(12), 1211–1221.

Olfson, M., Weissman, M. M., Leon, A. C., Sheehan, D. V., & Farber, L. (1996). Suicidal ideation in primary care. *Journal of General Internal Medicine, 11*(8), 447–453.

Pignone, M., Gaynes, B. N., Rushton, J. L., Mulrow, C. D., Orleans, C. T., Whitener, B. L., et al. (2002). *Screening for depression: Systematic evidence review no. 6.* Prepared by the Research Triangle Institute, University of North Carolina Evidence-Based Practice Center under Contract No. 290-97-0011. Rockville, MD: Agency for Healthcare Research and Quality.

Schulberg, H. C., Lee, P. W., Bruce, M. L., Raue, P. J., Lefever, J. J., Williams, J. W. Jr., et al. (2005). Suicidal ideation and risk levels among primary care patients with uncomplicated depression. *Annals of Family Medicine, 3*(6), 523–528.

Simon, G. E., & VonKorff, M. (1995). Recognition, management and outcomes of depression in primary care. *Archives of Family Medicine, 4*(2), 99–105.

Sobieraj, M., Williams, J., Marley, J., & Ryan, P. (1998). The impact of depression on the physical health of family members. *British Journal of General Practice, 48*(435), 1653–1655.

Titler, M. G., Kleiber, C., Steelman, V. J., Rakel, B. A., Budreau, G., Everett, L. Q., et al. (2001). The Iowa Model of Evidence-Based Practice to Promote Quality Care. *Critical Care Nursing Clinics of North America, 13*(4), 497–509.

United States Preventive Services Task Force. (2002). Screening for depression: Recommendations and rationale. *Annals of Internal Medicine, 136*(10), 760–764.

United States Preventive Services Task Force. (2004). Screening for suicide risk: Recommendation and rationale. *Annals of Internal Medicine, 140*(10), 820–821.

Valenstein, M., Vijan, S., Zeber, J. E., Boehm, K., & Buttar, A. (2001). The cost-utility of screening for depression in primary care. *Annals of Internal Medicine, 134*(5), 345–360.

Veterans Administration/Department of Defense. (2002). *Management of major depressive disorder (MDD) in adults in the primary care setting, initial assessment and treatment.* Retrieved January 25, 2006, from http://oqp.med.va. gov/cpg/cpg.htm

Waldrep, D. A., Cozza, S. J., & Chun, R. S. (2004). XIII. The impact of deployment on the military family. From the National Center for Post-Traumatic Stress Disorder. *Iraq War Clinician Guide.* Retrieved August 29, 2006, from http://www.ptsd.va.gov/ professional/manuals/manual-pdf/iwcg/iraq_ clinician_guide_ ch_13.pdf

TRANSLATING THE DIABETES PREVENTION PROGRAM TO PRIMARY CARE

A Pilot Study

Robin Whittemore • Gail Melkus • Julie Wagner •
James Dziura • Veronika Northrup • Margaret Grey

(whittemore et al.; 2009)

EDITOR'S NOTE

Additional information provided by the authors expanding this article is on the editor's Web site at
http://www.nursing-research-editor.com.

▶ **Background:** Research on the translation of
efficacious lifestyle change programs to prevent
type 2 diabetes into community or clinical settings
is needed.

▶ **Objective:** The objective of this study was to
examine the reach, implementation, and efficacy
of a 6-month lifestyle program implemented in
primary care by nurse practitioners (NPs) for adults
at risk of type 2 diabetes.

▶ **Methods:** The NP sites ($n = 4$) were randomized
to an enhanced standard care program (one NP
and one nutrition session) or a lifestyle program
(enhanced standard care and six NP sessions).
These NPs recruited adults at risk of diabetes from
their practice ($n = 58$), with an acceptance rate of
70%.

▶ **Results:** The program reached a diverse, obese,
and moderately low income sample. The NPs
were able to successfully implement the protocols. The average length of the program was 9.3
months. Attendance was high (98%), and attrition
was low (12%). The NPs were able to adopt the
educational, behavioral, and psychosocial strategies of the intervention easily. Motivational interviewing was more difficult for NPs. Mixed-model

repeated-measures analysis indicated significant
trends or improvement in both groups for nutrition
and exercise behavior. Participants of the lifestyle
program demonstrated trends for better high-
density lipoprotein (HDL) and exercise behavior
compared with the enhanced standard care participants. Twenty-five percent of lifestyle participants
met treatment goals of 5% weight loss compared
with 11% of standard care participants.

▶ **Discussion:** A lifestyle program can be implemented in primary care by NPs, reach the targeted
population, and be modestly successful. Further
research is indicated.

▶ **Key Words:** diabetes prevention · nurse practi-
tioner· translation research

Type 2 diabetes (T2D) is emerging as a public
health epidemic of the 21st century, with
approximately 17 million persons affected in
the United States. Ethnic minority persons
have a disproportionate risk and are twice as
likely as are non-Hispanic White persons of
similar age to develop T2D (Centers for
Disease Control and Prevention [CDC],

2004), and T2D is the leading cause of blindness, renal failure, and nontraumatic amputation in adults in the United States. In addition, T2D increases the risk of cardiovascular disease and stroke twofold to fourfold (CDC, 2004). These complications often occur concomitantly and contribute to extensive disability, personal suffering, and significant societal costs. In the United States, the economic costs associated with diabetes in 2007 were estimated to be $174 billion (American Diabetes Association, 2008). Therefore, the greatest opportunity in addressing the personal and societal burden of T2D is to prevent the progression of the disease.

Recent evidence demonstrates that individuals at risk of T2D can be identified, and T2D can be delayed, if not prevented, through lifestyle change programs. International trials have demonstrated a 31%–58% reduction in the incidence of T2D for adults with impaired glucose tolerance (IGT) who participated in lifestyle change programs of weight reduction and physical activity compared with that for a control group (Pan et al., 1997; Tuomilehto et al., 2001). Most recently, the diabetes prevention program (DPP), a large clinical trial in the United States with an ethnically diverse sample of adults, provided evidence on the dramatic decrease in progression from IGT to T2D with a lifestyle change program (Knowler et al., 2002).

The DPP intervention protocol was based on behavioral science theories and included the following components: a provider-partnership model of care, education, behavioral support (i.e., goal setting and problem solving), and motivational interviewing (Diabetes Prevention Research Group, 1999). Research supports that education, goal setting, and problem solving are effective in changing health-related behaviors (Foster, Makris, & Bailer, 2005; Nothwehr & Yang, 2007). Motivational interviewing is a collaborative counseling method for enhancing motivation to change by exploring and resolving ambivalence when individuals are having difficulty meeting mutually determined treatment goals (Rollnick, Miller, & Butler,

2007). Motivational interviewing has demonstrated efficacy in a wide range of health promotion interventions, including interventions to promote nutrition and physical activity (Resnicow et al., 2002; West, DiLillo, Bursac, Gore, & Greene, 2007). These components provided the conceptual framework for the lifestyle program protocol of this pilot study. *Conceptual framework*

Results from lifestyle change trials emphasize the importance of lifestyle in the prevention of T2D. A strong correlation was seen between the ability to prevent T2D and the degree to which participants made the recommended lifestyle changes (Tuomilehto et al., 2001). Also encouraging from a translational perspective was that the lifestyle change goals that contributed to diabetes prevention in these studies were quite modest. Participants were counseled to lose 5%–7% of body weight, reduce fat intake to <30%, reduce saturated fat intake to <10%, increase fiber intake to 15 g/1000 kcal, and exercise for 30 minutes 5–7 days per week. Making these modest lifestyle changes also reduced the magnitude of cardiac risk factors of participants (e.g., hypertension; Tuomilehto et al., 2001). The challenge is how to provide research-based lifestyle change programs to at-risk populations that are aligned with current healthcare systems. The DPP was a proof-of-principle study demonstrating the ability to delay T2D with lifestyle change and therefore provided extreme measures to promote lifestyle change (e.g., frequent sessions and free sneakers) that are not translated easily into community or clinical settings.

Approaches to translate DPPs into different settings have been investigated. A systematic review of community-based interventions to prevent or delay T2D (nine studies of adults) reported variable treatment models with very modest improvements in outcomes. Most studies in this review used one-group designs and were not based on the DPP, and few measured plasma glucose or insulin resistance (IR; Satterfield et al., 2003). More recently, group-based lifestyle programs translating the DPP to the community have demonstrated preliminary efficacy in terms of participants meeting weight loss goals (Laatikainen et al., 2007; Seidel, Powell, Zgibor, Siminerio, & Piatt, 2008) and improving glucose tolerance (GTT) and lipid profiles (Laatikainen et al., 2007) in one-group designs. Experimental research evaluating the translation of the DPP into community or clinical settings is indicated. The lessons learned from previous translational research that were applied in the development of the protocol for this study are highlighted in a table at the Editor's Web site at http://www.nursing-research-editor.com.

Primary care represents a setting to screen at-risk adults and implement interventions to prevent T2D. Primary care practitioners typically provide healthcare for a large percentage of the population and have the ability to follow up with patients over time. In addition, many primary care practitioners have established relationships with patients, which may enhance the delivery and receptivity of the recommended lifestyle changes. However, lifestyle change counseling has been reported to be difficult to accomplish in many primary care settings. Providers have reported pessimism about the motivation of patients to change their lifestyles, skepticism about the efficacy of brief lifestyle change counseling, limited time to provide lifestyle change counseling, limited training on effective counseling techniques, and low reimbursement rates (Kristeller & Hoerr, 1997; Larme & Pugh, 1998).

Nurse practitioners (NPs) represent an ideal health professional to implement lifestyle change counseling in primary care. There are currently more than 85,000 certified registered NPs in the United States; the majority (77%) are certified in family or adult specialties (American Academy of Nurse Practitioners, 2002). They have been reported to be particularly cost effective in preventive care because of their expertise in counseling, health education, and case management (Hummel & Pirzada, 1994). In providing care to adults with T2D, NPs were more likely to provide health education about nutrition, weight, and exercise compared with physicians (Lenz,

Mundinger, Hopkins, Lin, & Smolowitz, 2002). In addition, many NPs provide healthcare for individuals who would be otherwise underserved (Fairbanks, Montoya, & Viens, 2001). Therefore, NPs are health professionals with access to adults at risk of T2D and the expertise to implement a DPP.

Designing studies to test the translation of a research-based program (with established efficacy in clinical trials) into the healthcare setting requires consideration of broad processes and outcomes of care. The RE-AIM (reach, efficacy, adoption, implementation, and maintenance) model was the organizing framework of this study as it was developed for use in evaluating the effectiveness of health behavior programs in terms of public health significance (Glasgow, Vogt, & Boles, 1999). The major premise of the model is that public health impact of programs requires more than efficacy. Programs must also reach a diverse sample, representative of the population at risk. They must be appealing to healthcare providers and realistic to adopt in specific practice settings. Programs must also be able to be implemented as intended. Finally, programs must be maintained by both the individual and the clinical setting. These dimensions, involving both individual and organizational factors, interact to determine the overall population-based impact of a program.

The purpose of this pilot study was to test the translation of the DPP modified specifically for NPs to deliver in the context of primary care. Specific aims of the study were (a) to modify the DPP collaboratively with NPs for implementation in primary care; (b) to evaluate the reach, implementation, and preliminary efficacy of a 6-month lifestyle program provided in primary care by NPs for adults at risk of diabetes on clinical (weight change, waist circumference, IR, and lipids), behavioral (nutrition and exercise), psychosocial (depressive symptoms), and participant satisfaction outcomes compared with those of enhanced standard care; and (c) to evaluate the effects of 5% weight loss on clinical, behavioral, and psychosocial outcomes.

■ Methods

DESIGN

A mixed-method design was used to modify a lifestyle change program for primary care and to evaluate the processes and outcomes associated with implementing the program in NP practices. The study had two distinct phases: Phase I was an interpretive and participatory method with the purpose of modifying the intervention protocol for easier implementation in the NP practices. Phase II was a prospective clinical trial pilot study with cluster randomization and repeated measures to evaluate the reach, implementation, and preliminary efficacy of the modified lifestyle program.

SAMPLE

A convenience sample of four NP primary care practice sites were recruited from a regional practice-based research network for NPs in New England through a mailed invitation (22% response rate). Nonrespondent NPs declined because of ongoing research, having limited patients able to speak English, or lack of time. The network had 68 members; 80% were certified as family NPs (56%) or adult NPs (24%) providing care for ethnically and racially diverse adults. A cluster randomization procedure using a computerized table of random numbers randomized four sites: two sites into the lifestyle change program and two sites into an enhanced standard care program. Each site had a different distribution of NPs working with study participants (Sites 1 and 3 had 2 NPs for the duration of the study; Site 2 had 1 NP; and Site 4 had 2 NPs, with the second NP replacing the first one due to illness).

PROCEDURE

The NPs recruited a convenience sample of 58 adults at risk of T2D from their practices (31 treatment and 27 control group participants).

The sample size for this pilot study was determined by a power analysis, recruiting 20% of what would be necessary for a clinical trial testing the intervention. Inclusion criteria were (a) age of 21 years or older; (b) medically stable and safe to exercise; (c) at risk of IGT, metabolic syndrome, or T2D; and (d) able to speak English. Potential participants were considered at risk if they were overweight or obese (body mass index [BMI] $\geq$25 kg/m^2) and were 65 years or older. Adults younger than 65 years and overweight or obese were also considered at risk if they had any other risk factor for T2D (family history of T2D, history of gestational diabetes or giving birth to a baby $\geq$9 lb, of an ethnic group at high risk of T2D, hypertension, or lipid abnormalities of high triglycerides and low-density lipoproteins [LDL] and low high-density [HDL] lipoproteins). Exclusion criteria included current participation in a commercial diet program or treatment of IGT with metformin. Approval was obtained from all institutional review boards associated with the study. *review Board*.

INTERVENTIONS

Enhanced Standard Care. After informed consent was obtained and baseline data were collected, all participants (regardless of group assignment) received culturally relevant written information about diabetes prevention, a 20- to 30-minute individual session with their NP on the importance of a healthy lifestyle for the prevention of T2D, and a 45-minute individual session with a nutritionist hired for the study. The goals of the standard care approach were similar to the DPP and represented the current treatment recommendation for individuals at risk of T2D. Specifically, participants were encouraged to follow a healthy diet (limit calories, fat, and processed foods), to lose 5%–7% of their initial weight through diet and exercise, and to increase their exercise gradually, with a goal of at least 30 minutes of exercise (e.g., walking) 5 days per week.

Training for NPs at the sites randomized only to enhanced standard care and study nutritionists consisted of a 2-hour education session reviewing the study protocols. Monthly meetings were conducted to discuss any implementation questions.

Lifestyle Change Program. The lifestyle change program for this pilot study was based on the protocol for the DPP (Diabetes Prevention Research Group, 1999). The goals for this program were identical to enhanced standard care, yet the approach was more intensive and based on behavioral science evidence which recognizes the difficulty inherent in diet and exercise lifestyle change. The lifestyle change program for this study provided (a) culturally relevant education on nutrition, exercise, and T2D prevention; (b) behavioral support in collaboratively identifying lifestyle change goals and problem-solving barriers to change; and (c) motivational interviewing when participants were unable to achieve lifestyle goals. These components were identical to those utilized in the DPP. Training for NPs at the sites randomized to the lifestyle program consisted of training on the enhanced standard care protocol, self-study (reading and a 45-minute DVD on motivational interviewing), two 2-hour workshops on motivational interviewing (before study and at 3 months), a 2-hour education session reviewing the lifestyle program protocols, and monthly meetings with the primary investigator. Consultation with an expert on motivational interviewing was available throughout the study. Study nutritionists provided nutrition sessions at all sites and were blinded to the site assignment.

The NPs who worked at the lifestyle program sites participated in the modification process of the lifestyle protocol, which was aimed at maintaining key elements of the DPP while simultaneously enhancing the ability to implement the protocol in their practice settings. The changes made to the DPP protocol for this study were a reduction of the number of in-person sessions from 16 over 6 months to 6 in-person sessions and 5 telephone sessions over 6 months and the revision of some content to be provided for participants to complete at home. The reduction in time was based on the NP's consideration of cost and time constraints of primary care. In-person sessions were structured to be provided in a 20-minute office visit. All educational content of the DPP was provided; however, content was abbreviated, and the nutritional content was revised slightly. The lifestyle protocol used in this study is provided in Table 1. Over the 6 months of the intervention, participants were to receive approximately 3 hours of in-person NP support and 1 hour of NP telephone support in contrast to 12–16 hours of individual sessions in the DPP core curriculum.

Outcome Measures. Data were collected at the individual (participant) and organizational (NP and site) levels at scheduled time points throughout the study to evaluate the reach, implementation, and preliminary efficacy of the lifestyle program. All data were collected by trained research assistants blinded to group assignment, with the exception of GTT, IR, and lipids, which were collected by experienced laboratory personnel at each site and sent to one laboratory for analysis.

Reach. Recruitment rates were documented for each NP practice. Demographic and clinical data (e.g., age, gender, socioeconomic status, ethnicity, and health history) were collected using a standard form.

Implementation. Participant measures of implementation consisted of attendance, attrition, and a satisfaction survey. The satisfaction survey was a 7-item summated scale modified from the Diabetes Treatment Satisfaction Survey (Bradley, 1994) to evaluate a DPP. Adequate internal consistency has been reported with the original scale ($\alpha = .82$) and was demonstrated with the modified scale in this study ($\alpha = .86$).

Organizational measures of implementation consisted of NP and nutrition session documentation forms which were created with components of each session itemized. The percentage of protocol implementation

Table 1. Lifestyle Protocol

Session	Topic
NP Session 1A	Welcome to the Lifestyle Balance Program; highlighted study goals: 7% weight loss and 150 minutes of weekly physical activity
NP Session 1B	Healthy Eating Part I; emphasized the importance of a regular meal pattern and eating slowly; used the food guide pyramid as a model for healthy eating and compared personal eating patterns with these recommendations; recommended specific low-fat, low-calorie substitutes at each level of the food pyramid
Take home	Healthy Eating Part II; more information on low-fat, healthy eating using culturally relevant recipes and information
NP Session 2	Get Started Being Active Part I; discussed physical activity and importance to weight loss; helped participants learn to set incremental exercise goals
Take home	Get Started Being Active Part II; more information on the benefits of exercise and how to exercise safely
NP Session 3	Tip the Calorie Balance; discussed the fundamental principle of energy balance and what it takes to lose 1–2 lb per week
Take home	Take Charge of What's Around You; introduced the principle of stimulus control and ways to identify cues in the home environment that lead to unhealthy food and activity choices
NP Session 4A	Talk Back to Negative Thoughts; practiced identifying common patterns of self-defeating, negative thoughts, and ways to counter these thoughts with positive statements
NP Session 4B	The Slippery Slope of Lifestyle Change; stressed that slips are normal and that learning to recover quickly is the key to success
Take home	Four Keys to Healthy Eating Out; introduced four basic skills for managing eating away from home: anticipating and planning ahead, having positive assertion, having stimulus control, and making healthy food choices
NP Session 5	You Can Manage Stress; highlighted the importance of coping with stress, including stress caused by the lifestyle program
Take home	Make Social Cues Work for You; presented strategies for managing problem social cues, for example, being pressured to overeat, and helped participants learn social cues to promote healthy behaviors
NP Session 6	Ways to Stay Motivated Part I; enhanced motivation to maintain behavior change by reviewing participants' personal reasons for joining the lifestyle program and by recognizing personal successes thus far
Take home	Ways to Stay Motivated Part II

Note. NP = nurse practitioner.

was calculated by dividing the number of protocol items by the number of protocol items completed per session. The NPs were also interviewed at 3 and 6 months to address issues of implementation.

Efficacy. Efficacy data were collected on clinical outcomes (weight loss, waist circumference, IR, and lipid profiles), behavioral outcomes (nutrition and exercise), psychosocial outcomes (depressive symptoms), and participant satisfaction. All data were collected at baseline, 3 months, and 6 months, with the exception of laboratory data which were collected at baseline and 6 months and the satisfaction survey which was collected at 6 months. Efficacy data collection measures and times were based on the DPP study and modified for the short duration of this pilot study.

Weight loss was the primary outcome and was calculated as the percentage of weight loss from baseline to 6 months. IR was an additional primary clinical outcome. After an 8-hour fast, participants had fasting insulin and glucose levels drawn, ingested a standard glucose load (75 g), and had insulin and glucose drawn at 120 minutes. The IR was assessed using the homeostasis model assessment (HOMA) which has been shown to be a good approximation ($r = .35$, $p < .05$) of more complex tests (metabolic clearance rate for glucose [fasting insulin {μ/IU/ml} × fasting glucose {mmol/l} / 22.5]; Wallace, Levy, & Matthews, 2004). Glucose at 120 minutes was used to assess GTT. Waist circumference and lipid profiles were secondary clinical outcomes. Waist circumference was measured by positioning a tape measure snugly midway between the upper hip bone and the uppermost border of the iliac crest. In very overweight participants, the tape was placed at the level of the umbilicus (Klein et al., 2007). Lipid profiles (LDL, HDL, total cholesterol, and total triglycerides) were determined using fasting venous blood.

Diet and exercise health-promoting behaviors were measured with the exercise and nutrition subscales of the Health-Promoting Lifestyle Profile II (eight and nine items,

respectively) which has items constructed on a 4-point Likert scale and measures patterns of diet and exercise behavior (Walker, Sechrist, & Pender, 1987). This instrument has been used in diverse samples and demonstrates adequate internal consistency ($r = .70$ to .90 for subscales; Jefferson, Melkus, & Spollett, 2000). The alpha coefficients for the exercise and nutrition subscales in this study were .86 and .76, respectively. Data on approximate minutes per week of exercise were also collected.

Psychosocial data were collected on depressive symptoms, as measured by the Center for Epidemiologic Studies-Depression Scale (CES-D), a widely used scale (Radloff, 1977). The CES-D consists of 20 items that address depressed mood, guilt or worthlessness, helplessness or hopelessness, psychomotor retardation, loss of appetite, and sleep disturbance. Each item is rated on a scale of 0 to 3 in terms of frequency during the past week. The total score may range from 0 to 60, with a score of 16 or more indicating impairment. High internal consistency, acceptable test–retest reliability, and good construct validity have been demonstrated (Posner, Stewart, Marin, & Perez-Stable, 2001). The alpha coefficient was .93 for the CES-D in this sample.

DATA ANALYSIS

Data were entered into databases (Microsoft Access or Excel) via an automated Teleform (Cardiff, Vista, CA) system. Mean substitution was employed for missing data of individual items on instruments (up to 15%). If more than 15% of items were missing (rare), the subscale or scale was coded as missing data. Descriptive statistics were calculated using frequency distributions and appropriate summary statistics for central tendency and variability (using SAS, Cary, NC). The two groups were compared on major variables to make certain that the cluster random assignment equally distributed the sample. Variables unequally distributed were controlled for in subsequent analyses.

Reach and implementation were analyzed with descriptive statistics and content analysis of NP interviews and process notes. The hypothesis that at-risk adults who received the lifestyle change program would demonstrate better clinical, behavioral, and psychosocial outcomes than those of at-risk adults who received an enhanced standard care control program was tested using an intent-to-treat repeated-measures mixed-modeling procedure (PROC MIXED, SAS). Each model had fixed effects (group assignment, income, race, month, and month by group interaction, with age as a covariate) and random effects (intercept and site for dependent variables with two evaluation time points; intercept, site, and month for dependent variables with three evaluation points). The main effect of time was estimated, which described the average monthly change in outcomes across both groups, as well as treatment by time interaction, which compared the rates of monthly change between treatment and control groups. Because it was possible that significant main effects or interaction effects would not be found due to the sample size, identification of trends of significance (e.g., $p < .20$) and effect sizes were examined. Participant satisfaction was analyzed with t test analysis.

■ Results

REACH

Fifty-eight participants were enrolled in April–August 2006, and the study ended in September 2007. There was a 70% response rate to in-person recruitment at NP practices and a 12% attrition rate at 6 months (Figure 1). Those who did not complete the study were younger, had higher BMI, and had lower LDL ($p < .05$). Reasons for attrition included competing life demands such as medical issues ($n = 4$), moved or lost to follow-up ($n = 2$), or preference for alternative treatment ($n = 1$).

The sample represented diverse (45% White), primarily women (92%), obese, and moderately low income adults at risk of T2D (Table 2). Thirty-three percent of the sample reported increased depressive symptoms. There were no statistically significant differences between groups at baseline on clinical, behavioral, or psychosocial variables. There were more Black participants in the treatment group in contrast to more Hispanic participants in the control group ($p = .01$). More participants in the treatment group had moderately low income compared with low income in the control group ($p = .01$).

IMPLEMENTATION OF THE INTERVENTION

Attendance for in-person sessions was high at 96%. Completion of telephone calls for the lifestyle program was problematic, with only a 37% success rate because of difficulty scheduling and making telephone appointments (both providers and participants). Implementation of the lifestyle program took 9.3 months compared with the outlined protocol of 6.5 to 7 months because of NP illnesses, rescheduling of participant appointments, and the end-of-the-year holidays. The protocols for in-person sessions were implemented with moderately good success. Implementation of the standard care NP protocol was 80%, implementation of the standard care nutrition protocol was 92%, and NP implementation of the lifestyle protocol was 76%. The NPs of the lifestyle program reported confidence in the ability to implement the educational and behavioral strategies of goal setting and problem solving. All NPs reported that motivational interviewing was the most challenging aspect of the protocol to implement. The NPs reported difficulty in building motivation to change and in helping participants see that their behavior was inconsistent with personal values and goals; however, they worked consistently at improving their skills for the duration of the study. The NPs requested additional training and expert consultation throughout the

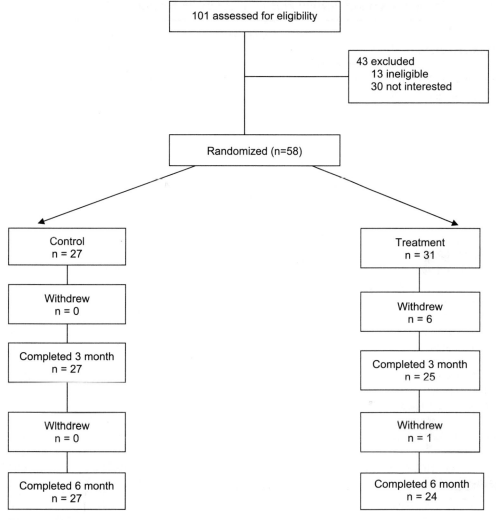

Figure 1. Consort table.

course of the study. Protocol implementation increased over time. One factor that contributed to difficulty implementing the protocol was time as NPs were encouraged to complete sessions in 20 minutes to maintain their office schedule. The NPs reported that study participants often discussed psychosocial issues within the context of lifestyle change (e.g., stress of job), and this sometimes precluded the ability to complete all aspects of the protocol. In this situation, participants

were encouraged to complete the session content at home using the standardized education handouts.

PRELIMINARY EFFICACY OF THE INTERVENTION

Clinical Outcomes. Results of the mixed-model analyses for all outcomes are reported in Table 3. Participants in the lifestyle program

Table 2. Characteristics of Participants at Baseline by Treatment Group

Characteristic	Treatment (*n* = 31)	Control (*n* = 27)	*p*
Age (years), *M* (SD)	48.2 (12.4)	43.2 (13.2)	.1415[a]
Gender, *n* (%)			
Male	3 (50.0)	3 (50.0)	1.0000[b]
Female	28 (53.8)	24 (46.2)	
Race, *n* (%)			
White	15 (57.7)	11 (42.3)	.0116[b]
Black	14 (70.0)	6 (30.0)	
Hispanic	2 (16.7)	10 (83.3)	
Income ($), *n* (%)			
<19,999	1 (9.1)	10 (90.9)	.0176[b]
20,000–39,999	12 (70.6)	5 (29.4)	
40,000–59,999	7 (58.3)	5 (41.7)	
60,000–99,999	7 (70.0)	3 (30.0)	
100,000 and greater	4 (50.0)	4 (50.0)	
Clinical variables			
HOMA[c]	5.6 (3.1)	5.7 (5.4)	.5942[a]
Glucose 120 minutes (mg/dl)	119.1 (40.9)	109.8 (36.1)	.3670[a]
LDL (mg/dl)	123.0 (38.0)	109.7 (33.4)	.1164[a]
HDL (mg/dl)	48.6 (13.1)	43.7 (11.0)	.1295[a]
BMI (kg/m^2)	40.0 (9.0)	37.4 (7.0)	.2262[a]
Waist (in.)	45.3 (7.8)	42.6 (6.9)	.1720[a]
Behavioral variables			
Physical activity	1.8 (0.5)	1.9 (0.6)	.7747[a]
Minutes of exercise per week	139.7 (191.3)	129.5 (139.7)	.8162[a]
<150 minutes, *n* (%)	22 (57.9)	16 (42.1)	.4130[b]
Nutrition (HPLP range 0–4)	2.4 (0.6)	2.4 (0.5)	.6695[a]
CES-D (range 0–60)	12.1 (10.7)	14.9 (13.6)	.3890[a]
≥16 total score, *n* (%)	10 (52.6)	9 (47.4)	1.0000[b]

Note. HOMA = homeostasis model assessment; LDL = low-density lipoprotein; HDL = high-density lipoprotein; BMI = body mass index; HPLP = health-promoting lifestyle profile; CES-D = Center for Epidemiologic Studies-Depression Scale.
[a]Student's *t* test.
[b]Fisher's exact test.
[c]Log-transformed for analysis.

demonstrated trends for greater percentage of weight loss (*p* = .08) and higher HDL levels (*p* = .21) over participants in the enhanced standard care program. Mean percentage of weight change from baseline between the two groups is shown in Figure 2. At 6 months, 25% of lifestyle participants achieved a weight loss goal of 5% compared with 11% of standard care participants. The HOMA levels demonstrated a trend to increase over time in both groups (*p* = .11). There were no significant

Table 3. Estimates of Monthly Change in Outcome in Treatment and Control Groups

Characteristic	Control Group Rate of Change	Treatment Group Rate of Change	p^a	p^b	Group Effect Size at 6 Months
Clinical variables					
Percentage change in weight	0.13	−0.42	.45	.08	.33
HOMA[c]	0.02	0.01	.11	.61	.14
Glucose 120 minutes (mg/dl)	1.50	0.28	.30	.48	.03
Insulin 120 minutes (μU/ml)[c]	0.01	−0.03	.59	.29	.05
LDL (mg/dl)	−0.14	0.07	.94	.87	.28
HDL (mg/dl)	0.17	0.60	.03	.21	.24
BMI (kg/m^2)	−0.02	−0.03	.55	.97	.11
Waist (in)	−0.03	−0.19	.33	.35	.28
Behavioral variables					
Physical activity	0.05	0.10	<.0001	.08	.24
Nutrition	0.04	0.03	.001	.63	.02
CES-D (range 0–60)	−0.01	−0.34	.40	.42	.01

Note. HOMA = homeostasis model assessment; LDL = low-density lipoprotein; HDL = high-density lipoprotein; BMI = body mass index; CES-D = Center for Epidemiologic Studies-Depression Scale.
[a]*p* value for main effect of time (month) across both groups.
[b]*p* value for interaction of treatment and time (month).
[c]Log-transformed for analysis.

differences or trends with respect to other clinical variables.

Behavioral Outcomes. Participants in both groups demonstrated improvement over time in nutrition behavior (*p* = .001). Both groups also demonstrated a significant monthly increase in exercise behavior (*p* = .001), with lifestyle participants demonstrating trends toward greater improvement in exercise (*p* = .08; Figure 3). The percentage of participants meeting the exercise goal of 150 minutes per week increased in the lifestyle group from 29% at baseline to 46% at 6 months and was relatively stable in the enhanced standard care group (39% to 40% at 6 months).

Psychosocial and Satisfaction Outcomes. Although there was a decrease in depressive symptoms over time, this change was not significant. Participants of the lifestyle program

were more satisfied with the program compared with the standard care participants (*t* = 2.06; *p* = .048).

EFFECT OF 5% WEIGHT LOSS ON CLINICAL OUTCOMES

Mixed-model analysis comparing participants with 5% weight loss, regardless of group assignment, with participants who did not achieve 5% weight loss supported the beneficial effect of weight loss with respect to a decrease or a decreasing trend in HOMA (*p* = .10), GTT (*p* = .02), insulin at 120 minutes (*p* = .001), LDL (*p* = .10), triglyceride (*p* = .14), and cholesterol (*p* = .07; Table 4). Both groups improved their exercise (*p* = .001) and nutrition behaviors (*p* = .001), with a greater rate of increase in exercise among participants who achieved 5% weight loss (*p* = .01).

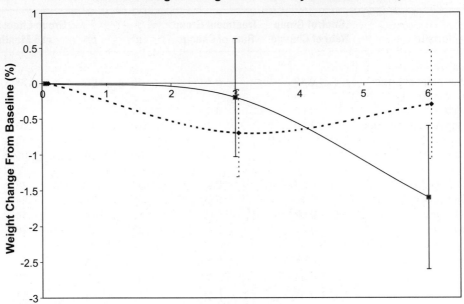

Figure 2. Weight change from baseline (%) by group. Dotted line = control group; Solid line = the treatment group.

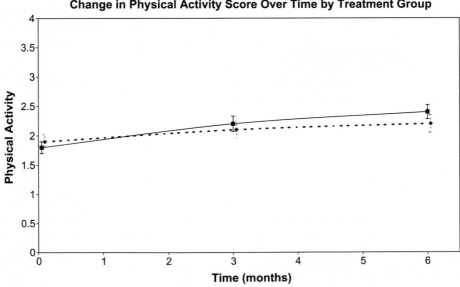

Figure 3. Exercise change from baseline (HPLP) by group. Dotted line = control group; Solid line = the treatment group.

Table 4. Estimates of Monthly Change in Outcomes in Group with 5% Weight Loss at 6 Months Versus Group with <5% Weight Loss at 6 Months

Characteristic	Rate of Change in <5% Weight Loss Group	Rate of Change in 5% Weight Loss Group	p[a]	Group Effect Size at 6 Months
Clinical variables				
HOMA[b]				
Glucose 120 minutes (mg/dl)	0.02	−0.03	.10	0.45
Insulin 120 minutes (μU/ml)[b]	1.94	−2.98	.02	0.64
LDL (mg/dl)	0.02	−0.14	.0001	1.43
HDL (mg/dl)	0.34	−2.38	.10	0.50
Triglyceride (mg/dl)[b]	0.45	−0.02	.30	0.44
Cholesterol (mg/dl)	0.003	−0.03	.14	0.59
Waist (in.)	0.78	−3.22	.07	0.59
Behavioral variables	−0.07	−0.24	.38	0.24
Physical activity	0.05	0.15	.01	0.87
Nutrition (HPLP range 0–4)	0.03	0.04	.62	0.29
CES-D (range 0–60)	−0.14	−0.53	.46	0.17

Note. HOMA = homeostasis model assessment; LDL = low-density lipoprotein; HDL = high-density lipoprotein; HPLP = health-promoting lifestyle profile; CES-D = Center for Epidemiologic Studies-Depression Scale.
[a]p value for interaction of treatment and time (month).
[b]Log-transformed for analysis.

▪ Discussion

Results of this study support the feasibility of implementing a DPP by NPs in a primary care setting to adults at risk of T2D. Study participants were primarily women, of diverse race or ethnicity, obese, sedentary, of low to moderately low income, and with increased depressive symptoms, which is representative of adults at risk of T2D. There were some differences with respect to race or ethnicity and income between groups, which were due to the geographical location of NP practices. More importantly, the reach of the intervention to diverse racial and ethnic groups and to adults with low and moderately low income needs to be highlighted as racial and ethnic differences in rates of obtaining routine preventive care have been documented (Kirk et al., 2005). Although public health interventions are being advocated increasingly to reduce health disparities, continued attention

to the implementation of interventions in the community settings is indicated (Liburd & Vinicor, 2003). The NPs clearly reach this targeted population, providing culturally relevant care within indigenous community structures. The provision of culturally relevant care for diverse ethnic and racial groups appears critical to improved health outcomes in the prevention and management of chronic illnesses (Campbell et al., 2007; Whittemore, 2007).

Successful reach and implementation of study protocols are important results of this study. There was high attendance for in-person sessions and low attrition, critical elements to improving diabetes prevention efforts in vulnerable populations. Previous research implementing behavioral or psychological intervention research into primary care has demonstrated high attrition (30%–40%) and considerable implementation issues (Zayas, McKee, & Jankowski, 2004). Although there were some notable issues in the implementation of study protocols in this study (i.e., difficulty completing telephone sessions, longer duration of program, and frequent rescheduling of participant appointments), protocol implementation of in-person sessions was very good. The NPs were able to implement successfully an enhanced standard care and a lifestyle program aimed at T2D prevention within the context of primary care (i.e., 20-minute sessions) and without considerable training. Future dissemination of this program will be facilitated as NPs in both groups reported high levels of confidence in implementing the educational and behavioral strategies subsumed within the programs. Motivational interviewing was the only behavioral strategy that NPs in the lifestyle program expressed lack of confidence. The finding that NPs were able to implement many aspects of a lifestyle program easily is important as lifestyle counseling has been reported to be difficult to implement by primary care physicians.

Preliminary efficacy results of the lifestyle program indicate modest improvements with respect to clinical and behavioral outcomes. Twenty-five percent of lifestyle participants achieved a 5% weight loss goal compared with 11% of participants in standard care. These results were obtained with a lifestyle program of much shorter duration than that of the DPP (4 vs. 12–16 hours), which is considerably less costly and potentially more acceptable to practitioners and participants. Weight loss of 5%–7% in adults at risk of T2D improves GTT and has been shown consistently to reduce the risk of T2D (Colman et al., 1995; Rana, Li, Manson, & Hu, 2007). Modest weight loss was a strong predictor of T2D risk reduction in the DPP, with a 16% reduction in diabetes risk per kilogram of weight loss (Hamman et al., 2006).

Both lifestyle and standard care participants demonstrated improvements in diet and exercise behavior over time, additional behaviors shown to decrease T2D risk (Hamman et al., 2006). However, lifestyle participants demonstrated a trend toward greater improvements in exercise behavior. This finding is important as increasing exercise has been the primary

behavior associated with risk reduction for T2D, often in combination with weight loss. In the DPP, diabetes risk decreased as nutrition, exercise, and weight loss goals were met. Increased physical activity helped to sustain weight loss, and for those participants not meeting the weight loss goal at 1 year, it helped to lower diabetes risk (Hamman et al., 2006). Exercise decreases glucose-stimulated insulin production, increases insulin sensitivity, and decreases abdominal adiposity, all risk factors for IGT and T2D (Bloem & Chang, 2008; Pratley et al., 2000). In a prospective study with adults at risk of T2D, a protective effect of exercise was observed, even in adults with high BMI and glucose levels (Hu et al., 2004).

More than 50% of all Americans are not engaging in regular exercise or physical activity, and 25% reported no leisure-time physical activity (Zoeller, 2007). Participants in this study were not physically active at baseline, with only 34% reporting an exercise goal of 150 minutes per week. Thus, lifestyle programs that provide at-risk adults with strategies to initiate and maintain exercise safely are critical to T2D prevention. The increased intensity of the lifestyle program in this study appears to have enhanced participants' ability to engage in exercise.

Nutrition behaviors also play an important role in T2D risk reduction. Both groups in this study improved nutrition behaviors over time. Providing educational and behavioral strategies on nutrition and physical activity is a foundational aspect to DPPs. Meeting nutritional goals has been associated with weight loss maintenance, which has been shown to improve diabetes risk factors (Avenell et al., 2004). Strategies to support weight loss and insulin sensitivity are important in T2D prevention. The beneficial effect of weight loss in adults at risk of diabetes was supported in this study as participants with a 5% weight loss demonstrated clinically significant improvements on important clinical outcomes of glucose, IR, and lipids and exercise behavior.

Although this was a pilot study focused on the reach, implementation, preliminary efficacies, inadequate power precludes strong conclusions or clinical implications. Clearly, NPs represent a healthcare provider able to provide a DPP within the context of primary care. The targeted population of diverse adults at risk of T2D was reached, NPs were able to implement the intervention components, and modest efficacy was achieved. Systems of care were complex and unique to each practice, and successful implementation required research support, primarily with scheduling of appointments.

Future research will be aimed at increasing the intensity of the intervention while considering the structure and processes of primary care. Eliminating telephone sessions, providing additional in-person sessions, addressing increased depressive symptoms, encouraging family participation at sessions, and developing a maintenance component to the program are revisions that are currently in progress. Previous research strongly supports increasing the intensity of behavioral interventions to increase the potential for weight reduction and maintenance (Norris et al., 2004). The challenge remains to identify the settings and sessions required. Typically, NPs provide ongoing follow-up care for adults at risk of T2D; thus, a maintenance component to this lifestyle program appears feasible. In addition, enhanced motivational interviewing training for NPs is also indicated. Strategies to simplify the implementation process for primary care office personnel are also being explored.

CONCLUSION

With the increasing prevalence of obesity and T2D risk, many adults would benefit from a preventive intervention. Yet, intensive lifestyle interventions are not implemented easily in the current healthcare system. Research is needed to evaluate less intensive interventions that take into consideration issues of reach and implementation and intervention efficacy. Results demonstrate a collaborative process of translating the DPP into the primary care setting, with NPs taking part in shaping and implementing the intervention protocol. Although this was a small pilot study from one geographical area, with a relatively short program duration, preliminary results with respect to reach, implementation, and efficacy support further development and testing of this lifestyle program.

Robin Whittemore, PhD, is Associate Professor; and Gail Melkus, EdD, is Independence Foundation Professor of Nursing, Yale School of Nursing, New Haven, Connecticut.
Julie Wagner, PhD, is Assistant Professor, Division of Behavioral Sciences and Community Health, University of Connecticut Health Center, Farmington.
James Dziura, PhD, is Biostatistician; and Veronika Northrup, MPH, is Biostatistician, Yale Center for Clinical Investigation, New Haven, Connecticut.
Margaret Grey, DrPH, is Dean and Annie Goodrich Professor of Nursing, Yale School of Nursing, New Haven, Connecticut.

Accepted for publication September 16, 2008.
This study was supported by a grant from National Institutes of Health/National Institute of Diabetes and Digestive and Kidney Diseases (R34DK070594). NIH/NCRR/CTSA Program Grant # UL1 RR024139.
The members of the clinical team were the following: Nanette Alexander, MSN, APRN; Alison Beale, RD; Diane Bussolini, RD; Elizabeth Magenheimer, MSN, APRN; Ulrike Muench, MSN, APRN; Karen Stemler, MS, APRN; Elizabeth Visone, APRN; Stephanie Wilborne, MSN, APRN; and Stacie Zibel, MS, APRN. The members of the clinical team were the following: Jo Cecille Demarest, MS, project director; Amy Triche, BA; Monika Haugstetter, BS; Felicia Lucas, BSN; Alyssa Roman, BA; and Leah Swalley, BS, research assistants; Tony Ma, PhD, data manager; Siobhan Thompson, MPH, director of research administration, Center for Self and Family Management of Vulnerable Populations; and Judith Wylie-Rosett, EdD, RD, consultant.

Corresponding author: Robin Whittemore, PhD, Yale School of Nursing, 100 Church Street South, New Haven, CT 06536-0740 (e-mail: robin.whittemore@yale.edu).

REFERENCES

American Academy of Nurse Practitioners. (2002). *Annual report 2002.* Retrieved April 22, 2003, from http://www.aanp.org

American Diabetes Association. (2008). Economic costs of diabetes in the US in 2007. *Diabetes Care, 31*(3), 1–20.

Avenell, A., Broom, J., Brown, T. J., Poobalan, A., Aucott, L., Stearns, S. C., et al. (2004). Systemic review of the long-term effects and economic consequences of treatments for obesity and implications for health improvement. *Health Technology Assessment, 8*(21), 1–182.

Bloem, C. J., & Chang, A. M. (2008). Short-term exercise improves beta-cell function and insulin resistance in older people with impaired glucose tolerance. *Journal of Clinical Endocrinology and Metabolism, 93*(2), 387–392.

Bradley, C. (1994). Diabetes treatment satisfaction questionnaire. In C. Bradley (Ed), *Handbook of psychology and diabetes* (pp. 111–132). Melbourne, Australia: Harwood Academic Publishers.

Campbell, M. K., Hudson, M. A., Resnicow, K., Blakeney, N., Paxton, A., & Baskin, M. (2007). Church-based health promotion interventions: Evidence and lessons learned. *Annual Review of Public Health, 28,* 213–234.

Centers for Disease Control and Prevention. (2004). *National diabetes fact sheet: General information and national estimates of diabetes in the United States, 2000.* Atlanta, GA: Author.

Colman, E., Katzel, L. I., Rogus, E., Coon, P., Muller, D., & Goldberg, A. P. (1995). Weight loss reduces abdominal fat and improves insulin action in middle-aged and older men with impaired glucose tolerance. *Metabolism, 44*(11), 1502–1508.

Diabetes Prevention Research Group. (1999). Design and methods for a clinical trial in the prevention of type 2 diabetes. *Diabetes Care, 22*(4), 623–634.

Fairbanks, J., Montoya, C., & Viens, D. C. (2001). Factors influencing the recruitment and retention of nurse practitioners into rural, underserved, and culturally diverse areas. *American Journal for Nurse Practitioners, 5,* 21–31.

Foster, G. D., Makris, A. P., & Bailer, B. A. (2005). Behavioral treatment of obesity. *American Journal of Clinical Nutrition, 82* (1 Suppl.), 230S–235S.

Glasgow, R. E., Vogt, T. M., & Boles, S. M. (1999). Evaluating the public health impact of health promotion interventions: The RE-AIM framework. *American Journal of Public Health, 89*(9), 1322–1327.

Hamman, R. F., Wing, R. R., Edelstein, S. L., Lachin, J. M., Bray, G. A., Delahanty, L., et al. (2006). Effect of weight loss with lifestyle intervention on risk of diabetes. *Diabetes Care, 29*(9), 2102–2107.

Hu, G., Lindstrom, J., Valle, T. T., Eriksson, J. G., Jousilahti, P., Silventoinen, K., et al. (2004). Physical activity, body mass index, and risk of type 2 diabetes in patients with normal or impaired glucose regulation. *Archives of Internal Medicine, 164*(8), 892–896.

Hummel, J., & Pirzada, S. (1994). Estimating the cost of using non-physician providers in an HMO: Where would the savings begin? *HMO Practice, 8*(4), 162–164.

Jefferson, V. W., Melkus, G. D., & Spollett, G. R. (2000). Health promotion practices of young Black women at risk for diabetes. *Diabetes Educator, 26*(2), 295–302.

Kirk, J. K., Bell, R. A., Bertoni, A. G., Arcury, T. A., Quandt, S. A., Goff, D. C., Jr., et al. (2005). A qualitative review of studies of diabetes preventive care among minority patients in the United States, 1993–2003. *American Journal of Managed Care, 11*(6), 349–360.

Klein, S., Allison, D. B., Heymsfield, S. B., Kelley, D. E., Leibel, R. L., Nonas, C., et al. (2007). Waist circumference and cardiometabolic risk: A consensus statement from Shaping America's Health: Association for Weight Management and Obesity Prevention; NAASO, The Obesity Society; the American Society for Nutrition and the American Diabetes Association. *Obesity, 15*(5), 1061–1067.

Knowler, W. C., Barrett-Connor, E., Fowler, S. E., Hamman, R. F., Lachin, J. M., Walker, E. A., et al. (2002). Reduction in the incidence of type 2 diabetes with lifestyle intervention or metformin. *New England Journal of Medicine, 346*(6), 393–403.

Kristeller, J. L., & Hoerr, R. A. (1997). Physician attitudes toward managing obesity: Differences among six specialty groups. *Preventive Medicine, 26*(4), 542–549.

Laatikainen, T., Dunbar, J. A., Chapman, A., Kilkkinen, A., Vartiainen, E., Heistaro, S., et al. (2007). Prevention of type 2 diabetes by lifestyle intervention in an Australian primary health care setting: Greater Green Triangle (GGT) diabetes prevention project. *BMC Public Health, 7,* 249.

Larme, A. C., & Pugh, J. A. (1998). Attitudes of primary care providers toward diabetes: Barriers to guideline implementation. *Diabetes Care, 21*(9), 1391–1396.

Lenz, E. R., Mundinger, M. O., Hopkins, S. C., Lin, S. X., & Smolowitz, J. L. (2002). Diabetes care processes and outcomes in patients treated by nurse practitioners or physicians. *Diabetes Educator, 28*(4), 590–598.

Liburd, L. C., & Vinicor, F. (2003). Rethinking diabetes prevention and control in racial and ethnic communities. *Journal of Public Health Management Practice, Suppl.,* S74–S79.

Norris, S. L., Zhang, X., Avenell, A., Gregg, E., Bowman, B., Schmid, C. H., et al. (2004). Long-term effectiveness of weight-loss interventions in adults with pre-diabetes: A review. *American Journal of Preventive Medicine, 28*(1), 126–139.

Nothwehr, F., & Yang, J. (2007). Goal setting frequency and the use of behavioral strategies related to diet and physical activity. *Health Education Research, 22*(4), 532–538.

Pan, X. R., Li, G. W., Hu, Y. H., Wang, J. X., Yang, W. Y., An, Z. X., et al. (1997). Effects of diet and exercise in preventing NIDDM in people with impaired glucose tolerance: The Da Qing IGT and Diabetes Study. *Diabetes Care, 20*(4), 537–544.

Posner, S. F., Stewart, A. L., Marin, G., & Perez-Stable, E. J. (2001). Factor variability of the Center for Epidemiological Studies Depression Scale (CES-D) among urban Latinos. *Ethnicity & Health, 6*(2), 137–144.

Pratley, R. E., Hagberg, J. M., Dengel, D. R., Rogus, E. M., Muller, D. C., & Goldberg, A. P. (2000). Aerobic exercise training-induced reductions in abdominal fat and glucose-stimulated in responses in middle-aged and older men. *Journal of American Geriatrics Society, 48*(9), 1055–1061.

Radloff, L. S. (1977). The CES-D scale: A self-report depression scale for researching the general population. *Applied Psychological Measurement, 1,* 385–401.

Rana, J. S., Li, T. Y., Manson, J. E., & Hu, F. B. (2007). Adiposity compared with physical Inactivity and risk of type 2 diabetes in women. *Diabetes Care, 30*(1), 53–58.

Resnicow, K., DiIorio, C., Soet, J. E., Ernst, D., Borrelli, B., & Hecht, J. (2002). Motivational interviewing in health promotion: It sounds like something is changing. *Health Psychology, 21*(5), 444–451.

Rollnick, S., Miller, W. R., & Butler, C. C. (2007). *Motivational interviewing in health care.* New York, Guilford Press.

Satterfield, D. W., Volansky, M., Caspersen, C. J., Engelgau, M. M., Bowman, B. A., Gregg, E. W., et al. (2003). Community-based lifestyle interventions to prevent type 2 diabetes. *Diabetes Care, 26*(9), 2643–2652.

Seidel, M. C., Powell, R. O., Zgibor, J. C., Siminerio, L. M., & Piatt, G. A. (2008). Translating the diabetes prevention program into an urban medically underserved community: A nonrandomized prospective intervention study. *Diabetes Care, 31*(4), 684–689.

Tuomilehto, J., Lindstrom, J., Eriksson, J. G., Valle, T. T., Hamalainen, H., Illanne-Parrika, P., et al. (2001). Prevention of type 2 diabetes mellitus by changes in lifestyle among subjects with impaired glucose tolerance. *New England Journal of Medicine, 344*(18), 1343–1350.

Walker, S. N., Sechrist, K. R., & Pender, N. J. (1987). The Health-Promoting Lifestyle Profile: Development and psychometric characteristics. *Nursing Research, 36*(2), 76–81.

Wallace, T. M., Levy, J. C., & Matthews, D. R. (2004). Use and abuse of HOMA modeling. *Diabetes Care, 27*(6), 1487–1495.

West, D. S., DiLillo, V., Bursac, Z., Gore, S. A., & Greene, P. G. (2007). Motivational Interviewing improves weight loss in women with type 2 diabetes. *Diabetes Care, 30*(5), 1081–1087.

Whittemore, R. (2007). Culturally competent interventions for Hispanic adults with type 2 diabetes: A systematic review. *Journal of Transcultural Nursing, 18*(2), 157–166.

Zayas, L. H., McKee, M. C., & Jankowski, K. R. (2004). Adapting psychosocial intervention research to urban primary care environments: A case example. *Annals of Family Medicine, 2*(5), 504–508.

Zoeller, R. F. (2007). Prescribing physical activity for cardiovascular and metabolic health. *American Journal of Lifestyle Medicine, 1*(2), 99–102.

THE ARM

There Is No Escaping the Reality for Mothers of Children With Obstetric Brachial Plexus Injuries

Cheryl Tatano Beck

▶ **Background:** Shoulder dystocia is considered the obstetric nightmare. A potentially devastating complication of shoulder dystocia to the infant is obstetric brachial plexus injury (OBPI). Between 20% and 30% of infants with OBPI experience residual functional deficits.

▶ **Objective:** The objective of this study was to investigate mothers' experiences caring for their children who have an OBPI.

▶ **Methods:** Colaizzi's phenomenology was the method used to examine the phenomenon of mothers' caring for their children with an OBPI. A recruitment notice was placed on the Web site of the United Brachial Plexus Network. Twenty-three mothers comprised the convenience sample. Eleven mothers participated in the study over the Internet, and 12 mothers were interviewed in person. Each mother was asked to describe in as much detail as she wished her experiences caring for her child with an OBPI.

▶ **Results:** Six themes emerged to describe mothers' experiences caring for their children with an OBPI: (a) In an Instant: Dreams Shattered; (b) The Arm: No Escaping the Reality; (c) Tormented: Agonizing Worries and Questions; (d) Therapy and Surgeries: Consuming Mothers' Lives; (e) Anger: Simmering Pot Inside; and (f) So Much to Bear: Enduring Heartbreak.

▶ **Conclusions:** The results of this phenomenological study helped to make visible the daily struggle and enduring heartache of mothers who care for their children with OBPI.

▶ **Key Words:** brachial plexus injury · phenomenology · shoulder dystocia

In one newborn's crib in the nursery was a little sign that said, "my left wing is broken so please lay me on my side." Shoulder dystocia is considered the obstetric nightmare (Langer, Berkus, Huff, & Samueloff, 1991). Morris (1955) described this frightening scene as a hush comes over the delivery room after the infant is born and the affected arm hangs limply from the shoulder. The incidence of shoulder dystocia ranges from 0.2% to 3% of vaginal deliveries, and recurrence of shoulder dystocia ranges from 11.9% to 16.7% (Gherman et al., 2006). A potentially devastating complication of shoulder dystocia to the infant is obstetric brachial plexus injury (OBPI), which results from a traction injury to the nerve plexus during delivery.

The incidence of OBPI ranges from 1.2% (Chauhan et al., 2007) to 3.3% (Mollberg, Wennergren, Bager, Ladfors, & Hagberg, 2007). In a recent nationwide study in the United States, the reported mean and standard error of the incidence of OBPI were 1.51 ± 0.02 cases per 1,000 live births (Foad, Mehlman, & Ying, 2008). These statistics were based on more than 11 million births in 1997, 2000, and 2003 recorded in the Kids' Inpatient Database. This is a nationwide public database that is part of the Healthcare Cost and Utilization Project sponsored by the Agency for Health Care Research and Quality. Documented risk factors for brachial plexus injuries (BPIs) include shoulder dystocia, gestational diabetes, women with shorter stature and greater body mass index, birth weight of infants >4,000 grams, prolonged second stage of labor, instrumental vaginal deliveries, and increased number or types of maneuvers used to deliver the shoulder (Chauhan et al., 2007; Dyachenko et al., 2006; Foad et al., 2008; Mehta, Blackwell, Bujold, & Sokol, 2006; Mollberg et al., 2007).

Most infants with OBPI exhibit complete recovery. Mollberg et al. (2007) reported 83.9% recovery at 18 months of age; Noetzel, Park, Robinson, and Kaufman (2001) reported that 66% of infants recovered full strength by 6 months of age and 66% by 16 months (Hoeksma et al., 2004). Rates of permanent BPI, however, are reported to be up to 34% (Hoeksma et al., 2004). In the systematic review of Pondaag, Malessy, van Dijk, and Thomeer (2004), they reported that 20%–30% of infants with OBPIs experience residual functional deficits. The purpose of this phenomenological study was to investigate mothers' experiences caring for their children who had an OBPI.

▪ Parental Experiences of OBPI

Only three quantitative studies were located that were focused on parents of children with BPIs. In the United Kingdom, Bellew and Kay (2003) investigated whether poor communication or reactive grief played the more prominent role in determining parents' reactions. Forty-four parents completed an 11-item questionnaire about early experiences related to giving birth to a child with an OBPI. This sample was divided into two groups: parents whose children's injury required nerve surgery ($n = 18$) and parents whose children had a mild injury that did not require surgery ($n = 26$). Reactions of both groups were remarkably similar. Parents chose the following adjectives to describe how they felt when they received the diagnosis of their child's OBPI: "upset/grief, anger, shock, protective, confused, helpless, and disbelief" (p. 340). One third of the parents

felt that they had been given "too little" information. Findings revealed parents' dissatisfaction with how their early experiences had been managed by healthcare clinicians. For example, one mother stated, "the paediatrician informed me it was my fault for not pushing hard enough" (p. 341). Information parents received shortly after birth was confusing and at times contradictory. Bellew and Kay concluded that there was support for difficulties in communicating bad news and not for the reactive grief hypothesis.

Adjustment of mothers of children with BPIs was examined in Australia (McLean, Harvey, Pallant, Bartlett, & Mutimer, 2004). Resistance factors such as optimism, social support, family functioning, and risk factors such as the severity of injury and disability-related stress were measured with a battery of instruments. Resistance and risk factors accounted for 30% of the variance in maternal adjustment. Nineteen percent of the mothers reported poor adjustment to having a child with an OBPI. Mothers' stress and adjustment were moderated by their optimism.

Parents' use of and satisfaction with the Internet in obtaining materials on OBPIs and those materials' influence on parents' decision making were assessed in 122 completed surveys (Shah, Kuo, Zurakowski, & Waters, 2006). Eighty-nine percent ($n = 108$) of the sample reported searching the Internet for BPI information on causes, symptoms, treatment and surgical options, physicians or surgeons, and hospitals. Satisfaction with the information obtained was reported by 98% of the parents. More than 50% of the sample made clinical decisions based on the Internet information.

These three quantitative studies focused on the involvement of poor communication and reactive grief in parents' reactions to an OBPI, resistance and risk factors in maternal adjustment to this birth injury, and parents' use of and satisfaction with the Internet to learn about OBPI. In these studies, information was gathered via a battery of questionnaires. Missing from the literature is an insider's glimpse of what it is like for mothers to care for these children on a daily basis. Understanding mothers'

> Missing from the literature is an insider's glimpse of what it is like for mothers to care for these children on a daily basis.

experiences is necessary for clinicians to develop appropriate interventions to assist these women. This literature review did not, however, reveal any qualitative studies examining mothers' experiences caring for their children with an OBPI.

■ Methods

RESEARCH QUESTION

What is the experience of mothers caring for their children with OBPIs?

RESEARCH DESIGN

Colaizzi's (1973, 1978) phenomenological method was chosen to investigate the phenomenon of mothers caring for their children with BPIs. Colaizzi's method has its origins in the philosophy of phenomenology. Drawing from Husserl's (1962) philosophy of pure phenomenology as description, Heidegger's (1962) interpretive phenomenology, and Merleau-Ponty's (1962) existential phenomenology, Colaizzi's method includes elements of both descriptive and interpretive phenomenology. Colaizzi (1978) proposed that, to investigate human experience, one must use "a method which neither denies experience nor denigrates it or transforms it into operationally defined behavior; it must be, in short, a method that remains with human experience as it is experienced, one which tries to sustain contact with experience as it is given" (p. 53). Colaizzi's method supports Heidegger's philosophical stance "to let that which shows itself be seen from itself in the very way in which it shows itself from itself" (p. 58).

Husserl (1962) emphasized the need to bracket one's natural attitude to allow the phenomenon to show itself. He called this process *complete reduction*. Colaizzi, however, supports Merleau-Ponty's (1962) belief that complete reduction is not possible. Following Merleau-Ponty's existential phenomenology, Colaizzi (1978) proposed that phenomenologists start their research study by investigating their own presuppositions about the investigated phenomenon to identify their beliefs, attitudes, and hypotheses regarding the phenomenon. It is a personal, phenomenonological reflection. Colaizzi does not, however, have the researchers' bracket or set aside their presuppositions as Husserl would have them do. Colaizzi instead advises researchers to use their presuppositions to formulate their research questions.

DATA COLLECTION

After receiving approval from the university's institutional review board, two methods of data collection were used to obtain mothers' descriptions of their experiences caring for their children with OBPIs: the Internet and in-person interviews. Data collection continued for 2 years and 2 months, from October 2005 to December 2007.

The Internet. A recruitment notice was placed on the Web site of the United Brachial Plexus Network (UBPN, www. ubpn.org), a registered not-for-profit organization that strives to inform, support, and unite families and those concerned with BPIs and their prevention worldwide. Mothers who were interested in obtaining more information about the study e-mailed the researcher directly. In response to women's e-mails, the researcher sent as an attachment an information sheet and directions for participating in the study. Mothers sending their stories to the researcher via the Internet implied their informed consent. Eleven women participated in the study via the Internet. One of these mothers in addition sent via regular postal mail her journal that she diligently wrote in during the first year of her daughter's life.

In-Person Interviews. Twelve women were interviewed individually in person by the researcher at a biennial UBPN camp in Seattle. The camp combined fun activities and educational programs that were planned for every member of the family. The camp provided a chance to meet and share time face-to-face with others who knew what these families have to live with every day since the injury occurred. The families learned more about what it means to live with such an injury not only from healthcare professionals but also from each other.

All interviews were tape-recorded and transcribed verbatim. The same opening interview statement was used in both the Internet and in-person interviews: "Please describe for me in as much detail as you can your experiences caring for your child with a BPI. Include all of your thoughts and feelings that you wish to share about these experiences."

SAMPLE

Twenty-three mothers of children with OBPIs comprised this convenience sample from the United States. The age of the women ranged from 25 to 47 years ($M = 37.75$ years). The age of their children with an OBPI ranged from 3 months to 10 years old. Nineteen women (83%) were married, 3 women were divorced (13%), and 1 mother was single (4%). Eighteen women were Caucasian (79%), and 1 each was Hispanic (4%), Asian (4%), and Black (4%). Two women did not provide any information on their ethnicity. Regarding education, 2 mothers had doctoral degrees (9%), 4 had master's degrees (17%), 7 women held bachelor's degrees (30%), 3 had associate degrees (13%), 3 mothers reported partial college (13%), 2 mothers had high school diplomas (9%), and 2 women did not report their education level.

DATA ANALYSIS

Colaizzi's (1978) written protocol analysis was used to analyze the mothers' descriptions of their experiences caring for their children with an OBPI. His procedural steps for data analysis overlap, and the sequencing of these steps is flexible (Figure 1). A significant statement is

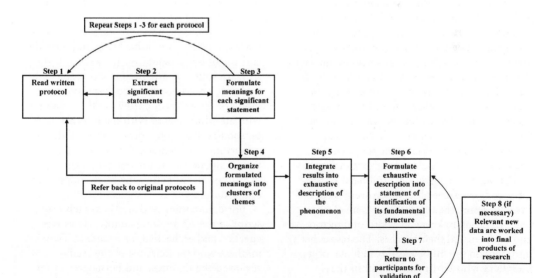

Figure 1. Colaizzi's procedural steps in phenomenological data analysis.

the unit of analysis. Colaizzi defined significant statements as "phrases or sentences that directly pertain to the investigated phenomenon" (p. 59).

For each significant statement that was extracted from the mothers' descriptions, the researcher attempted to spell out its meaning. Colaizzi (1978) termed this step as *formulating meanings*. Next, all the formulated meanings were organized into clusters of themes. These results were integrated into an exhaustive description, which in turn was condensed into as clear a statement as possible of the identification of mothers' experiences caring for their children with an OBPI. The researcher returned to two of the participants as the final validating step of the findings.

QUALITY ENHANCEMENT STRATEGIES

Strategies used to enhance the quality and integrity of this qualitative research study are discussed according to the organizational framework of Polit and Beck (2007): data generation, data coding and analysis, and presentation of findings. Throughout this qualitative inquiry, the researcher kept a reflective journal and in-depth field notes. Notations were made regarding, for example, the researcher—participant relationship, effects of the researcher's presence on the data collected, and the researcher's reactions to the participants' experiences. Throughout data analysis, the researcher referred to her field notes to help ensure that she was remaining faithful to the participants' descriptions. Careful documentation of the researcher's decision trail was made throughout the inquiry.

During data generation, prolonged engagement and persistent observation were used. For over 2½ years, the researcher was involved in UBPN, getting to know its board of directors and mothers and their families. The researcher's introduction to UBPN was through one of its members who had participated in the researcher's earlier study on birth trauma (Beck, 2004a). In 2005, the researcher was invited to present her research findings on

birth trauma and its resulting posttraumatic stress disorder (Beck, 2004b) at the UBPN's biennial camp. After her presentation, the researcher conducted a debriefing session with the mothers at the camp. Two years later, the researcher was invited to present her latest research on the anniversary of birth trauma (Beck, 2006) at their biennial camp. A powerful debriefing session was again held with the mothers. As Lincoln and Guba (1985) noted, "If prolonged engagement provides scope, persistent observation provides depth" (p. 304). The researcher's time spent at both camps, where entire families of children with BPIs spend a long weekend together in fun activities and educational sessions, provided invaluable persistent observation.

When conducting each interview, the researcher used what Colaizzi (1978) termed *imaginative listening.* Here, the researcher strives to be totally present to the participants as they describe their experiences of the phenomenon, their gestures, and nuances of speech. Colaizzi called for the researcher to be aware that the participant is so much more than just a data source. The participant "is exquisitely a person, and the full richness of a person and his verbalized experiences can be contacted only when the researcher listens to him with more than just his ears; he must listen with the totality of his being and with the entirety of his personality" (p. 64).

Data source triangulation was employed to develop a comprehensive description of mothers' experiences caring for their children with an OBPI. Use of both the Internet and personal, one-on-one interviews provided an opportunity to evaluate that a consistent picture of the phenomenon emerged. Saturation of data occurred before the final sample size of 23 mothers.

For data coding and analysis, each transcript of the 12 audiotaped interviews was checked and rechecked for accuracy. Two mothers who participated in the study reviewed the findings, and both agreed that the results captured their experiences. One woman wrote, "Wow! You've done it! You've been able to capture the essence of the overwhelming and heartbreaking experience within the OBPI community." Also kept was a detailed audit trail of each step in Colaizzi's (1978) data analysis method. The researcher maintained documentation of all her methodological decisions. Regarding presentation of findings, each theme was illustrated with multiple quotes from the mothers.

■ Results

Data analysis revealed 252 significant statements, which were organized into six themes describing mothers' experiences caring for their children with an OBPI (Figure 2). These themes were all part of the whole experience of mothers and therefore overlap at times. For mothers, their dreams of giving birth to a perfect infant were shattered in an instant as the baby's arm hung limply from the shoulder in the delivery room. From that moment on, there was no escaping the reality of an OBPI for mothers. This birth injury permeated all aspects

of mothers' lives. Their days were filled with the grueling routine of therapy and multiple surgeries. Mothers were tormented with anger, worry, and questions about their children's OBPI. In the end, there was so much heartache for mothers to bear as the permanency of their child's birth injury became apparent.

In their descriptions, mothers tended to just use the term *BPI* instead of OBPI. All the women in the study, however, cared for children with an OBPI. BPIs that do not occur at birth are termed BPI.

THEME 1. IN AN INSTANT: DREAMS SHATTERED

Mothers' dreams of a beautiful birthing experience and of enjoying their precious newborns were shattered, and that is something they never will be able to get back. A mother disclosed that, "I almost feel as if a part of me died on the day I gave birth. Isn't that ironic? . . . My baby was birthed with BPI. Her arm just dangled, severely curled up, twisted and withdrawn like a wilted vine!"

The injuries often were minimized by healthcare providers. Mothers were instructed just to pin the sleeve of the T-shirt to the baby's chest and were reassured that the baby would be fine in a month or so. The baby has a "95% chance of recovering" was heard frequently, along with "Just give it time to heal. The nerves are just shocked. These things heal on their own fairly quickly."

Some women felt that they were made to feel as if the injury were their own fault to take the blame away from the clinician who delivered the baby. For example,

> The next day after the delivery, the doctor called, and he sent flowers. When he came to my room to see how I was, I said, "did you hear about the baby's arm?" He said, "yeah, that's what happens when you refuse a C-section!"

Another woman shared,

> One of the most emotional and maddening parts of this journey is the reality that this injury should have never happened. It is preventable! The people who harm your baby for life just

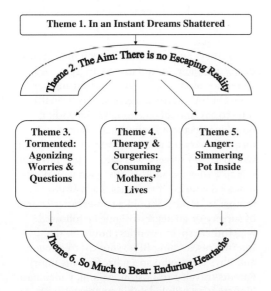

Figure 2. The linking of the six themes describing mothers' experiences caring for children with obstetric brachial plexus injuries.

walk away with no apology and offer no support. They walk away blaming you and your body, the shape of your pelvis, your inability to push effective, the size of your baby, your weight gain, etc. I was led to believe that I was the reason my child was injured and my body was inadequate because "your pelvis was too small." The medical profession took no responsibility whatsoever, and there was no accountability.

These early interactions immediately after delivery fueled mothers' mistrust of the medical community.

THEME 2. THE ARM: NO ESCAPING THE REALITY

The arm: So much was lost that first year of life as all eyes were focused on the injury. The infant was so much more than an arm, but that was forgotten at times. It almost became the injury first and then the child as mothers were constantly examining the injured arm, looking, watching, and obsessing to see flickers of improvement. As one mother revealed, "It was very hard. Everyone was so concerned about her arm that every other part of motherhood was taken away."

During that first year of life, mothers struggled to succeed in seeing their infants as a whole child when they were so focused on the arm. One mother divulged,

I used to tell people that, in my mind's eye, when I thought of my son as a baby, I saw the big, looming arm attached to a little baby's body. And as he grew, the body got bigger, and the arm got smaller. I would close my eyes to see a proportional child.

Mothers never got a break from the constant reminder. As a child gets older, one mother remarked,

Even when you would like to think you can finally begin to put this horrible injury behind you, the reality is, you can't. For now, before my very eyes, there is increasing deformity in my son's arm as he grows. The constant visual reminder of his injury is something I can never escape. I am forced to see what was done to him every single day. I am forced to watch him struggle and get very frustrated with his arm and his limitations. I have to hear the sobbing in bed at night when I walk in his room to find him crying because of the stabbing pain of pins and needles he is experiencing, the throbbing, or the deep aching he describes in his arm. The weeping because someone teased him at school for something he couldn't do, how weak he was, or how he looked different with his smaller and more withered looking arm.

THEME 3. TORMENTED: AGONIZING WORRIES AND QUESTIONS

Mothers constantly questioned themselves. Were they doing enough therapy for their child? Were they doing too much therapy? Were they doing the correct therapy? Was what they were doing sufficient to give their child the best possible chance to have a normal life? Table 1 is a list of some examples of these gnawing worries and questions as the children grow older and start school.

Mothers of children with an OBPI struggled daily with the unknowing. There was no standard protocol that should be followed. This was a source of distress, frustration, and self-doubt that continued to plague mothers over the years. Each surgeon, for instance, would think his or her way was the best. In the end, the final decision rests on the shoulders of the parents.

Mothers agonized over scheduling surgery or not for their child. How many surgeries were too many surgeries? After putting her child through seven surgeries, was it finally time to say enough is enough? Depending on which doctor was consulted, the recommended course of treatment varied. One doctor would say no surgery was needed, just physical therapy, whereas another physician would recommend a series of surgeries. How was a mother to decide? Should a conservative course of surgery or an aggressive one be followed?

Mothers spent countless hours on the Internet researching BPIs, surgical treatments, and physicians who specialized in this injury. Parents traveled to Boston, Miami, Cincinnati, Houston, and Philadelphia to consult with surgeons about the best plan of treatment of their child.

Table 1. The List is Endless: So Many Worries, So Many Questions as the Child Grows

Will the other children at school bully and laugh at my child?

What does the future hold for my child?

Will my child be able to drive a car?

How will the injury affect my child's self-esteem?

What limitations will my child have?

Will anyone want to date my child when he or she gets older?

At school, will my child be known as the kid with the arm?

Who will take care of my child when I die? Who will pick up this torch to carry it?

Where is the trade-off? Keeping up the intense therapy or allowing your child to socialize after school?

What will be the effects on my child's academic performance?

Am I doing enough so that my child gets as much functional use of his or her arm as possible?

At school, will my child be able to reach up to his or her locker?

How will my child go through the cafeteria line and get his or her lunch?

At day care, is my child using his or her affected arm enough?

Do other children advertently hurt my child at day care?

Will my child be an outcast because he or she is different?

How will my child manage a backpack while he or she tries to get on and off the school bus?

THEME 4. THERAPY AND SURGERIES:

Consuming Mothers' Lives. As one mother remarked, "BPI moms deserve to be on permanent disability to take care of their children." Therapy sessions literally took over a mother's life. During the early years, a mother's daily schedule was ruled by a range of motion and stretching exercises. In Table 2 can be found a typical day's schedule for one mother whose child had an OBPI.

A snapshot of this demanding, never-ending routine was provided by another mother:

When all I wanted was to be happy and just enjoy my precious newborn, I was doing therapy around the clock, and literally I was, since the exercises needed to be done every 2–3 hours even through the night as recommended by our doctor. Therapy included frequent range of motion exercises on his shoulder, arm, elbow, wrist, and fingers, along with prolonged stretching. Therapy also involved multiple electrical stimulation treatments applied daily at home using sticky electrodes which were hard to pull off the skin and several wires running over his arms, shoulder, and little back to stimulate the dying muscles. There was the sensory therapy as well and massage since my son, like many BPI kids, had some serious sensory integration issues.

The immersion in this loving dedication to their child's OBPI with all the therapy and surgeries took a definite toll on the women. As this mother reflected,

You ignore that you have other children, and you forget that you are even married. Since you live and breathe BPI, you have nothing to talk about with anyone, and your friends aren't really your friends unless they have a child with a BPI.

Some women did not devote any time to allowing themselves to heal physically or emotionally from the traumatic delivery that

Table 2. Example of a Typical Day in the Life of a Mother Caring for Her Youg Child With an OBPI

7:00 p.m.–7:30 p.m.	Eat dinner
7:30 p.m.–8:15 p.m.	Range of motion stretches to both arms, scar massage to both legs and neck, reaching exercises to improve range, biceps exercise to strengthen right biceps, wash and dry both legs and right arm with mild soap, apply Cica-Care silicon strips to scars on legs and wrap with ACE bandages, apply electrode pads to right biceps and deltoid (for nighttime threshold therapy), change batteries in TES machine, hook machine to wires and fasten to her waist with belt pack, and put her in bed
7:30 a.m.–8:00 a.m.	Change diaper, remove electrode pads from right arm, check for redness, rub skin beneath electrodes with lotion, unwrap ACE bandages from legs, remove Cica-Care strips, scar massage to both legs and neck
8:00 a.m.–8:30 a.m.	Breakfast. She tries to help feed with spoon, but lack of supination and external rotation makes this very hard. I must hold her to give her a bottle like a newborn as she cannot externally rotate either arm to hold a bottle to her mouth.
8:30 a.m.–9:00 a.m.	She plays with toys while I eat.
9:00 a.m.–9:15 a.m.	Range of motion stretches to both arms
9:15 a.m.–9:30 a.m.	She and I play with her toys together.
9:30 a.m.–10:00 a.m.	She and I continue to play with her toys together, but I put an arm-restraint brace on her during this time. I restrain her left arm to encourage her to use her right arm. The brace holds her left arm bent at the waist, with her left hand held at midline and exposed for use. This is to encourage her to bring her right hand to midline for bilateral play.
10:00 a.m.–10:30 a.m.	Brace is off, and depending on her mood, we can either take a walk around the neighborhood, continue to play with toys, read, or watch a video. I try to incorporate sensory awareness into this time, with touching different textures, and so forth.
10:30 a.m.–10:45 a.m.	Snack time. I try to make snack time as much of a therapy as I can without her knowing it.
10:45 (11:00) a.m.–12:30 p.m.	Nap
12:30 p.m.–1:00 p.m.	Diaper change, scar massage to both legs and neck, range of motion to both arms
1:00 p.m.–1:30 p.m.	Lunch. She helps me feed her with a spoon. I feed her a bottle.
1:30 p.m.–4:30 p.m.	Playtime, errand time, visiting-grandparents-and-great-grandparents time, playgroup time (depending on the day). Everything around her playtime is geared toward being therapy without her realizing it. She hears "use both hands please" at least 30 times a day.

(continued)

Table 2. *(Continued)*

4:30 p.m.–4:45 p.m.	Snack time (same as earlier snack time)
4:45 p.m.–5:15 p.m.	Catnap
5:15 p.m.–7:00 p.m.	My husband is home, and he and my daughter play together. Sometimes they go for walks or play outside. He is also mindful to make sure she does not forget about her right arm and to encourage her to use it for more tasks.
7:00 p.m.–picks up at beginning of schedule	We have occupational therapy every Monday morning from 8:30 a.m. to 9:30 a.m. and physical therapy every Wednesday morning from 8:30 a.m. to 9:30 a.m.

Note. For clarification purposes, it is easier to start with bedtime the night before. OBPI = obstetric brachial plexus injury.

resulted in the OBPI. These women lost themselves in the OBPI. For example, some women delayed for years their own surgery needed to repair a cystocele or rectocele that resulted from the difficult delivery of their infant. Mothers always put their children's surgeries before their own. One mother felt that the anonymous post (Table 3) she saw on a BPI message board sums up the life of a mother caring for her child with an OBPI.

THEME 5. ANGER: SIMMERING POT INSIDE

As one mother shared,

> When I first realized my baby was injured, I was lost. I replaced the lost feeling with the determination to learn everything about this injury. I thought that being proactive with the education meant that I dealt with the emotion, "I am fine." Not fine. Something was unresolved. There was anger and a frustration that I could not get a handle on. I wasn't out of control, but I felt like a simmering pot inside, and so I focused more on stretching, physical therapy, occupational therapy, speech . . . I learned and I moved forward, never looking back. Behind me was what she couldn't do, in front of me was what she would accomplish. Go forward, always forward. I couldn't look inward either. Inside was that simmering pot, always threatening to boil over.

The festering emotion of anger was pervasive in mothers. Mothers were so angry that

this lifelong injury was preventable. Anger was directed at the obstetricians, nurses, and the hospital "who allowed this brachial plexus injury to occur . . . What has tested my sanity

Table 3. Anonymous Post on the United Brachial Plexus Network Message Board That Sums Up the Life of a Mother Caring for a Child With an Obstetric Brachial Plexus Injury

I am so tired!

Tired of fighting insurance

Tired of fighting doctors

Tired of fighting for therapy

Tired of fighting my child to wear splints, braces, machines, and having scars

Tired of being judged by doctors, therapists, other parents, and teachers

Tired of pretending that I am all right

Tired of feeling like it will never be better

Tired of fighting just to make it through another day

Tired of thinking that I have 30+ years of this to go. When does a break ever happen?

There is no true recourse, no empowerment

more than anything has been all the lies and downright deceit in the medical birth records and at dispositions. All the lies and deceit haunt me and make me feel so disempowered."

One mother used the image of a scab to illustrate how she keeps her anger under wraps. All of a sudden something would happen that will take the scab off, and she felt anger in every part of her being for what had been done to her innocent child:

> You see your child suffer, and tears can no longer be contained inside you. She can't take her sister's hand-me-down jeans because it takes her too long to take the button and zipper down in the school bathroom because she might have an accident. So you search for stylish elastic pants.

After the first year, some women felt like that they began to come to terms with their anger. At some point was the need to close down the hurt and anger and start to work through these distressing emotions so that they could hopefully move on. The emotional part of caring for children with an OBPI was especially challenging for mothers. With all the emotions they were filled with and had to contend with, mothers tried so hard to keep a positive attitude in front of their children at all times. Mothers felt that they needed to be the strong one and help their children believe that they can overcome any obstacles.

Mothers need to heed the advice by one woman whose child with OBPI was now a grown adult. Her sage words to mothers of younger children were, "If you are fine, your children will perceive you as fine, then your children will be fine." One mother shared that "I keep hoping that my daughter heals, I heal. I keep hoping that the simmering pot will become still."

THEME 6. SO MUCH TO BEAR: ENDURING HEARTBREAK

The OBPI is lifelong and so is the heartache that accompanies it:

As a mother, your child's heartache is your heartache times 100. People like to tell you time will heal, and I used to try to convince myself of that as well. But the truth is, time never truly heals a permanent brachial plexus injury, and time never heals a mom's broken heart either.

Another woman affirmed,

> I think that children and mothers dealing with BPI should be treated as if they are one entity, one being, because the mother feels as if the injury has occurred to her as much as to the child. I know that as a mother, I feel very vulnerable, maybe it is because the injury happens at birth, which is a very emotional moment, maybe it is because the mother must invest so much time and energy on the child's recovery. No matter what the reason, both parties are injured. The mother's injury is invisible, a manifestation of the child's very visible trauma.

One mother articulated a theory she has for why mothers seem to have an extra layer of pain and heartache over injury:

> There is a deeper reason this injury is harder for mothers to deal with. We are the only people alive who actually experienced our children using both of their arms equally. While you are pregnant, you can very clearly feel both arms punching with equal strength. Since our children were too young to form memories, they can't remember using both of their arms equally. So this leaves us mothers completely alone in the memory of a child with two fully functional arms. It is always harder to accept the loss of something known.

As another woman shared,

> Being a mother of an OBPI could bring as much heartache as it does joy. I cannot tell you how often I come home from playgroups or even the nursery at church and sob until I feel like my body is breaking. It is hard to watch my innocent little girl try to do the same things the other babies do but fail.

Heartache was watching their little ones constantly tripping and hurting themselves because they have no natural swing in their impaired arm, and they could not break falls very well, if at all. Heartache was watching their children split their chin, chip a new baby tooth, and get terrible sores that never seemed to heal from frequent falls. As one mom poignantly put it, "All felt like a dagger to my heart."

■ Discussion

The six themes that emerged from the 23 mothers' stories confirmed and illuminated the findings of the three earlier quantitative studies on parental experiences with an OBPI. Bellew and Kay (2003) reported that anger was one of the adjectives parents chose to describe how they felt when they received their child's diagnosis. This emotion certainly came out loud and clear in the theme of mothers feeling as though they were a simmering pot of anger. Parents in the study of Bellew and Kay also shared their dissatisfaction with how they were informed of the injury. The theme that focused on mothers' dreams shattering in an instant confirmed this finding.

McLean et al. (2004) found that 19% of the mothers in their sample reported stress and poor adjustment to having a child with an OBPI. All the themes in this current study provided an insider's glimpse into just how grueling the daily routine for mothers can be. The theme of agonizing questioning and worrying spoke to mothers searching the Internet for help answering their never-ending questions about an OBPI. This finding supports research (Shah et al., 2006) that over 89% of the parents in their sample obtained information on OBPI from the Internet.

Implications for clinical practice can be derived from each of the six themes. Specific nursing interventions can be developed to target the never-ending struggles that mothers have to contend with in caring for their children with an OBPI, as illuminated in each theme. For instance, based on the first theme of shattered dreams, one intervention can focus on grief work for mothers. As revealed in the second theme of no escaping the reality of the arm, women need support and reminders to help them see their children as whole children and not just the injury. In the third theme, mothers struggled with the unknowing due to the lack of a standard protocol to follow

with an OBPI. Needed are development of educational materials, such as treatment options; a list of healthcare professionals who specialize in OBPI; and helpful hints for the daily care of children with this birth injury. The fourth theme, which disclosed how surgeries and therapy consumed mothers' lives, provides a glimpse of how other members of the family can be impacted by this birth injury. Support groups for siblings of children with an OBPI can be created in a local area or online if there are not enough siblings living in a certain locality. Women's festering anger that emerged in the fifth theme calls for interventions to help these women deal with their anger. For the sixth and final theme of enduring heartbreak, one intervention can center on respite care that could provide a lifeline to these heartbroken, stressed, and overtaxed women. Perhaps some of the respite care could provide precious time for the mothers to concentrate on themselves for once, and, for instance, some women could get the long overdue surgery needed to repair damage due to the physically traumatic childbirth they endured.

A suggestion for further qualitative research is a grounded theory study to discover the basic social–psychological problem that mothers of children with an OBPI experience and the process that they use to cope with or resolve this basic problem. Although women repeatedly remarked that they could not change what happened that fateful day of their child's birth, they could give their child the best possible chance in life. That was what they were working toward every day. Mothers were consumed by this as they felt the heavy weight of being their child's true advocate, the coordinator of the benefits, the primary caregiver, the proxy therapist, and in the end the one most responsible for success or failure. Expanding the demographic profile in research of mothers caring for children with an OBPI to include a more diverse sample regarding ethnicity and education will help to increase the transferability of the findings.

LIMITATIONS

It should be noted that, even with using both data sources, a limitation of this study was the fact that most of the sample consisted of White, well-educated women. The transferability of the findings may be limited to this sample profile.

Cheryl Tatano Beck, DNSc, CNM, FAAN, is Professor, School of Nursing, University of Connecticut, Storrs.

Accepted for publication February 23, 2009. This article is dedicated to the women whose courage and profound generosity made it possible to learn about mothers' experiences caring for children with brachial plexus injuries. Thank you to the board of directors of the United Brachial Plexus Network for their unwavering support and enthusiastic assistance with this research project. Thank you also to Mary Grace Amendola for her dedication and detailed care in transcribing the interviews.
Corresponding author: Cheryl Tatano Beck, DNSc, CNM, FAAN, University of Connecticut, 231 Glenbrook Road, Storrs, CT 06269- 2026 (e-mail: Cheryl.beck@uconn.edu).

REFERENCES

Beck, C. T. (2004a). Birth trauma: In the eye of the beholder. *Nursing Research, 53*(1), 28–35.

Beck, C. T. (2004b). Post-traumatic stress disorder due to childbirth: The aftermath. *Nursing Research, 53*(4), 216–224.

Beck, C. T. (2006). The anniversary of birth trauma: Failure to rescue. *Nursing Research, 55*(6), 381–390.

Bellew, M., & Kay, S. P. (2003). Early parental experiences of obstetric brachial plexus palsy. *Journal of Hand Surgery, 28*(4), 339–346.

Chauhan, S. P., Cole, J., Laye, M. R., Choi, K., Sanderson, M., Moore, R. C., et al. (2007). Shoulder dystocia with and without brachial plexus injury: Experience from three centers. *American Journal of Perinatology, 24*(6), 365–371.

Colaizzi, P. (1973). *Reflection and research in psychology: A phenomenological study of learning.* Dubuque, IA: Kendall/Hunt Publishing.

Colaizzi, P. (1978). Psychological research as the phenomenologist views it. In R. Valle & M. King (Eds.), *Existential phenomenological alternatives for psychology* (pp. 48–71). New York: Oxford University Press.

Dyachenko, A., Ciampi, A., Fahey, J., Mighty, H., Oppenheimer, L., & Hamilton, E. F. (2006). Prediction of risk for shoulder dystocia with neonatal injury. *American Journal of Obstetrics and Gynecology, 195*(6), 1544–1549.

Foad, S. L., Mehlman, C. T., & Ying, J. (2008). The epidemiology of neonatal brachial plexus palsy in the United States. *Journal of Bone and Joint Surgery, 90*(6), 1258–1264.

Gherman, R. B., Chauhan, S., Ouzounian, J. G., Lerner, H., Gonik, B., & Goodwin, T. M. (2006). Shoulder dystocia: The unpreventable obstetric emergency with empiric management guidelines. *American Journal of Obstetrics and Gynecology, 195*(3), 657–672.

Heidegger, M. (1962). *Being and time.* New York: Harper & Row Publishers.

Hoeksma, A. F., ter Steeg, A. M., Nelissen, R. G., van Ouwerkerk, W. J., Lankhorst, G. J., & de Jong, B. A. (2004). Neurological recovery in obstetric brachial plexus injuries: An historical cohort study. *Developmental Medicine and Child Neurology, 46*(2), 76–83.

Husserl, E. (1962). *Ideas: General introduction to pure phenomenology.* New York: MacMillan.

Langer, O., Berkus, M. D., Huff, R. W., & Samueloff, A. (1991). Shoulder dystocia: Should the fetus weighing greater than or equal to 4000 grams be delivered by cesarean section? *American Journal of Obstetrics and Gynecology, 165*(4 Pt. 1), 831–837.

Lincoln, Y. S., & Guba, E. G. (1985). *Naturalistic inquiry.* Newbury Park, CA: Sage.

McLean, L. A., Harvey, D. H. P., Pallant, J. F., Bartlett, J. R., & Mutimer, K. L. A. (2004). Adjustment of mothers of children with obstetric brachial plexus injuries: Testing a risk and resistance model. *Rehabilitation Psychology, 49*(3), 233–240.

Mehta, S. H., Blackwell, S. C., Bujold, E., & Sokol, R. J. (2006). What factors are associated with neonatal injury following shoulder dystocia? *Journal of Perinatology, 26*(2), 85–88.

Merleau-Ponty, M. (1962). *Phenomenology of perception.* NewYork: Humanities Press.

Mollberg, M., Wennergren, M., Bager, B., Ladfors, L., & Hagberg, H. (2007). Obstetric brachial plexus palsy: A prospective study on risk factors related to manual assistance during the second stage of labor. *Acta Obstetricia et Gynecologica Scandinavica, 86*(2), 198–204.

Morris, W. I. C. (1955). Shoulder dystocia. *Journal of Obstetrics and Gynaecology of the British Empire, 62*(2), 302–306.

Noetzel, M. J., Park, T. S., Robinson, S., & Kaufman, B. (2001). Prospective study of recovery following neonatal brachial plexus injury. *Journal of Child Neurology, 16*(7), 488–492.

Polit, D. F., & Beck, C. T. (2007). *Nursing research: Generating and assessing evidence for nursing practice* (8th ed.). Philadelphia: Lippincott Williams & Wilkins.

Pondaag, W., Malessy, M. J., van Dijk, J. G., & Thomeer, R. T. (2004). Natural history of obstetric brachial plexus palsy: A systematic review. *Developmental Medicine and Child Neurology, 46*(2), 138–144.

Shah, A., Kuo, A., Zurakowski, D., &Waters, P. M. (2006). Use and satisfaction of the Internet in obtaining information on brachial plexus birth palsies and its influence on decision-making. *Journal of Pediatric Orthopedics, 26*(6), 781–784.

WHY DO ELDERS DELAY RESPONDING TO HEART FAILURE SYMPTOMS?

Corrine Y. Jurgens • Linda Hoke • Janet Byrnes • Barbara Riegel

▶ **Background:** Elders with heart failure (HF) are at risk for frequent hospitalizations for symptom management. Repeated admissions are partly related to delay in responding to HF symptoms. Contextual factors such as prior illness experiences and social/emotional factors may affect symptom interpretation and response. The Self-Regulation Model of Illness guided this study as it acknowledges the dynamic nature of illness and influence of contextual factors and social environment on the interpretation and response to symptoms.

▶ **Objective:** The purpose of this study was to describe contextual factors related to symptom recognition and response among elders hospitalized with decompensated HF.

▶ **Methods:** A mixed-methods design was used. The HF Symptom Perception Scale (physical factors), Specific Activity Scale (functional performance), and Response to Symptoms Questionnaire (cognitive/emotional factors) were administered to participants aged ≥65 years. Symptom duration and clinical details were collected by interview and chart review. Open-ended questions addressing the symptom experience, including the context in which symptoms occurred, were audiotaped, transcribed, analyzed, and compared across cases to inform the quantitative data.

▶ **Results:** The convenience sample ($n = 77$) was 48% female, 85.7% were non-Hispanic White, and mean age was 75.9 years ($SD = 7.7$ years). Functional performance was low (81% class III/IV).

The most frequently reported symptoms were dyspnea, dyspnea on exertion, and fatigue. Median duration of early symptoms of HF decompensation was 5 to 7 days, but dyspnea duration ranged from 30 minutes to 90 days before action was taken. Longer dyspnea duration was associated with higher physical symptom distress ($r = .30$) and lower anxiety ($r = -.31$). Sensing and attributing meaning to early symptoms of HF decompensation were problematic.

▶ **Discussion:** The physical symptom experience and the cognitive and emotional response to HF symptoms were inadequate for timely care seeking for most of this older aged sample.

▶ **Key Words:** delay · elders · heart failure · symptom management

Heart failure (HF) is the most common admission diagnosis in the United States for persons over 65 years of age (Thomas & Rich, 2007), with readmission often occurring within 60 days of discharge (Moser, Doering, & Chung, 2005). Among Medicare beneficiaries, there were 673,600 discharges for HF in 2003 at a cost of $4.4 billion (Rosamond et al., 2008). These frequent hospitalizations are costly and contribute to poor-quality life for patients with HF (Rodriguez-Artalejo et al., 2005). Hospital admission typically is due to escalating symptoms of fluid overload. In one study, it was estimated that as many as 57% of admissions are potentially preventable with adequate self-care, which includes medication adherence and monitoring for symptom changes (Schiff, Fung, Speroff, & McNutt, 2003).

Part of the reason for repeated admissions is that patients delay responding to their HF symptoms. This delay may be related to poor symptom recognition. Various contextual factors such as prior illness experience, social situations, or the environment where symptoms are experienced may influence symptom response. Therefore, the purpose of this study was to describe contextual factors related to symptom recognition and response among elders hospitalized with decompensated HF.

A factor complicating symptom monitoring is the physical subtlety of early-warning symptoms of HF decompensation. Early symptoms, such as fatigue and dyspnea with activity, are typically ambiguous, nonspecific, and insidious, which may impede their recognition as significant and related to HF. Elders, in particular, are known to discount the early symptoms of decompensated HF, such as fatigue or shortness of breath, as normal aging (Leventhal & Prohaska, 1986; Miller, 2000; Patel, Shafazand, Schaufelberger, & Ekman, 2007). The interpretation and response to symptoms also are known to be affected by the social and emotional context in which they occur (Burnett, Blumenthal, Mark, Leimberger, & Califf, 1995; Horowitz, Rein, & Leventhal, 2004).

SYMPTOM RECOGNITION AS A COMPONENT OF SELF-CARE

Self-care has been defined as a naturalistic decision-making process involving the choice of behaviors that maintain physiologic stability (*maintenance*) and the response to symptoms when they occur (*management*; Riegel et al., 2004). Symptom recognition is key to effective self-care. Patient education is the primary intervention used to promote symptom recognition, as most investigators assume that failed self-care is due to a lack of knowledge.

Patients are taught to monitor their symptoms daily with the assumption that they will notify the provider for a sudden weight gain or take other definitive actions (e.g., an extra diuretic) to avoid hospitalization. Unfortunately, few patients monitor their symptoms routinely, and those who do often are unsure about how to interpret them (Carlson, Riegel, & Moser, 2001; Ni et al., 1999).

Patients' perceptions of symptoms have been correlated with the decision to seek care, to self-manage the symptoms, or to do nothing (Cameron, Leventhal, & Leventhal, 1993; Horowitz et al., 2004; Leventhal & Prohaska, 1986). Symptoms perceived to be less serious or those that incur little anxiety are more likely to result in delay of timely medical attention (Burnett et al., 1995; Dracup & Moser, 1997; Horowitz et al., 2004). Studies of patients hospitalized with decompensated HF suggest that patients typically endure increasing symptoms over days or weeks before seeking care (Evangelista, Dracup, & Doering, 2000, 2002; Friedman, 1997; Goldberg et al., 2008; Jurgens, 2006). Prior research has shown that in persons with HF, the factors associated with longer delay are younger age, male gender, African American race, multiple presenting symptoms, presenting with dyspnea and edema, a gradual onset of symptoms, higher symptom distress, absence of HF history, symptom onset between 12 midnight and 6 a.m., care by a primary care physician, and higher or worse New York Heart Association (NYHA) class (Goldberg et al, 2008; Evangelista et al., 2000, 2002; Jurgens, 2006).

A hospitalization for HF in the prior 6 months increases the risk of cardiovascular-related death or HF hospitalization by 73% (Pocock et al., 2006). As yet, there are no published reports as to whether delay in seeking care for decompensated HF also negatively affects morbidity and mortality; however, we assume that appropriate self-care leading to early intervention in the course of an exacerbation may avert hospitalization. Furthermore, to the best of our knowledge, there are no published studies specifically examining contextual factors affecting elders hospitalized with decompensated HF.

CONCEPTUAL FRAMEWORK

The Self-Regulation Model of Illness guided this study as it describes symptoms in a manner beyond a simple physical experience (Cameron et al., 1993; Cameron & Leventhal, 2003). Symptoms are multidimensional with physical, cognitive, and emotional components that translate into how individuals variably feel, think, and emotionally respond when symptoms arise (Figure 1). The Self-Regulation Model of Illness also incorporates the physical symptom experience within the context of an individual's experience both past and present including the social environment or situation in which it occurs. The model thus acknowledges the dynamic nature of illness, care seeking, and the influence of contextual factors and the social environment on the interpretation and response to symptoms.

According to the Self-Regulation Model of Illness, the response to illness occurs as a result of a person's perceptions of his/her illness or symptoms. Furthermore, response to illness is influenced by one's abstract knowledge or semantic memory about the illness (such as risk for illness), previous experiences with comorbid or episodic illness, and beliefs about the consequences and controllability of the illness. As such, prior illness experience provides a source of contextual knowledge with which one can begin to label symptoms.

Illness perceptions are developed via two parallel pathways (cognitive and emotional). A cognitive representation is the assessment of a health threat and is embedded in the personal and social context in which one lives. Forming a cognitive representation includes determining the identity (labeling), perceived cause(s), timeline (is it acute or chronic?), consequences (how serious), and controllability/curability of the symptom or illness. The cognitive representation begins when one is first aware of a change in somatic state. Sensing symptoms or declining functional status prompts the assessment of possible causes. An emotional representation is the affective response to the change in somatic

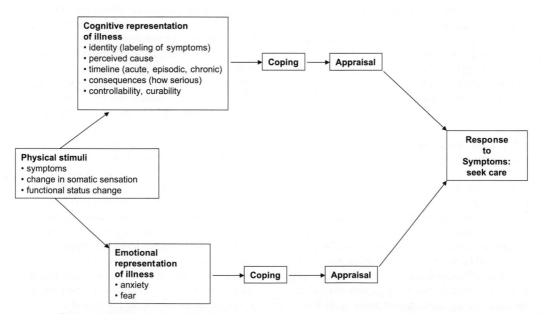

Figure 1. Self-regulation model of illness.

sensation and its subsequent cognitive representation. The intensity of the emotional response like anxiety or fear affects the response to symptoms and coping with the threat of illness. Coping could involve waiting to see what happens and delaying seeking care or calling for help. Professional and social relationships influence the way one copes with illness. Potential resources for help could include either medical or lay (e.g., family members or friends) consultation. Lastly is the evaluation phase in which the health threat and the effect of the coping plan is assessed.

We propose that delay in seeking care is due to the difficulty that HF patients experience in discerning the quality and meaning of their symptoms. Heart failure causes a multitude of symptoms, and comorbid conditions add to the number of symptoms experienced. Hypertension, coronary artery disease, chronic lung disease, and depression are common (Ceia et al., 2004; Dahlstrom, 2005; Masoudi & Krumholz, 2003). In addition, various contextual factors such as prior illness or symptom experience, social situation, or environment where the symptoms are experienced may affect symptom interpretation. The influence of contextual factors on recognition and response to acute HF symptoms is as yet unknown. Therefore, the specific aims of this study were to (a) describe the experience of and the cognitive and emotional response to the symptoms of decompensated HF, (b) determine the influence of sociodemographic, clinical, cognitive, emotional, and social contextual factors on symptom duration during this time, and (c) describe self-care behaviors prior to seeking care for decompensated HF.

■ Methods

A mixed-methods design with an emphasis on the quantitative data (QUANT/qual) was used to address the specific aims. In the quantitative component, an exploratory descriptive design was used to examine the duration of those symptoms before care seeking, patient responses to symptoms of decompensated HF, and self-care behaviors. Qualitative methods were used to elicit narrative accounts of the symptom perception process and to explore the contextual factors that influenced the process, thereby enhancing the quantitative data.

SAMPLE

A convenience sample of adult men and women hospitalized in an emergency department or as inpatients with a diagnosis of decompensated HF was recruited at tertiary care hospitals in Philadelphia and New York. In addition to conducting a power analysis to determine sample size, the feasibility of conducting a mixed-method study (QUANT/qual) was considered. Guidelines for sample size vary from 15 (Stevens, 1996) to approximately 40 (Cohen & Cohen, 1983) participants per predictor for multiple regression analysis. The exploratory nature of the study, together with the ability to meet the aims, was factored into the determination of the sample of 77 participants.

Participants were enrolled if they were 65 years of age or older, cognitively intact, medically stable, able to read or understand English fluently, and provided written informed consent. The diagnosis of HF was confirmed using the Framingham criteria (Ho, Anderson, Kannel, Grossman, & Levy, 1993). The Framingham criteria use the presence of two major criteria (e.g., neck vein distention, rales, and S3 gallop) or one major and two minor criteria (e.g., extremity edema, dyspnea on exertion, and pulmonary vascular congestion by chest x-ray) to diagnose HF. Participants were enrolled within 3 days of admission to limit problems with ability to recall their illness experience. Participants also had to be living independently in the community and able to manage their illness by self-care. The study protocol was reviewed and approved by the institutional review boards at Stony Brook University and the University of Pennsylvania. All participants signed an informed consent agreement.

PROCEDURE AND MEASURES

Heart Failure Somatic Perception Scale.

The Heart Failure Somatic Perception Scale was used to assess perceived symptom distress associated with the current hospitalization for HF (Jurgens, Fain, & Riegel, 2006). The scale, derived from the Framingham Diagnostic Criteria (Ho et al., 1993) and the literature, has 17 items that address symptom occurrence and perceived symptom severity on a 4-point Likert scale ranging from 0 = "not at all" to 3 = "extremely, could not have been worse" (possible range 0–51). The scale items are summative; higher scores indicate higher perceived distress.

The original questionnaire consisted of 12 items. Content validity was confirmed by nurse scientists in HF and expert HF nurse clinicians. Theta reliability for nonparallel items was 0.71 (Jurgens et al., 2006). Five additional items were added for this study; two items target the HF symptoms of nocturia and increased abdominal girth. Also, as patients often decrease their activity to accommodate escalating symptoms, making these symptoms difficult to capture, additional alternate items measuring dyspnea, fatigue, and dyspnea on exertion were added. For example, dyspnea on exertion was addressed by asking about difficulty with usual activities because of shortness of breath. The added alternate item asks if getting dressed made it hard to breathe. In consideration of the addition of more than one item assessing the symptoms cited above, items were no longer discrete and Cronbach's α was used to assess reliability. In the current study, the Cronbach's α for the 17-item version was .80.

Response to Symptoms Questionnaire.

The Response to Symptom Questionnaire (revised; Dracup & Moser, 1997) was used to assess cognitive, emotional and social contextual factors affecting symptom response. The questionnaire addresses the following variables from the conceptual model: (a) the context in which the symptoms occurred, (b) affective or emotional response to symptoms,

(c) cognitive response to symptoms (e.g., symptom appraisal), (d) response of others to the symptoms, and (e) the perceived severity of the symptoms in general. Instrument authors evaluated content validity, but reliability has not been reported (Dracup & Moser, 1997). The questionnaire was developed using single items to assess various contextual factors affecting response to acute myocardial infarction symptoms (Burnett et al., 1995). It was modified for use in patients with HF by the primary author. Questions on the process of seeking care were deleted (e.g., where they were when the symptoms were first noticed, who was with them, and self-care attempts). These were written as open-ended questions for the qualitative interview. Wording was changed from *heart attack* to *heart failure* as appropriate. The revision was evaluated for content validity by nursing experts in cardiac research and clinical practice. The items use a 5-point Likert scale to address how patients responded cognitively, emotionally, or behaviorally to their symptoms (e.g., 1 = "not at all anxious" to 5 = "extremely anxious"). Theta reliability, appropriate for questionnaires with discrete nonparallel items (Carmines & Zeller, 1979), was 0.72 for the 15 items used in the current study.

NYHA Functional Class and Specific Activity Scale.

Functional status can be affected by symptom burden and was measured in two ways. The NYHA functional class (range = class 1 to 4) on the day of admission was determined from review of the medical record or by interview if it was not documented in the admission physical examination. A higher class indicates worse functional ability. In addition, the participant's typical functional level when not acutely ill was measured using the Specific Activity Scale (Goldman, Hashimoto, Cook, & Loscalzo, 1981). This scale produces metabolic units based on common daily activities. Similar to the NYHA classes, this scale categorizes patients into one of four classes, with higher class indicating worse functional ability.

Charlson Comorbidity Index. To examine potential differences in symptom distress related to comorbid illnesses at the time of enrollment, the Charlson Comorbidity Index was assessed (Katz, Chang, Sangha, Fossel, & Bates, 1996). Responses were weighted and indexed into one of three comorbidity categories (low, moderate, or high) according to the published method. Scores can range from 0 to 34, although every patient in this study had a score of at least 1 because they were all diagnosed with HF. Validity of the scale was demonstrated by the instrument authors when comorbidity category was shown to predict mortality, complications, healthcare resource use, length of hospital stay, discharge disposition, and cost (Charlson, Pompei, Ales, & MacKenzie, 1987; Katz et al., 1996).

Interview. Sociodemographic and clinical data were collected through interview and review of the medical record. The content of the interview is outlined in Table 1. Symptom duration before hospitalization was used as a measure of the time taken to assess and respond to the symptoms of HF decompensation. Symptom duration was calculated in hours from the time a participant was first aware of symptoms until arrival at the hospital. The precise time of symptom onset was determined by participants with a use of calendar to assist recall. Once a particular time frame such as a weekend, social event, appointment, or holiday was identified, symptom duration was explored in relation to that day and time. Although this technique is subject to recall bias, Dempsey, Dracup, and Moser (1995) found that with careful questioning, patients are able to pinpoint the time of onset quite specifically. Prodromal or subacute symptoms were quantified in addition to the symptoms that were more acute in nature. Chronic symptoms were quantified from the time they increased in severity over the participant's baseline. Omnipresent chronic symptoms that did not vary in severity were recorded as present, but the duration was not quantified for the

Table 1. Content of Interview

Sociodemographic data	Occupation Marital status Living arrangement Education Income level
History related to HF	Year of HF diagnosis Number of previous HF-related hospitalizations Use of emergency medical services Medication history Participation in HF clinic
Symptoms	Symptom presence, duration, severity Symptom pattern (gradual or sudden onset) Decision to seek care (self or other person)
Factors affecting decision to seek care	Open-ended questions "Tell me more about the time leading up to this hospitalization." "What did you do when you first noticed your symptoms?" "What did you think was causing your symptoms?"

Note. HF=5 heart failure.

analysis. Participation in an HF clinic was documented to assess for ongoing disease management and access to information and support.

Upon completion of preliminary demographic and clinical data collection, open-ended questions were used to identify contextual factors affecting the process and decision to seek care. Individuals were asked to describe factors including but not limited to social/situational factors such as location when symptoms were noticed; contact with and response of family, friends, or health providers; and self-care behaviors. All interviews were conducted in the participant's hospital room and averaged an hour in duration. The audiotaped sessions were transcribed verbatim and augmented with field notes and participant observations.

DATA ANALYSIS

The relationship between duration of HF symptoms, perceived symptom distress, and cognitive and emotional factors was explored using Pearson correlations. Hierarchical regression was used to identify predictors of duration of dyspnea in three steps. A priori predictors of interest included age, gender (male = 1, female = 0), and perceived symptom severity. The HF Somatic Perception Scale score was used to reflect the physical symptom experience as depicted in the Self-Regulation Model of Illness. Contextual factors in the regression included the cognitive (perceived seriousness of symptoms) and emotional (anxiety) response to symptoms. Gender and age were entered in the first step, followed by perceived symptom distress. Anxiety and perceived seriousness were entered together in the last step. Logarithmic transformation was used to normalize the distribution of symptom duration for analysis. Median duration versus the mean is reported as extreme outliers skew interpretation of the data.

To assess for multicollinearity, correlations between the predictor variables were inspected. The highest correlation was between anxiety and perceived seriousness ($r = .635$). Although high, the correlation did not meet the cut-point for multicollinearity, predetermined as a linear correlation of greater than .8 (Allison, 1999). Tolerance for each independent variable ranged from .527 to .974, which is above the point of .40 considered problematic when assessing multicollinearity (Allison, 1999). Quantitative data were analyzed using the Statistical Package for the Social Sciences software version 14.0 (Chicago, Illinois).

Over 1,000 pages of qualitative data were analyzed using content analysis with Atlas.ti version 5.0.67 (Berlin, Germany) to identify cognitive, emotional, and contextual factors affecting the process and decision to seek care (Ayres, Kavanaugh, & Knafl, 2003; Denzin & Lincoln, 2000). First, data were analyzed using a priori codes based on the Self-Regulation Model of Illness (physical stimuli, cognitive appraisal, emotional response, and social factors). Voluntary explanations from explorations of self-care behaviors before admission and the Response to Symptoms Questionnaire were described. Repetitive themes were clustered into subgroups, labeled into meaningful categories and discussed with a coinvestigator. Then, across-case comparison analysis was conducted between those participants with and without a previous HF-related hospitalization by constructing a matrix of common experiences among the participants. This analysis was an iterative process whereby the researcher moved back and forth between individual cases and across cases to track variability of themes (Ayres et al., 2003). The final step in the data analysis was integration of the quantitative and qualitative data.

Methodological rigor of the qualitative analysis was maintained through an audit trail, periodic debriefing with a coinvestigator, and discussions with colleagues knowledgeable about HF self-care and mixed-methods research techniques. An audit trail of process and analytic memos and coding books was maintained to support the credibility of the study.

■ Results

STUDY SAMPLE

Participants ($n = 77$; Table 2) were enrolled over a 19-month period from October 2004 until May 2006. A prior HF-related hospital admission was reported by 72% of the sample, with a median duration since diagnosis of

Table 2. Sociodemographic and Clinical Characteristics (*n* = 77)

Variable	*n* (%)
Gender	
Men	40 (51.9)
Women	37 (48.1)
Race/Ethnicity	
Non-Hispanic White	66 (85.7)
Black	9 (11.7)
Hispanic	1 (1.3)
Other	1 (1.3)
Marital status	
Married	37 (48.1)
Widowed	34 (44.2)
Divorced, separated, never married	6 (7.8)
Education	
Less than 12 years	18 (23.4)
High school diploma	34 (44.2)
Some college/associate degree	7 (9.1)
Baccalaureate degree	10 (13)
Graduate degree	8 (10.4)
Total household income in past year	
Less than $10,000	10 (13)
$10,000–$24,999	24 (31.2)
$25,000–$39,999	10 (13)
$40,000–$54,999	7 (9.1)
$55,000 or greater	12 (15.6)
Do not know	12 (15.6)
Declined to answer	2 (2.6)
Comorbid illness	
Coronary artery disease	54 (70.1)
Hypertension	55 (72)
Diabetes	31 (40.3)
Charlson comorbidity category	
Low	36 (46.8)
Moderate	33 (42.9)
High	8 (10.4)
Specific Activity Scale—functional performance	
Class 1	1 (1.3)
Class 2	14 (18.2)
Class 3	39 (50.6)
Class 4	23 (29.9)

5 years (*SD* = 5.2 years). Functional capacity was low, with 81% of the participants classified as class 3 or 4 on the Specific Activity Scale. All participants completed the quantitative and qualitative procedures, although 13 tapes were unusable because of errors in the recording process (e.g., incorrect tape speed and equipment malfunction). Nineteen potential participants declined enrollment, citing reasons such as not wanting to sign a consent, not wanting to take the time, or lack of interest. Those who declined did not differ significantly from the 77 participants on any demographic or clinical characteristic.

PHYSICAL STIMULI: SYMPTOMS

Dyspnea, dyspnea on exertion, and fatigue were the most frequently reported symptoms (Table 3). Dyspnea duration had a range of 30 minutes to 90 days, with nearly half reporting dyspnea for greater than 3 days before admission. Only a minority of participants (*n* = 8; 11.8%) reported experiencing dyspnea for longer than 2 weeks before admission. Mean perceived symptom (Table 4) was significantly correlated with dyspnea duration (r = .30, p = .013). There were no significant differences in symptom distress scores in relation to age, gender, or Charlson

Table 3. Symptom Frequency and Duration Before Hospital Admission (*n* = 77)

Symptoms	*n* (%)	Median Duration (Days)
Dyspnea	68 (88)	3
Dyspnea on exertion	59 (77)	5
Fatigue	52 (68)	7
Edema	33 (43)	7
Orthopnea	27 (35)	3.4
Weight gain	26 (34)	9
Chest pain	25 (32)	1

Table 4. Mean Scores of Physical, Cognitive, and Emotional Response Measures (*n* = 77)

	Mean (*SD*)
Symptom distress	
Heart Failure Somatic Perception Scale	19.6 (8.5)
Cognitive responses	
Seriousness of symptoms	2.92 (1.24)
Perceived control related to symptoms	2.36 (1.22)
Emotional responses	
Anxiety related to symptoms	2.84 (1.28)
Fear of consequences of seeking help	1.79 (1.24)
Embarrassment related to seeking help	1.35 (.91)

Comorbidity category. Most participants (79%) made the decision themselves to seek care in response to their symptoms rather than being encouraged by others to do so.

COGNITIVE RESPONSE TO SYMPTOMS

Analysis of the Response to Symptoms Questionnaire revealed that over half of the sample did not know the symptoms of HF (56%) or realize their importance. Nearly 87% of the sample believed their symptoms to have some degree of seriousness, but most (80%) waited for the symptoms to go away. The correlation of dyspnea duration and perceived seriousness approached significance ($r = -.23, p = .06$). Slightly over half (50.6%) were reluctant to trouble anyone for help. Interestingly, 54% believed that they had little to no control over their symptoms.

Qualitative analysis revealed that over half had no idea what was causing their symptoms. Approximately a third misattributed their symptoms to conditions unrelated to their heart (e.g., upper respiratory infections, travel, arthritis, and emotional stress). "I knew I was getting short of breath. I had no idea that this had anything to do with the heart. I thought it was the lungs." For some, the accumulation of additional HF symptoms triggered care seeking but not necessarily the identification of their symptoms as HF related. A 68-year-old woman had symptoms of increasing dyspnea, fatigue, and edema before seeking care, stating:

> It had gone on for a few months where I just couldn't do some of the physical things I used to do. Like, um, walk a mile. . . . When I got these shortness of breath attacks, I would attribute it more to anxiety than to the heart. I was slower than my usual self. My feet were swollen, too, but that's been going on for years. This time my abdomen was swollen too. On Friday, I couldn't get out of my car so I called a friend [to take her to the hospital].

Among those with a previous HF-related admission (*n* = 53), a group one might assume would be more knowledgeable, 10 participants had no idea as to what was causing their symptoms. Further analysis of this subgroup identified comorbid illness such as chronic lung disease and obesity, incorrect symptom attribution (e.g., a cold or physical exertion), and a gradual progression of symptom severity as factors hampering the identification of their HF symptoms. An 82-year-old man with dyspnea and fatigue gradually increasing over a 2- to 3-month period said he used a treadmill daily. The number of steps on the treadmill had recently decreased, but he was not concerned. The change in his functional status lacked meaning for him in relation to his heart, and his wife initiated care seeking. Other participants did not recognize or define their physical decline as valid symptoms. One participant stated, "Fatigue is not a symptom," and another said, "I'm not tired, I'm just slowing down." Interestingly, attribution of symptoms specifically to advanced age was not a common theme in this older aged sample.

EMOTIONAL RESPONSE TO SYMPTOMS

Emotional response to symptoms was measured using items from the Response to

Symptoms Questionnaire. The duration of the early symptoms of HF (dyspnea on exertion, fatigue, edema, and weight gain) was unrelated to anxiety or fear at their onset. Dyspnea (vs. dyspnea on exertion) and anxiety were significantly related once dyspnea became more omnipresent; dyspnea and anxiety were inversely related ($r = -.31$, $p = .012$), indicating that a longer duration of dyspnea before hospital admission was associated with lower anxiety. Weight gain and fear produced a similar relationship ($r = -.63$, $p = .001$). There was no significant relationship between dyspnea duration and fear ($r = .03$, $p = .80$). A single item rating general symptom intensity on a scale of 0 ("no symptoms") to 10 ("worst symptoms experienced") was weakly correlated with fear ($r = .28$, $p = .012$). Only 28 (36.3%) participants experienced fear in relation to their symptoms, with 76.6% reporting no fear or being mildly fearful. The narrative accounts were consistent with the quantitative findings. Participants cited a variety of reasons for lack of fear or anxiety regarding their symptoms. A 69-year-old man stated, "I have shortness of breath 'cause I've had a heart attack and bypass, so a lot of problems . . . I wasn't alarmed by it." A 66-year-old man was not fearful about his several days of dyspnea until he noticed leg swelling.

SOCIAL FACTORS AND RESPONSE TO SYMPTOMS

Social factors, as assessed with the Response to Symptoms Questionnaire, were not a predominant influence on symptom response; 84% denied feeling embarrassed to seek care. Likewise, 87% denied that social plans factored into their decision to delay or seek care. Few (19%) reported delaying care because they were waiting for family to arrive, and less than one third reported delaying care because of wanting to avoid hospitalization.

The qualitative data offered explanations for delay in care seeking. Participants reported not wanting to inconvenience, disturb, or communicate their symptoms to their family

or friends: "I didn't want to alarm my wife." "I didn't want to 'wake/bother' my daughter." As a result of these reasons, some participants who were acutely short of breath waited until morning to call for help. Among those who wished to avoid hospitalization, various reasons cited included caregiver responsibilities, prior negative hospital experiences, and financial concerns. One participant with outstanding medical bills reported, "I'm not anxious to come to the hospital because it's very expensive. I want to leave something to my children."

The influence of family factored into care-seeking decisions in approximately 25% of the sample. In some cases, participants were unaware of their symptoms of dyspnea or decreased activity tolerance and their family initiated seeking care. For example, one family noticed that the participant was short of breath with activity for 2 weeks before hospitalization. This 81-year-old woman was unaware of her dyspnea until 5 days before admission, when it was increasingly severe. Her daughter observed her distress and made the decision to seek care, saying, "Momma, do you know you're not breathing well?" Another participant reported not knowing why he was in the hospital and said, "If my wife went out and bought some groceries, and she wanted me to carry them into the house, I would carry them and start puffing. I wasn't helping around the house lately, so my wife called the doctor and moved up the appointment." A gradual increase in symptom severity, followed by adaptation by pacing activities, impeded some patients in recognizing the importance of their symptoms until their families intervened.

INFLUENCE OF CONTEXTUAL FACTORS ON DYSPNEA DURATION

The hierarchical regression model explained 29% of the variance in duration of dyspnea before seeking care (Table 5). Three of the five predictors contributed significantly ($p \leq .03$) to the explained variance. Male

Table 5. Hierarchical Regression Predictors for Duration of Dyspnea ($n = 68$)

Predictor	B	SE	Standard β	p
Age	0.056	0.028	.235	.053
Gender	1.141	0.427	.311	.01
Physical factor Symptom distress	0.074	0.024	.347	.003
Cognitive factor Seriousness	−0.061	0.234	−.039	.795
Emotional factor Anxiety	−0.464	0.215	−.323	.035

$R = .539, R^2 = .29.$

gender, higher symptom distress, and lower anxiety were associated with a longer duration of dyspnea. Older age approached significance, with a $p = .053$.

SELF-CARE MANAGEMENT BEHAVIORS

The qualitative data revealed the use of alternative strategies than those routinely suggested to HF patients. Few ($n = 4$) took an extra dose of their diuretic. One explained, "I'm already on medication." Others described energy conservation measures such as resting, sitting up, or sleeping in a recliner as temporarily sufficient for improving symptoms. "I control my symptoms by not going up and down stairs." Several participants tried various medications not typically used for treating symptoms of HF, including aspirin, sublingual nitroglycerin, acetaminophen, inhalers, cold remedies, and higher doses of oxygen. Some simply took deep breaths, tried to calm themselves, or prayed. None of the participants reported decreasing their sodium or fluid intake in response to escalating symptoms.

■ Discussion

Sensing and attributing meaning to the early symptoms of HF decompensation were prob-lematic for participants in this older aged sample. Many participants interpreted their symptoms in the context of a less threatening condition or illness and were not alarmed enough to seek care. Poor symptom recognition resulted in nearly half of the participants experiencing dyspnea for 3 days or more before hospitalization for decompensated HF, a finding consistent with those of others (Evangelista et al., 2000, 2002; Friedman, 1997; Goldberg et al., 2008; Jurgens, 2006). Symptoms increased gradually, generating little anxiety or fear, and participants were hesitant to bother others about their symptoms. According to the Self-Regulation Model of Illness, responding to symptoms is an iterative process. The process begins with *sensing* a somatic change in physical status, which initiates an attempt to label the sensation, assessing its cause, applying a coping strategy, and evaluating the effect of the strategy. If the strategy is ineffective, the symptom or sensation is relabeled or the cause is reevaluated and another coping strategy is tried. In this study, some participants were physically unaware of their escalating symptoms, which may be an important factor in symptom response. There is growing evidence that HF is associated with changes in cognitive function, which may impair symptom perception and the ability to make self-care decisions (Alves et al., 2005; Woo, Macey, Fonarow, Hamilton, & Harper, 2003). The physical symptom experience is clearly an insufficient stimulus for a timely process of seeking care.

The cognitive representation or labeling of HF symptoms was also problematic and negatively affected timely care seeking in this sample. Congruent with prior HF studies of both inpatients and outpatients (Horowitz et al., 2004; Patel et al., 2007), the cognitive representation of symptoms was either absent or incorrect for many participants trying to *interpret* the meaning of their symptoms. Resources for identifying and interpreting current symptoms (lay sources, family, and healthcare providers) were inadequate for timely care for many of the participants.

Most striking was the lack of an emotional response (e.g., anxiety) to the early symptoms of HF decompensation, which further compromised an effective response. One explanation may be that patients with HF view symptoms individually as opposed to being related to one another. As such, symptoms such as dyspnea with activity and fatigue are unlikely to cause concern and are more easily dismissed as unimportant or unworthy of medical attention. Patients also appear to decrease activity to accommodate symptoms such as dyspnea associated with walking. Elders who lead generally sedentary lives may not perform activities that incur dyspnea or fatigue, making these nonspecific symptoms less noticeable.

Similar to previous studies (Friedman, 1997; Jurgens, 2006), prior experience with an HF-related hospital admission did not assure accurate labeling of symptoms or timely self-care. Although a definition of what constitutes delay in treatment for decompensated HF has not been established, these elders waited long enough that emergency hospitalization was necessary for symptom management. Few intentionally ignored their symptoms or avoided hospitalization, but knowledge about HF and symptom recognition abilities were poor. Those most likely to delay seeking care were men, those with higher symptom distress, and those with lower anxiety.

Confirming the study by Patel et al. (2007), the social influence of family had both positive and negative outcomes in relation to timely medical attention. Several participants reported reluctance to disturb family members despite significant respiratory distress. In other cases, the family members were instrumental in initiating access to treatment. Educating both patient and family regarding the significance and necessity of early intervention for escalating symptoms is important.

STUDY STRENGTHS AND LIMITATIONS

The results of the study are strengthened by the mixed-methods design. Detailed narrative accounts of the symptom perception process added depth to the analysis and interpretation of the results by illustrating the highly variable and often incorrect interpretations of the meaning of symptoms. The complexity of the contextual factors affecting the process that patients with HF use to make self-care decisions would be overlooked if the analysis was based on quantitative data alone.

Limitations to the generalizability of these results include the relatively small and largely White sample. The sample size was robust for the qualitative data but was limited for the quantitative analysis. The richness of the qualitative data was limited by interviewing and equipment use skills of the research assistants in some cases. Lastly, the quantitative analysis of emotional factors such as fear, anxiety, and embarrassment in relation to symptom duration was limited by the use of single items from the Response to Symptoms Questionnaire. Although summated scores from multiple-item scales are commonly used for such analyses (e.g., to measure anxiety), single-item scales are reported to generate valid measures and are, in some cases, superior to multiple-item scales (Gardner, Cummings, Dunham, & Pierce, 1998).

■ Conclusion

The window of opportunity to treat the early symptoms of HF decompensation is hampered by the difficulty that patients experience in sensing and interpreting the meaning of these symptoms. The lack of an emotional response to symptoms decreases the likelihood of instituting timely self-care management strategies or seeking medical guidance. Educating patients in HF self-care might be more effective if the meaning of their symptoms were clearer. Strategies for helping patients to evaluate their symptoms are in need of further study.

Corrine Y. Jurgens, PhD, RN, ANP-BC, FAHA, is Clinical Associate Professor, Stony Brook University, New York, and John A. Hartford Postdoctoral Fellow, University of Pennsylvania, Philadelphia.

Linda Hoke, PhD, RN, APN-BC, CCNS, CRRN, is Clinical Nurse Specialist, Hospital of the University of Pennsylvania, Philadelphia.

Janet Byrnes, MS, RN, ANP, is Assistant Director of Nursing, Stony Brook University Medical Center, New York.

Barbara Riegel, DNSc, RN, FAAN, FAHA, is Professor, University of Pennsylvania, Philadelphia.

Accepted for publication January 30, 2009.

Funding for this study was provided by the John A. Hartford Foundation Building Academic Geriatric Nursing Capacity Scholarship Program.

The authors gratefully acknowledge the scholarly support of Dr. Neville Strumpf and the faculty of the University of Pennsylvania's Hartford Center of Geriatric Nursing Excellence.

Corresponding author: Corrine Y. Jurgens, PhD, RN, ANP-BC, FAHA, School of Nursing, Stony Brook University, HSC L2-223, Stony Brook, NY 11794-8240 (e-mail: corrine.jurgens@stonybrook.edu).

REFERENCES

Allison, P. D. (1999). *Multiple regression: A primer.* Thousand Oaks, CA: Pine Forge Press.

Alves, T. C., Rays, J., Fraguas, R. Jr., Wajngarten, M., Meneghetti, J. C., Prando, S., et al. (2005). Localized cerebral blood flow reductions in patients with heart failure: A study using 99mtchmpao spect. *Journal of Neuroimaging, 15,* 150–156.

Ayres, L., Kavanaugh, K., & Knafl, K. A. (2003). Within-case and across-case approaches to qualitative data analysis. *Qualitative Health Research, 13,* 871–883.

Burnett, R. E., Blumenthal, J. A., Mark, D. B., Leimberger, J. D., & Califf, R. M. (1995). Distinguishing between early and late responders to symptoms of acute myocardial infarction. *American Journal of Cardiology, 75,* 1019–1022.

Cameron, L., Leventhal, E. A., & Leventhal, H. (1993). Symptom representations and affect as determinants of care seeking in a community-dwelling, adult sample population. *Health Psychology, 12,* 171–179.

Cameron, L. D., & Leventhal, H. (Eds.). (2003). *The self-regulation of health and illness behavior.* London: Routledge.

Carlson, B., Riegel, B., & Moser, D. K. (2001). Self-care abilities of patients with heart failure. *Heart & Lung, 30,* 351–359.

Carmines, E. G., & Zeller, R. A. (1979). *Reliability and validity assessment.* Beverly Hills, CA: Sage Publications.

Ceia, F., Fonseca, C., Mota, T., Morais, H., Matias, F., Costa, C., et al. (2004). Aetiology, comorbidity and drug therapy of chronic heart failure in the real world: The EPICA substudy. *European Journal of Heart Failure, 6,* 801–806.

Charlson, M. E., Pompei, P., Ales, K. L., & MacKenzie, C. R. (1987). A new method of classifying prognostic comorbidity in longitudinal studies: Development and validation. *Journal of Chronic Diseases, 40,* 373–383.

Cohen, J., & Cohen, P. (1983). *Applied multiple regression/correlation analysis for the behavioral sciences* (2nd ed.). Hillsdale, NJ: Lawrence Erlbaum Associates.

Dahlstrom, U. (2005). Frequent non-cardiac comorbidities in patients with chronic heart failure. *European Journal of Heart Failure, 7,* 309–316.

Dempsey, S. J., Dracup, K., & Moser, D. K. (1995). Women's decision to seek care for symptoms of acute myocardial infarction. *Heart & Lung, 24,* 444–456.

Denzin, N., & Lincoln, Y. (Eds.). (2000). *Handbook of qualitative research* (2nd ed.). Thousand Oaks, CA: Sage Publications.

Dracup, K., & Moser, D. K. (1997). Beyond sociodemographics: Factors influencing the decision to seek treatment for symptoms of acute myocardial infarction. *Heart & Lung, 26,* 253–262.

Evangelista, L. S., Dracup, K., & Doering, L. V. (2000). Treatment-seeking delays in heart failure patients. *Journal of Heart and Lung Transplantation, 19,* 932–938.

Evangelista, L. S., Dracup, K., & Doering, L. V. (2002). Racial differences in treatment-seeking delays among heart failure patients. *Journal of Cardiac Failure, 8,* 381–386.

Friedman, M. M. (1997). Older adults' symptoms and their duration before hospitalization for heart failure. *Heart & Lung, 26,* 169–176.

Gardner, D. G., Cummings, L. L., Dunham, R. B., & Pierce, J. L. (1998). Single-item versus multiple-item measurement scales: An empirical comparison. *Educational and Psychological Measurement, 58,* 898–915.

Goldberg, R. J., Goldberg, J. H., Pruell, S., Yarzebski, J., Lessard, D., Spencer, F. A., et al. (2008). Delays in seeking medical care in hospitalized patients with decompensated heart failure. *American Journal of Medicine, 121*, 212–218.

Goldman, L., Hashimoto, B., Cook, E. F., & Loscalzo, A. (1981). Comparative reproducibility and validity of systems for assessing cardiovascular functional class: Advantages of a new specific activity scale. *Circulation, 64*, 1227–1234.

Ho, K. K. L., Anderson, K. M., Kannel, W. B., Grossman, W., & Levy, D. (1993). Survival after the onset of congestive heart failure in Framingham heart study subjects. *Circulation, 88*, 107–115.

Horowitz, C. R., Rein, S. B., & Leventhal, H. (2004). A story of maladies, misconceptions, and mishaps: Effective management of heart failure. *Social Science & Medicine, 58*, 631–643.

Jurgens, C. Y. (2006). Somatic awareness, uncertainty, and delay in care-seeking in acute heart failure. *Research in Nursing & Health, 29*, 74–86.

Jurgens, C. Y., Fain, J. A., & Riegel, B. (2006). Psychometric testing of the heart failure somatic awareness scale. *Journal of Cardiovascular Nursing, 21*, 95–102.

Katz, J. N., Chang, L. C., Sangha, O., Fossel, A. H., & Bates, D. W. (1996). Can comorbidity be measured by questionnaire rather than medical record review? *Medical Care, 34*, 73–84.

Leventhal, E. A., & Prohaska, T. R. (1986). Age, symptom interpretation, and health behavior. *Journal of the American Geriatric Society, 34*, 185–191.

Masoudi, F. A., & Krumholz, H. M. (2003). Polypharmacy and comorbidity in heart failure. *BMJ, 327*, 513–514.

Miller, C. L. (2000). Cue sensitivity in women with cardiac disease. *Progress in Cardiovascular Nursing, 15*, 82–89.

Moser, D. K., Doering, L. V., & Chung, M. L. (2005). Vulnerabilities of patients recovering from an exacerbation of chronic heart failure. *American Heart Journal, 150*, 984.e7–984.e13.

Ni, H., Nauman, D., Burgess, D., Wise, K., Crispell, K., & Hershberger, R. E. (1999). Factors influencing knowledge of and adherence to self-care among patients with heart failure. *Archives of Internal Medicine, 159*, 1613–1619.

Patel, H., Shafazand, M., Schaufelberger, M., & Ekman, I. (2007). Reasons for seeking acute care in chronic heart failure. *European Journal of Heart Failure, 9*, 702–708.

Pocock, S. J., Wang, D., Pfeffer, M. A., Yusuf, S., McMurray, J. J., Swedberg, K. B., et al. (2006). Predictors of mortality and morbidity in patients with chronic heart failure. *European Heart Journal, 27*, 65–75.

Riegel, B., Carlson, B., Moser, D. K., Sebern, M., Hicks, F. D., & Roland, V. (2004). Psychometric testing of the self-care of heart failure index. *Journal of Cardiac Failure, 10*, 350–360.

Rodriguez-Artalejo, F., Guallar-Castillon, P., Pascual, C. R., Otero, C. M., Montes, A. O., Garcia, A. N., et al. (2005). Health-related quality of life as a predictor of hospital readmission and death among patients with heart failure. *Archives of Internal Medicine, 165*, 1274–1279.

Rosamond, W., Flegal, K., Furie, K., Go, A., Greenlund, K., Haase, N., et al. (2008). Heart disease and stroke statistics—2008 update: A report from the American Heart Association statistics committee and stroke statistics subcommittee. *Circulation, 117*, e25–e146.

Schiff, G. D., Fung, S., Speroff, T., & McNutt, R. A. (2003). Decompensated heart failure: Symptoms, patterns of onset, and contributing factors. *American Journal of Medicine, 114*, 625–630.

Stevens, J. (1996). *Applied multivariate statistics for the social sciences* (2nd ed.). Mahwah, NJ: Lawrence Erlbaum.

Thomas, S., & Rich, M. W. (2007). Epidemiology, pathophysiology, and prognosis of heart failure in the elderly. *Clinics in Geriatric Medicine, 23*, 1–10.

Vinson, J. M., Rich, M. W., Sperry, J. C., Shah, A. S., & McNamara, T. (1990). Early readmission of elderly patients with congestive heart failure. *Journal of the American Geriatric Society, 38*, 1290–1295.

Woo, M. A., Macey, P. M., Fonarow, G. C., Hamilton, M. A., & Harper, R. M. (2003). Regional brain gray matter loss in heart failure. *Journal of Applied Physiology, 95*, 677–684.

YOUNG WOMEN WITH TYPE 1 DIABETES' MANAGEMENT OF TURNING POINTS AND TRANSITIONS

Bodil Rasmussen • Beverly O'Connell • Patricia Dunning • Helen Cox

The authors used grounded theory to explore and develop a substantive theory to explain how 20 young women with type 1 diabetes managed their lives when facing turning points and undergoing transitions. The women experienced a basic social problem: being in the grip of blood glucose levels (BGLs), which consisted of three categories: (a) the impact of being susceptible to fluctuating BGLs, (b) the responses of other people to the individual woman's diabetes, and (c) the impact of the individual women's diabetes on other people's lives. The women used a basic social process to overcome the basic social problem by creating stability, which involved using three interconnected subprocesses: forming meaningful relationships, enhancing attentiveness to blood glucose levels, and putting things in perspective. Insights into the processes and strategies used by the women have important implications for provision of care and service delivery.

▶ *Keywords:* type 1 diabetes; women; transitions; turning points; grounded theory.

Diabetes is a significant chronic illness and a growing global public health problem. It represents a considerable personal and public burden (Commonwealth of Australia, 1999). In Australia, diabetes was nominated as the fifth National Health Priority in 1998. Diabetes affects more than 940,000 Australians over the age of 25 years, and it is estimated that there will be 1.23 million Australians with diabetes by the year 2010 (Dunstan et. al., 2001). Diabetes is the seventh leading cause of death in Australia and contributes significantly to morbidity, disability, poor quality of life, and loss of potential years of life (Australian Institute of Health and Welfare, 2004).

Individuals living with diabetes and their families and friends face many challenges. Researchers have argued that people with chronic illness handle their conditions in individual ways, often in isolation and with little information (Glasgow, Fisher, Anderson, & La Greca, 1999). Likewise, ill people adopt innovative ways of managing their lives, which

Authors' Note: This research was supported by a scholarship provided by Deakin University, Victoria, Australia. The research team thanks the participants for their time and willingness to share their experiences and Reality Check, a support group for young people with diabetes.

are often unnoticed by health professionals and relatives and friends (Paterson, 2001; Paterson, Thorne, Crawford, & Tarko, 1999; Rayman & Ellison, 2000). Learning to help people with a chronic illness is challenging for health professionals as more people develop chronic illnesses (Glasgow, Hiss, Anderson, & Friedman, 2001).

Life transitional processes have been a research focus for some years; however, more clarity about the concept is needed (Anderson & Wolpert, 2004; Liddle, Carlson, & McKenna, 2003). Although the literature from different disciplines raises germane questions about life course perspectives, there is limited information linking people's experiences of chronic illness to their life trajectory, or to identify what signifies a turning point for individuals (Charmaz, 1991; Moen, 1997). A turning point is defined as an event that results in a fundamental shift in the meaning, purpose, or direction of a person's life and must include a self-reflective awareness of or insight into the significance of the change (Clausen, 1995). Turning points can sometimes be predictable, but are often unpredictable, uncontrollable, and linked to a specific context (Gotlib & Wheaton, 1997). They can provoke transitions and change people's life courses in positive and negative directions. Transitions accommodate both the continuities and discontinuities in the life processes of humans and are invariably related to change and development (Chick & Meleis, 1986). Transitions have many characteristics, including how they are experienced, their developmental and growth value, and their function in linking people to their social context (Wheaton, 1990).

The current study was based on the findings from a pilot study that explored the experiences of young adults with type 1 diabetes when they accessed health services in Victoria, Australia (Rasmussen, Wellard, & Nankervis, 2001). In Rasmussen et al.'s study, the participants recounted that the transition from adolescence into young adulthood was difficult and complex. Female participants identified the transition into motherhood as being particularly difficult and stressful. They described lack

of services to support decision making in family planning and perinatal care as well as the ongoing difficulties associated with being a parent with diabetes. However, there is a paucity of evidence to verify and describe the strategies young women with type 1 diabetes use to address issues related to transition into motherhood. The findings of the pilot study were the basis for focusing exclusively on women in the current study.

The aim of the current study was to develop a substantive theory of how women with type 1 diabetes managed turning points and transitions in their lives.

■ Design and Methods

Grounded theory was used to address the study objectives. This involves seeking social processes within a given phenomenon about which little is known (Charmaz, 1995).

SETTING AND SAMPLE

The study was conducted in Victoria, Australia. Participants were women who volunteered for the study in response to an advertisement in Diabetes Australia newsletters and local diabetes support group Web sites. Ethics approval was obtained from Deakin University.

The initial sample comprised 20 women, age range 20 to 36 years, mean 28 years, who volunteered and consented to participate in the study. They had lived with diabetes for between 4 and 28 years, mean 17 years. Twelve women had no family history of type 1 diabetes. Five women had immediate family members with diabetes, and 3 had remote family members with diabetes. All of the women spoke English but came from Indian, Italian, and Greek backgrounds.

SAMPLING PROCEDURE

Both purposeful and theoretical sampling procedureswere used. Initially, as a part of the purposeful sampling procedure, women who had diabetes since childhood (between 5 and 11 years) were invited to participate. This age group was selected because they had more opportunities to experience transitions while living with diabetes. A total of 20 initial interviews were conducted.

Data analysis revealed a need for further theoretical sampling to assist with the development of the theory (Charmaz, 2000). Therefore, individual interviews were conducted with women who had experienced childbirth, relatives of young women with type 1 diabetes, and health professionals involved in managing diabetes of women with type 1 diabetes. Ten interviews were conducted in the theoretical sampling phase of the study.

DATA COLLECTION

The main source of data was formal interviews with 20 women; however, other sources were used such as informal interviews, relevant documents, newspapers, and nonverbal communication.

The interviews lasted between 30 and 140 minutes and were conducted over a period of 1½ years. These interviews were audiotaped. Immediately after each interview, the researcher recorded her observations and thoughts in a nonprioritized manner.

DATA ANALYSIS

The recorded interviews were transcribed verbatim by the first author, examined line by line, and coded using open coding techniques, which is the first stage of developing a theory (Glaser & Strauss, 1967). Theoretical coding was applied simultaneously and involved connecting the developing categories through open coding with emerging relationships between categories and their properties (Glaser, 1992). Constant comparative analysis was used throughout the study.

In the current study, the core category was the main problem experienced by the women

and was identified as being in the grip of blood glucose levels (BGLs). The core category was identified as the basic social problem, because it accounted for the greatest variation in the data, was related to all of the other categories in the data, and accurately described the problem the women experienced during transitional periods. The basic social process the women used to overcome the basic social problem was labeled "creating stability".

Throughout the study, memos were written by the first author to guide her in identifying links between categories, compare and identify differences in the data, develop new questions, and test assumptions. O'Connell and Irurita (2000) described a visual data analysis procedure, which was used to schematize the linkages between categories and the developing theory.

RIGOR AND CREDIBILITY

It has been argued that grounded theory involves methodological procedures that promote rigor and credibility (Silverman, 2001). Constant comparative analysis presented the first author with opportunities to confirm or deny her interpretation of data. Applying theoretical sampling also provided a flexible mode to verify information from multiple sources. Credibility was enhanced in the study by lengthy contact with the women, which Lincoln and Guba (1985) referred to as prolonged engagement, and Charmaz (2000) described as "sustained involvement with research participants" (p. 519).

The substantive theory in the study was validated through peer review throughout the research process. For example, national and international conference presentations where abstracts were peer reviewed, and the findings were evaluated by clinical and academic colleagues. In addition, the women in the study checked the researcher's interpretation of the data. These strategies were all very important assuring credibility (Glaser & Strauss, 1967).

■ Findings

CORE PROBLEM: BEING IN THE GRIP OF BLOOD GLUCOSE LEVELS (BGLs)

The findings revealed that the women experienced a basic social problem, which emerged from the understandings and meanings the women made of their transitional experiences. Although the experiences were based on individual perceptions, and the individual woman managed and responded differently to these experiences, it was possible to explicate a story line about a central phenomenon around which other categories were integrated with linked strategies. The basic social problem was identified and described as being in the grip of blood glucose levels (BGLs). Three subcategories emerged from the data as having the most impact on the women's experiences of turning points and transitions: (a) the impact of being susceptible to fluctuating BGLs, (b) the responses of other people to the woman's diabetes, and (c) the impact of the woman's diabetes on other people's lives.

IMPACT OF BEING SUSCEPTIBLE TO FLUCTUATING BGLs

Fluctuating BGLs profoundly affected the women's daily activities, their emotional responses to diabetes, and their responses to other people in their social networks and health professionals. The women were aware of the potential impact of hypo- and hyperglycemia on their physical, psychological, and social health. The long-term impact of diabetes was the major concern for the women, who stated that the "forever" aspect made it very difficult for them to acknowledge and accept that they had diabetes. There was an important distinction between acknowledging having diabetes and accepting it. However, acknowledgment was the beginning of the journey of transition toward acceptance, which started at the time of diagnosis, which was a turning point. Some women acknowledged

that diabetes was present, but integrating it into their self-perception and identity was a complex and often long process. The women developed many ways of coping with diabetes shortly after being diagnosed, but the transition to accepting diabetes as a part of their identity took years for some women.

The transition from perceiving themselves to be a "healthy person" to "a person with diabetes" was a major one with complex and long-term implications.

The fear of developing diabetes complications greatly affected their lives and made the women feel vulnerable, and intensified the grip of BGLs. The women described their fear of diabetes complications, in particular when circumstances in their lives changed and when they went through life transitions, such as leaving home or becoming a student, worker, partner, or mother.

Fearing Complications. In general, the women did not discuss long-term complications, such as developing renal, cardiovascular, or other comorbidities. Their primary fears related to four areas: (a) having an acute episode of ketoacidosis, (b) having a hypoglycemic episode, (c) developing eye complications, (d) and having complications during pregnancy.

Of the four areas, hypoglycemic episodes, or fear of developing hypoglycemia, had the most significant impact on the women's daily lives, in particular when imbalances in their blood glucose levels required acute hospitalization. The experience of being unconscious and waking up in a hospital, sometimes in intensive units, was referred to as a "wake-up call" or turning point, because it made the women realize they had sole responsibility for their diabetes management. These experiences made some women reconsider their diabetes management; for other women, it was the beginning of a transition in their lives. The women found it was extremely difficult to balance their social needs with the demands of their diabetes regimens during transitions.

> I felt scared, because I normally have good control, but during the first year of University, I just wanted to have fun. I'm not saying it is right to

live badly with that sort of behaviours, but I think that has to be factored in [when considering transition and diabetes].

Fluctuating BGLs and Entering the Workforce. The transition into the workforce raised other prominent issues for the women in terms of adjusting fluctuating BGLs. The women experienced difficulties trying to adjust their insulin requirements to accommodate their new lifestyles, as they were often unable to eat or inject when necessary because of unpredictable work schedules, not knowing how long a meeting would take, or not knowing when they would to be able to take a break and eat.

> It was the first job interview I had ever gone for, and thank goodness, I came straight out and said that I had type 1[diabetes] and no, no that will not a problem. They wanted 9-to-9 shifts and I actually ended up having a hypo. I ended up passing out behind the counter and knocking my head on the glass counter.

The women acted differently in each work situation, but the decision whether to disclose their diabetes was difficult for all of the women. The underlying factor that influenced disclosure was fear of unpredictable hypoglycemia, which often triggered the decision to disclose diabetes to help them feel safe at work.

Fluctuating BGLs During Pregnancy and in Transition to Motherhood. Planning and going through pregnancy made the grip of BGLs particularly tight. The women had to be more vigilant in their diabetes management. They attempted to keep their BGLs within the recommended level, which was lower than their usual blood glucose level and increased the potential for hypoglycemia. The women were anxious about the impact diabetes could have on their and their babies' health. The women often felt their previous knowledge of and skills in managing diabetes were inadequate to cope with "hypos" during pregnancy.

The women who had experienced the transition into motherhood found it was particularly complex because of the impact

of diabetes on their bodies and their lives in general. The women's fear of hypos increased dramatically because of the hormonal changes associated with pregnancy and lactation. Their fears became reality when they had hypos, some for the first time in their lives. Often these hypos occurred at unusual times, for example, overnight or when they least expected it. The women struggled to balance diabetes management, their own needs, and the needs of their babies. The feeling of being in the grip of BGLs was particularly tight during this transition.

RESPONSES OF OTHER PEOPLE TO THE INDIVIDUAL WOMAN'S DIABETES

The responses and reactions of other people to the woman's diabetes had a profound impact on their sense of being in control of their lives at the time of diagnosis, and had an ongoing and long-lasting effect on their lives. The responses and reactions from people in the women's social networks and health professionals affected how tightly or loosely the women felt the grip of BGLs. When the women felt the responses and reactions were negative, the grip was tight and exacerbated their sense of losing control of their diabetes and their lives in general.

Social Network. The women were not able to control the negative or unexpected responses of other people to their diabetes, which made them feel emotionally vulnerable, especially in the context of family and school communities and when people exhibited misconceptions and lack of understanding diabetes, especially differences between type 1 and type 2 diabetes.

Lack of knowledge and understanding about diabetes was consistently displayed in the wider community, particularly when people confused type 1 and type 2 diabetes. The confusion between the two types of diabetes had a major impact on the women and caused frustration, anger, and feelings of not being understood or of being judged by other people.

> They say diabetes and there are such misconceptions of the two types of diabetes. People often do not even realise that type 2 is a completely different thing or how you get type 1 or how you get type 2 and why you get it. It is very frustrating.

Health Professionals. The women realized the importance of having a good relationship with health professionals, especially during transitional periods, and tried to maintain good relationships. One of the most prominent issues the women raised was that health professionals tended to focus on their BGLs rather than on their personal issues. This exacerbated the women's sense of being in the grip of BGLs, especially when blood glucose monitoring dominated their interactions with health professional, and sometimes made them reluctant to continue consulting health professionals.

> I don't see a dietitian or anyone like that anymore. It was just always pointless. They did not really seem to be that concerned about how I was. They just wanted to look at my HbA1c. They just wanted to see the test result. If I was in what was considered as good control [blood glucose result], which is under nine, then "Good, see you later."

The women felt they were being judged on the basis of their blood glucose results. Indeed, a "bad girl" or "good girl" dichotomy emerged from the data. As one woman said, "There is definitely a good-bad girl association, you know, if your blood glucoses are good you are good, and if your glucoses are bad, you are bad. There is kind of stigma attached to people [with diabetes]."

Health professionals' comments about and constant gaze on the BGLs became deeply embedded in the women's mind-set and contributed to their perception of themselves as being either a "bad" girl or "good" girl. There was a shift from being "seen" as a bad girl by others "to feeling" they "were" bad girls, which exacerbated feelings of guilt if the women did not comply with their diabetes regimen.

IMPACT OF THE INDIVIDUAL WOMAN'S DIABETES ON OTHER PEOPLE'S LIVES

Diabetes affected other people's lives when the women went through transitions, because the changes occurring at these times also affected people in their social networks. The level of dependency had to be renegotiated with their social support people, in particular mothers, husbands, or partners. The women felt they were a burden to their families, which exacerbated the grip of BGLs. As one woman said, "I felt I was just being a burden to my husband and to my family and everybody else. That was really difficult for me to overcome."

Generally, the women perceived coping with diabetes was "a big ask" and identified a lack of support from health services for their partners. The women indicated their partners needed opportunities to share their experiences with other partners in similar situations. They said diabetes highlighted their dependence on their partners when they became mothers, and they found this dependency burdensome and frustrating.

The data analysis confirmed family members also felt they were in the grip of BGLs because of the impact diabetes had on their lives, and transitional times were particularly difficult for them too.

CREATING STABILITY: A BASIC SOCIAL PROCESS

The consequences of being in the grip of BGLs were complex, and the women applied interrelated processes to overcome the grip of BGLs. Certain patterns could be discerned in the processes and were identified as the basic social and psychological process labeled Creating Stability, which involved three interconnected subprocesses that tended to occur simultaneously: forming meaningful relationships; enhancing attentiveness to blood glucose levels (BGLs); and putting things in perspective.

Forming Meaningful Relationships. All of the women described personal interactions and social support as important factors that influenced how they stabilized their lives with diabetes. They reassessed their personal relationships with people in their social networks during transitional periods to overcome their sense of isolation, low self-esteem, and uncertainty.

Achieving a sense of belonging was a major aspect of creating stability. Being with other people with diabetes enhanced the women's self-confidence and was a major factor in their ability to achieve a sense of belonging, especially when the group consisted of people of their own age. Some of the women explained how, when they were young, they met other children at diabetes camps, which they felt contributed to their having a sense of belonging.

> I participated in camps as a child, which was a great way of growing up with peers and knowing that I wasn't all alone, because today when I mix with diabetes support people, some people say, oh, look I haven't known one other person with diabetes in my whole life.

One consistent source of frustration, and a dimension of being in the grip of BGLs, was other people's ignorance about diabetes. The women usually responded by "cutting them out" of their networks, for example, when people became "food" police: "I can say, 'Look, I can have it [chocolate cake], leave me alone'. I can do this, leave me alone, and I will cut them out. I tend to do it that way." By selectively drawing on supportive people, the women felt they had a higher degree of control, which enhanced stability in their lives.

The women needed to trust other people and sometimes to maintain anonymity to manage transitions well. Using Web sites and e-mails was a way of obtaining information anonymously and forming new, meaningful relationships when appropriate during transitions. The women's need for information constantly changed, and Web sites and e-mails were able to accommodate these changing needs quickly. The women indicated that sensitive issues, such as discriminatory behaviors in workplaces due to diabetes, stigma, contra-ception, and sexual issues, were easier to discuss anonymously.

Enhancing Attentiveness to Blood Glucose Levels. The women said they needed to feel prepared for unexpected events and situations by knowing how to manage their diabetes and recognize and respond to their body reactions quickly. For example, one woman said, "I guess relating it [uncertainty] to the diabetes thing, what do I know, do I need to take insulin with me, so I need to take it with me. Do I need to carry food?"

Learning to read body clues was generally the first measure the women took when taking control of their BGLs.

> You have got to know your own body and how different things affect it and how, you know, what to do to prevent the high sugar levels. Yes, vigilance, you got to, because some people when they exercise they go hypo, some people go high because of the adrenalin, you know.

The women experienced increased well-being when they had good blood glucose control. Improved well-being was important to their ongoing motivation and made them feel more assertive in getting what they needed to stay in control. One assertive action was to apply up-to-date medical technology to their diabetes management, for example, by using insulin pumps. The pumps made the women's day-to-day lives easier, reduced their fear of fluctuating BGLs, and increased their sense of control. The women said that reaching a stage where they were in full control was very difficult. Nevertheless, they explained, they could achieve a sense of balance and tried to create stability by putting things in perspective.

Putting Things in Perspective. The main difficulties the women experienced during transitions were associated with the demands of their new social roles that were often imposed by changes and the demands of diabetes management. Putting things in perspective helped the women achieve balance in their lives.

> Just do not let things stress you out too much. Try to keep it in perspective and try to maintain

balance. You might be having a real bad day with your diabetes, but you sort of learn to keep it in perspective. It is only a day and the next day will be a different day.

The women explained that putting things in perspective helped them accept life with diabetes. Accepting diabetes was a difficult journey for some women because it involved changing their self-perception, which became a part of the strategy of accepting diabetes and moving on. For example, one woman said, "That is the thing, it is when I decide and not when someone else, parents or friends or doctors, tell me to do something. It is when I decide for myself, that it is time for change."

The importance of having role models who managed diabetes very well, for example by not letting diabetes get in the way of their aspirations and goals in life, was a repeated theme raised by the women. The women said role models influenced how they perceived their opportunities and achievements, and helped them to put their difficulties into perspective.

I guess, the other people who had a big impact were the diabetic leaders on the camps—I looked up to them. I think, camp leaders are real positive role models. It is good to look up to someone who says, "I turned out all right," and this person, who could be a doctor, a nurse or a scientist or recreation team leader, and then say, "I can do that as well."

The women regarded their transitions as evaluation processes that enabled them to reevaluate their lives, including their life aims, goals, priorities, and perspectives. Diabetes affected the women's quality of life in different ways. The basic social problem described how some women felt diabetes reduced their quality of life. However, this study clearly indicates that the women's perceived quality of life was strongly associated with their sense of being in control of diabetes. The higher the women's perception of control was, the higher they rated their quality of life. According to one woman, "The pump definitely increased my quality of life. I have not had complications, but psychologically the pump is what has truly affected and changed my life for the better." Viewing diabetes in a more positive

light was clearly connected to hope of a cure and better treatment. The majority of the women placed great hope in stem cell and islet cell transplantations. One women moved interstate to be closer to "'where things happen' in diabetes research."

Melbourne is probably a good place to be when looking for cures and things. They are doing a lot of research and stem cell stuff. You feel, when you are in a country town and certainly when I was in [name of small town in NSW], I felt much, much further away from any talk about cures.

Hoping for a cure affected how the women created stability by applying other strategies to help them on a day-to-day basis, for example comparing diabetes to other illnesses and people they considered to be "worse off" than they, such as those with asthma, other chronic illnesses, or terminal illnesses. The women used the comparative strategy as a general coping mechanism that helped them put things in perspective and create stability.

CONSEQUENCES OF BEING IN THE GRIP OF BLOOD GLUCOSE LEVELS

There were many consequences of being in the grip of diabetes. The worst of these was when the women felt stuck or unable to adapt to changes associated with transitions. Despite the women's ability to identify opportunities to change their behavior, they still found it difficult. One woman said, "I could do things differently but for some reasons I just feel stuck."

Feeling stuck or unable to adapt to transitional changes was not always the outcome of being in the grip of BGLs. In general, the women said that they experienced different levels of control, which affected their emotions, their lives, their and health. When the women felt they had little control, they also felt a high level of vulnerability, uncertainty, and guilt.

The women explained that transitions caused instability in their lives. The women's sense of being unstable deeply affected other people in their social networks. Family members also experienced high levels of guilt, uncertainty, and the grip of BGLs. They could not escape diabetes either and also focused on the women's BGLs, particularly strongly during transitions.

The women explained that being in the grip of BGLs was reduced when they felt supported by people in their social networks. Turning points and transitions made the women appreciate and make better use of the resources and support around them. When social support was perceived to be good, the women experienced growing confidence and self-worth, which helped them to develop new skills and knowledge.

■ Discussion

In this study, transition represented a passage from one life phase to another, which embraced the elements of a process that consisted of change, perception, passage of time, and outcomes of transitions. The women referred to turning points, such as losing a job or getting divorced, as life events that caused instability in their lives. Some of the women's definitions concur in the literature, which describe life events in terms of crises (Erikson, 1968). Specifically related to women with chronic illnesses, some researchers have described transitions as processes or movements that occur in a nonlinear, cyclical way and potentially recur throughout the course of life (Ellison & Rayman, 1998; Kralik, 2002; Rayman & Ellison, 2004). The women in the current study also identified transition (e.g., becoming an adult or a mother) from a life course perspective.

The substantive theory provides unique insight into how the ever-present grip of BGLs made the management of turning points and transitions a complex social and psychological process in which the women constantly tried to stabilize their lives. The metaphor of being in the grip of BGLs illustrates the physical, psychological, and social impact of type 1 diabetes on young women. As a consequence of experiencing transitions, the women felt their lives were unbalanced, which made them feel vulnerable. Other researchers have established

that people with diabetes have a high sense of vulnerability (Weiss & Hutchinson, 2000), particularly during life course transitions (Seiffge- Krenke, 2001). In the current study, "stability" during transitions meant taking control and maintaining stable BGLs in changing social and psychological environments. However, to achieve stability, it was necessary for the women to enhance attention to BGLs, because stable BGLs allow them to feel more positive about their diabetes management. Paterson (2001) referred to this situation as one of the paradoxes in diabetes management, because "illnesses require attention in order not to have to pay attention to it" (p. 24) and fostering a shift in people's perception of a threat to control. The individual's perception of reality, not the reality itself, is the essence of how people respond (Paterson, 2001). As the personal and social context changes, people's perspectives shift in the degree to which illness is in the foreground or background of their reality. It is an ongoing, continuously shifting process in which people experience a complex dialectic between themselves and their world that contains elements of both illness and wellness. People's experience is depicted as an ever-changing perspective about illness that enables them to make sense of their experiences (Paterson, 2003).

During transitions, women with type 1 diabetes felt there was a constant gaze on their BGLs, which they found oppressive. It both helped and hindered successful transitions. The constant gaze was hindering when the women felt people's attention to their BGLs was judgmental, disrespectful, and ignorant. In contrast, when the women felt valued and involved in decisions about their care and treatment, they felt encouraged to disclose their concerns. The findings challenge health professionals to review their attitudes toward patients. Health professionals can help by paying attending to attributes of expertise in everyday diabetes management (Paterson & Thorne, 2000a; Thorne, Nyhlin, & Paterson, 2000), in particular, how people negotiate their assessment of risks, make comparative analysis of their previous experiences, seek explanations for changing in their BGLs, make choice of actions, and evaluate their decisions (Paterson & Thorne, 2000b).

The women found that disclosing their diabetes was particularly difficult in their work environment. They feared stigmatization and discrimination if they disclosed. If they did not disclose, on the other hand, they feared they would be blamed for "telling a lie" should their diabetes become apparent. They felt more at risk by nondisclosure, because their colleagues might not be able to assist them should they need it: for example, if they developed a "hypo."

The decision to disclose diabetes was a major source of internal conflict, which sometimes took years for people with diabetes to resolve (Hernandez, 1996). Charmaz (1991) noted that individuals with chronic illness attempt to control stigma by being highly selective about the individuals to whom they reveal their condition and rely on them to withhold the information from others. These measures also emerged in the current study. In some circumstances, disclosure increased support from selected individuals or groups (Charmaz, 1991; Joachim & Acorn, 2000). However, trying to pass as "normal" caused stress, because the individual worried about being found out as "calculated cheating" or "caught in a lie" (Thorne, Paterson, & Russell, 2003, p. 1345). There is a risk of being rejected and stigmatized, of having difficulty handling the responses of others, and of losing control (Charmaz, 1991). The current study further highlighted the importance of maintaining autonomy and staying anonymous about diabetes until the women chose to disclose it.

The concept of autonomy has been widely explored and is an important aspect of coping with diabetes. However, the association between autonomy and anonymity in the process of how young people with type 1 diabetes establish their networks has not been extensively explored, and neither has young people's perceptions of the impact of the responses of health professionals. Health professionals need to consider the triad

between autonomy, anonymity, and how their actions and responses affect young people with diabetes.

Forming meaningful relationships with people in their social networks, including health professionals, was essential to the women's management of transitions. Certain qualities were vital to forming meaningful relationships, especially with health professionals. The women sought health professionals who showed respect, empathy, recognition, autonomy, and, an important point, nonjudgmental attitudes. The study demonstrates that when the women felt supported and engaged in meaningful relationships, they were capable of and resourceful in managing diabetes during transitions. The values of honesty, trust, and openness were an integral part of useful communication with health professionals. When the women perceived health professional's attitudes to be judgmental, lacking in genuine concern for their well-being, and focused only on the BGLs rather than on the women's concerns, they chose not to listen to their health professional's advice or consult them again.

The current study indicates that health professionals need a higher degree of awareness of the impact their attitudes have on young adults with diabetes. Health professionals must be sensitive to the powerful influences their values and attitudes have on the self management decisions their patients make (Thorne, Nyhlin, et al., 2000). The current study also illuminated that during transitions, young women feel it is important to involve family members in management, particularly during pregnancy and early motherhood, when the women felt torn in two directions between their babies' needs and the requirement of their diabetes regimens. Managing motherhood and diabetes is a balancing act (Poirier-Solomon, 2002) and increased the women's dependence on their partners and mothers.

It was critical to the management of transitions that simultaneous to forming meaningful relationships, the women had to take control of their fluctuating BGLs. Unpredictable experiences, such as hypo- or hyperglycemia, called forth unknown and unused resources essential for generating positive ways of responding and adapting to new situations (Antonovsky, 1987). Responding to new situations in positive ways depends on the resources under direct individual control and the resources accessible from family, friends, or the community (Rayman & Ellison, 2004; Schlossberg, Waters, & Goodman, 1995). Manageability largely depends on people's experiencing a practical and physical sense of self empowerment in coping with their biology and threats to their health (Sanden-Eriksson, 2000). Manageability and self-empowerment also emerged in the current study, evidenced by the women's enhanced attentiveness to body clues and controlling their BGLs by using medical technology, such as modern blood glucose meters and insulin pumps.

In Ellison and Rayman's (1998) study among women with type 2 diabetes, engagement and ability to adjust diabetes management helped the participants to move on in the process where the diabetes was just a part of the life, not the whole life. Furthermore, the ability to reframe problems with a positive perspective required transformation (Paterson, 2001) and integration (Hernandez, 1996) of oneself in relation to diabetes management.

In this study, the women tried to remain positive and indicated that "things could have been worse." Comparative strategies helped the women put things in perspective and sustain or gain stability in their lives after turning points and during transitions. Comparing their situation with others was part of the normalization process the women used to help them to accept diabetes and move on. Making comparisons is a way of positioning oneself in terms of time, space, and relationship to others, and helps the individual adjust to his or her chronic illness (Dewar & Lee, 2000; Meleis, Sawyer, Im, Messias, & Schumacher, 2000). To feel integrated into the world again and included, and to reduce feelings of isolation, individuals must learn to live with new limits and find new ways to accommodate the transitional changes. In addition, the women in the current study indicated that positive role models gave them hope and were integral to the adjustment process.

PRACTICE IMPLICATIONS AND FURTHER RESEARCH

The substantive theory developed in this study has the potential to be used in future studies considering life transitions and decision-making situations that chronically ill people encounter, including people with asthma and epilepsy.

There is a need to explore further how health professionals can evaluate their communication strategies and be flexible in their communication with young people with type 1 diabetes. A shared decision making and understanding of attributes of expertise in everyday diabetes management process that develops an equal, respectful, and productive relationship between health professionals and women with diabetes needs to be adopted. Particular attention needs to be paid to the good girl–bad girl association. The study indicates that diabetes camps helped the women and their families cope with diabetes, and so health professionals need to support and encourage families to attend diabetes camps.

Health professionals and health policy makers need to take up the challenge to put more emphasis on the social and psychological issues associated with disclosing diabetes, especially in the context of stigma and discrimination in workplaces. The differences between type 1 and type 2 diabetes, and the impact the lack of understanding about the differences can have on young women with type 1 diabetes and their families, is also important and worth exploring in more depth. It is particularly important to support current and potential employers of young people with diabetes to enhance employers' understanding of diabetes and reduce discrimination in workplaces.

It is necessary to involve individuals with diabetes, and people in their social networks, in health service planning and resource allocation so their experiences and specific needs can be utilized to benefit young women with diabetes and to guide health professionals.

Bodil Rasmussen, PhD., is a lecturer at Deakin University, School of Nursing, Melbourne Campus, Burwood, Victoria, Australia.
Beverly O'Connell, PhD, is a professor at Southern Health and Deakin University, Melbourne, Victoria, Australia.
Patricia Dunning, PhD, is a professor at Deakin University, Melbourne, Victoria, Australia.
Helen Cox, PhD, is an emeritus professor at Deakin University, Melbourne, Victoria, Australia.

REFERENCES

Anderson, B. J., & Wolpert, H. A. (2004) A developmental perspective on the challenge of diabetes education and care during the young adult period. *Patient Education and Counseling, 53,* 347–352.

Antonovsky, A. (1987). *Unraveling the mystery of health: How people manage to stay well.* San Francisco: Jossey-Bass.

Australian Institute of Health and Welfare. (2004). *Australia's health 2004.* Canberra, Australia: Author.

Charmaz, K. (1991). *Good days, bad days: The self in chronic illness and time.* New Brunswick, NJ: Rutgers University Press.

Charmaz, K. (1995). Grounded theory. In J. A. Smith, R. Harré, & L. Van Langenhove (Eds.), *Rethinking methods in psychology* (pp. 27–49). London: Sage.

Charmaz, K. (2000). Grounded theory: Objectivist and constructivist methods. In N. K. Denzin & Y. Lincoln (Eds.), *Handbook in qualitative research* (2nd ed., pp. 509–535). Thousand Oaks, CA: Sage.

Chick, N., & Meleis, A. I. (1986). Transitions: A nursing concern. In P. Chinn (Ed.), *Nursing research methodology: Issues and implementation* (pp. 237–257). Rockville, MD: Aspen.

Clausen, J. A. (1995). Gender, contexts, and turning points in adults' lives. In P. Moen, G. H. Elder, & K. Luscher (Eds.), *Examining lives in context: Perspectives on the ecology of human development* (pp. 365–389). Washington, DC: American Psychological Association.

Commonwealth of Australia. (1999). *National diabetes strategy 2000–2004* (Australian Health Ministers' Conference). Canberra, Australia: Commonwealth Department of Health and Aged Care.

Dewar, A., & Lee, E. A. (2000). Bearing illness and injury. *Western Journal of Nursing Research, 22*(8), 912–926.

Dunstan, D, Zimmet, P., Welborn, T., Sieree, R. Armstrong, T., Atkins. R., et al. (2001). *Diabesity and associated disorders in Australia—2000: The accelerating epidemic.* Melbourne, Australia: International Diabetes Institute.

Lincoln, Y., & Guba, E. G. (1985). *Naturalistic inquiry.* Beverly Hills, CA: Sage.

Ellison, G., & Rayman, K. M. (1998) Exemplars' experiences of self-managing type 2 diabetes. *Diabetes Educator, 24,* 325–330. Erikson, E. (1968). *Identity: Youth and crisis.* New York: W. W. Norton.

Glaser, B. G. (1992). *Basics of grounded theory analysis.* Mill Valley, CA: Sociology Press.

Glaser, B. G., & Strauss, A. (1967). *The discovery of grounded theory.* Chicago: Aldine.

Glasgow, R. E., Fisher, E. B., Anderson, B. J., & La Greca, A. M. (1999). Behavioral science in diabetes: Contributions and opportunities. *Diabetes Care, 22*(5), 832–843.

Glasgow, R. E., Hiss, R. G., Anderson, R., & Friedman, N. M. (2001). Report of the health care delivery work group: Behavioral research related to the establishment of a chronic disease model for diabetes care. *Diabetes Care, 24*(1), 124–129.

Gotlib, I. H., & Wheaton, B. (1997). *Stress and adversity over the life course: Trajectories and turning points.* Cambridge, UK: Cambridge University Press.

Hernandez, C. A. (1996). Integration: The experience of living with insulin-dependent diabetes. *Canadian Journal of Nursing Research, 28,* 37–56.

Joachim, G., & Acorn, S. (2000). Living with chronic illness: The interface of stigma and normalization. *Canadian Journal of Nursing Research, 32*(3), 37–48.

Kralik, D. (2002). The quest for ordinariness: Transition experienced by midlife women living with chronic illness. *Journal of Advanced Nursing, 39,* 146–154.

Liddle, J., Carlson, G., & McKenna, K. (2004). Using a matrix in life transition research. *Qualitative Health Research, 14,* 1396–1417.

Meleis, A. I., Sawyer, L. M., Im, E., Messias, D. K., & Schumacher, K. (2000). Experiencing transitions: An emerging middle-range theory. *Advanced Nursing Science, 23*(1), 12–28.

Moen, P. (1997). Women's role and resilience: Trajectories of advantage and turning points? In I. H. Gotlib & B. Wheaton (Eds.), *Stress and adversity over the life course: Trajectories and turning points* (pp. 133–158). Cambridge, UK: Cambridge University Press.

O'Connell, B. O., & Irurita, V. (2000). Facilitating the process of theory development by creating visual data analysis trail. *Graduate Research in Nursing On-line Journals, 2*(1). Retrieved 23 October, 2003, from http://www.graduateresearch.com

Paterson, B. L. (2001). The shifting perspectives model of chronic illness. *Journal of Nursing Scholarship, 3*(1), 21–26.

Paterson, B. (2003). The koala has claws: Applications of the shifting perspectives model in research of chronic illness. *Qualitative Health Research, 13,* 987–994.

Paterson, B. L., & Thorne, S. E. (2000a). Developmental evolution of expertise in diabetes self-management. *Clinical Nursing Research, 4,* 402–419.

Paterson, B. L., & Thorne, S. E. (2000b) Expert decision making in relation to unanticipated blood glucose levels. *Research in Nursing & Health, 23*(2), 47–57.

Paterson, B. L., Thorne, S. E., Crawford, J., & Tarko, M. (1999). Living with diabetes as a transformational experience. *Qualitative Health Research, 9,* 786–803.

Poirier-Solomon, L. (2002). A balancing act: Managing motherhood and diabetes (women's health exchange). *Diabetes Forecast, 55*(11), 46–49.

Rasmussen, B., Wellard, S., & Nankervis, A. (2001). Consumer issues in navigating health care services for type 1 diabetes. *Journal of Clinical Nursing, 10,* 628–634.

Rayman, K. M., & Ellison, G. C. (2000). The patient perspective as an integral part of diabetes disease management. *Disease Management Health Outcomes, 1,* 5–12.

Rayman, K. M., & Ellison, G. C. (2004). Home alone: The experience of women with type 2 diabetes who are new to intensive control. *Health Care for Women International, 25,* 900–915.

Sanden-Erikson, B. (2000). Coping with type-2 diabetes: The role of sense of coherence compared with active management. *Journal of Advanced Nursing, 31*(6), 1393–1397.

Schlossberg, N. K., Waters, E. B., & Goodman, J. (1995). *Counseling adults in transition: Linking practice with theory* (2nd ed.). New York: Springer.

Seiffge-Krenke, I. (2001). *Diabetic adolescents and their families: Stress, coping, and adaptation.* Cambridge, UK: Cambridge University Press.

Silverman, D. (2001). *Interpreting qualitative data: Methods for analysing talk, text and interaction* (2nd ed.). London: Sage.

Thorne, S. E., Nyhlin, K. T., & Paterson, B. L. (2000). Attitudes towards patient expertise in chronic illness. *International Journal of Nursing Studies, 37*(4), 303–311.

Thorne, S. E., Paterson, B., & Russell, C. (2003). The structure of everyday self-care decision making in chronic illness. *Qualitative Health Research, 13*(10), 1337–1352.

Weiss, J., & Hutchinson, S. A. (2000). Warnings about vulnerability in clients with diabetes and hypertension. *Qualitative Health Research, 10,* 521–537.

Wheaton, B. (1990). Life transitions, role histories, and mental health. *American Sociological Review, 55,* 209–223.

RANDOMIZED CONTROLLED TRIAL OF A PSYCHOEDUCATION PROGRAM FOR THE SELF-MANAGEMENT OF CHRONIC CARDIAC PAIN

Michael H. McGillion • Judy Watt-Watson • Bonnie Stevens • Sandra M. LeFort • Peter Coyte • Anthony Graham

▶ **Abstract:** Cardiac pain arising from chronic stable angina (CSA) is a cardinal symptom of coronary artery disease and has a major negative impact on health-related quality of life (HRQL), including pain, poor general health status, and inability to self-manage. Current secondary prevention approaches lack adequate scope to address CSA as a multidimensional ischemic and persistent pain problem. This trial evaluated the impact of a low-cost six-week angina psychoeducation program, entitled The Chronic Angina Self-Management Program (CASMP), on HRQL, self-efficacy, and resourcefulness to self-manage anginal pain. One hundred thirty participants were randomized to the CASMP or three-month wait-list usual care; 117 completed the study. Measures were taken at baseline and three months. General HRQL was measured using the Medical Outcomes Study 36-Item Short Form and the disease-specific Seattle Angina Questionnaire (SAQ). Self-efficacy and resourcefulness were measured using the Self-Efficacy Scale and the Self-Control Schedule, respectively. The mean age of participants was 68 years, 80% were male. Analysis of variance of change scores yielded significant improvements in treatment group physical functioning [F = 11.75(1,114), P < 0.001] and general health [F = 10.94(1,114), P = 0.001] aspects of generic HRQL. Angina frequency [F = 5.57(1,115), P = 0.02], angina stability [F = 7.37(1,115), P = 0.001], and self-efficacy to manage disease [F = 8.45(1,115), P = 0.004] were also significantly improved at three months. The CASMP did not impact resourcefulness. These data indicate that the CASMP was effective for improving physical functioning, general health, anginal pain symptoms, and self-efficacy to manage pain at three months and provide a basis for long-term evaluation of the program.

▶ This trial was made possible in part by a Canadian Institutes of Health Research Fellowship (No. 452939) and a University of Toronto Centre for the Study of Pain Clinician-Scientist Fellowship.

▶ Portions of the CASMP first appeared in or are derived from the Chronic Disease Self-Management Program Leader's Master Trainer's Guide (1999). Those portions are Copyright 1999, Stanford University.

▶ **Key Words:** Chronic stable angina · self-management · randomized controlled trial · health-related quality of life

■ Introduction

Cardiac pain arising from chronic stable angina (CSA) pectoris is a cardinal symptom of coronary artery disease (CAD), characterized by pain or discomfort in the chest, shoulder, back, arm, or jaw.[1] CSA is a widespread clinical problem with a well-documented, major negative impact on health-related quality of life (HRQL), including pain, poor general health status, impaired role functioning, activity restriction, and reduced ability for self-care.[2-14] Limitations in current surveillance systems worldwide have precluded the examination of CSA prevalence in most countries. Available prevalence data estimate CSA prevalence at 6,500,000 (1999–2002) in the United States,[1] and 28/1000 men and 25/1000 women (April 2001–March 2002) in Scotland.[15] With the growing global burden of angina and CAD, nongovernmental organizations in Canada, the United States, and the United Kingdom have stressed the need for developments in secondary prevention strategies.[1,16,17] Current secondary prevention models largely target postacute cardiac event and/or coronary artery bypass patients and, depending on region, can be inaccessible to those with chronic symptoms.[18,19] Consequently, the vast majority of those with CSA and other CAD-related symptoms must manage on their own in the community. Moreover, these models focus predominantly on conventional CAD risk-factor modification to enhance myocardial conditioning and reduce ischemic threshold. However, cumulative basic science and clinical evidence point to the variability of cardiac pain perception for CSA patients, wherein pain can occur in the absence of myocardial ischemia, and conversely, ischemic episodes can be painless.[20-32] Given few alternatives, CSA patients revisit their local emergency departments when uncertain about how to manage their pain.[33,34] There is a critical need for a secondary prevention strategy with adequate scope and complexity to address CSA as a multidimensional ischemic and persistent pain problem, and to help CSA patients learn pain self-management strategies.[33]

Evidence from well-designed randomized controlled trials has demonstrated the effectiveness of psychoeducation for improving the self-management skills, HRQL, self-efficacy, and/or resourcefulness of persons with other chronic pains including arthritis and chronic noncancer pain.[35-37] Psychoeducation interventions are multimodal, self-help treatment packages that use information and cognitive-behavioral strategies to achieve changes in knowledge and behavior for effective disease self-management.[38] To date, the effectiveness of psychoeducation for enhancing CSA self-management is inconclusive.[39] Although a few small trials over the last decade have demonstrated positive effects to some degree related to pain frequency, nitrate use, and stress,[40-43] numerous methodological problems, particularly inadequate power and the lack of a standard intervention approach, have precluded the generalization of findings.[39] Moreover, more recent and robust psychoeducation trial research has been limited to patients with newly diagnosed angina.[44] Therefore, the purpose of this study was to evaluate the effectiveness of a standardized psychoeducation program, entitled the Chronic Angina Self-Management Program (CASMP), for improving the HRQL, self-efficacy, and resourcefulness of CSA patients.

■ Methods

STUDY DESIGN

This study was a randomized controlled trial. On completion of demographic and baseline measures, participants were randomly allocated to either 1) the six-week CASMP group or 2) the three-month wait-list control group; posttest study outcomes were evaluated at three months from baseline. A short-term follow-up period was chosen for this study as it was the inaugural test of the effectiveness of the CASMP and the basis for a future larger-scale trial, with long-term follow-up. Ethical approval for the study was received from a university in central Canada and three university-affiliated teaching hospitals.

STUDY POPULATION AND PROCEDURE

This study was conducted in central Canada over an 18-month period. The target population was CSA patients living in the community. Participants had a confirmed medical diagnosis of CAD, CSA for at least six months and were able to speak, read, and understand English. Individuals were excluded if they had suffered a myocardial infarction and/or undergone a coronary artery bypass graft in the last six months, had Canadian Cardiovascular Society (CCS) Class IV angina[45] and/or a major cognitive disorder. Participants were recruited from three university-affiliated teaching hospitals with large cardiac outpatient programs, allowing for timely subject referral. Three recruitment strategies found to be effective in prior psychoeducation trials with community-based samples were used.[36,37,46,47] First, clinicians at designated hospital recruitment sites identified eligible patients in the clinic setting. Second, study information was made available in participating clinicians' offices and hospital recruitment site newsletters. Third, the study was advertised in community newspapers.

Participant eligibility was initially assessed by a research assistant (RA) via telephone. Willing participants were then interviewed by the RA on-site to confirm eligibility and obtain informed consent. Demographic and baseline measures were completed on-site and participants were randomly allocated to either the six-week CASMP group, or the three-month wait-list control group. Randomization was centrally controlled using a university-based tamper-proof, computerized randomization service. Those randomized to the six-week intervention group were invited to participate in the next available program, whereas those randomized to usual care were told that they were in the three-month wait-list control group.

Usual care consisted of all nursing, medical, and emergency care services as needed; those allocated to the control group did not receive the CASMP during the study period.

Participants were contacted by the RA to schedule posttest data collection at three months from baseline. Assiduous follow-up procedures were used to minimize attrition; participants received up to three telephone calls and a follow-up letter regarding collection of their three-month follow-up data. Participants' completion of all study questionnaires was invigilated by the RA blinded to group allocation. Blinding was preserved by informing participants that their questions would be answered after they completed the questionnaire booklet and that a letter explaining their part in the next phase of the project was forthcoming. Those in the wait-list control group were offered entry into the next available CASMP once posttest measures were completed.

INTERVENTION

The CASMP is a standardized psychoeducation program given in two-hour sessions weekly, over a six-week period. The goal of the CASMP is to improve HRQL by increasing patients' day-to-day angina self-management skills. The CASMP is an adaptation of Lorig et al.'s Chronic Disease Self-Management Program (CDSMP, © 1999 Stanford University).[47–50] In 2004, McGillion et al. conducted a preliminary study to identify CSA patients' specific pain-related concerns and self-management learning needs.[33] With permission, the results of this study were used to adapt the CDSMP to make it directly applicable to CSA. The principal investigator (PI) was certified as a CDSMP "Master Trainer" at the Stanford Patient Education Research Center to ensure that all tenets of the adapted program were in accordance with the standardized CDSMP psychoeducation format.

The program was delivered by a Registered Nurse using a group format (e.g., 8–15 patients) in a comfortable classroom setting. Program sessions were offered both day and evening and participants were encouraged to bring a family member or friend if they wished. A facilitator manual specified the intervention protocol in detail to ensure consistent delivery of the CASMP across sessions. In addition, all sessions were audio taped and a random sample of these tapes (10%) was externally audited to ensure standard intervention delivery.

The CASMP integrates strategies known to enhance self-efficacy including skills mastery, modeling, and self-talk. Designed to maximize discussion and group problem solving, it encourages individual experimentation with various cognitive-behavioral self-management techniques and facilitates mutual support, optimism, and the self-attribution of success. Key pain-related content includes relaxation and stress management, energy conservation, symptom monitoring and management techniques, medication review, seeking emergency assistance, diet, and managing emotional responses to cardiac pain. Fig. 1 provides an overview of all content covered over the six-week course of the program.

Both the content and process components of the CASMP are grounded in Bandura's Self-Efficacy Theory, which states that self-efficacy is critical to improve health-related behaviors and emotional well-being and that one's self-efficacy can be enhanced through performance mastery, modeling, reinterpretation of symptoms, and social persuasion.[51,52] Throughout the program, participants worked in pairs between sessions to help one another to stay motivated, problem solve, and meet their respective self-management goals. A CASMP workbook was also provided for reinforcement of key material from each session.

MEASURES

Sociodemographic information and angina and related clinical characteristics were obtained via a baseline questionnaire developed for the trial. Braden's evidence-based Self-Help Model of Learned Response to Chronic Illness Experience guided our selection of trial outcomes.[53,54] Braden's model emphasizes human resilience and suggests that people can develop enabling skills to enhance their life quality when faced with the adversities of chronic illness.[53,54] Therefore, the primary outcome was life quality, conceptualized as CSA patients' HRQL. The secondary outcome was enabling skill, reflected by CSA patients' self-efficacy and resourcefulness to self-manage their pain.

Primary Outcome: HRQL. HRQL was measured using the Medical Outcomes Study 36-Item Short Form (SF-36).[55–57] The SF-36 is a comprehensive, well-established, and psychometrically strong instrument designed to capture multiple operational indicators of functional status including behavioral function and dysfunction, distress and well-being, self-evaluations of general health status.[58,59] Eight subscales are used to represent widely measured concepts of overall quality of life: physical functioning (PF), role limitations due to physical problems (RP), social functioning (SF), bodily pain (BP), mental health (MH), role limitations due to emotional problems (RE), vitality (VT), and general health perception (GH).[57] Raw SF-36 data were submitted to Quality-Metric Incorporated's 100% accurate online scoring service. Scoring was according to the method of summated ratings where items for each subscale are summed and divided by the range of scores. Raw scores were transformed to a 0-100 scale where higher scores reflect better functioning.[57] We also used norm-based scoring (NBS) where linear T-score transformations were performed to transform all scores to a mean of 50 and standard deviation (SD) of 10.[57,60] We chose the NBS method to allow our SF-36 scores to be readily comparable to current published SF-36 CSA population norms.[57] (Raw SF-36 scores available on request from the first author.) NBS also guards against subscale ceiling and floor effects; scores below 50 can be understood as below average.[57]

Reliability estimates for all eight SF-36 subscales have exceeded 0.70 across divergent patient populations including CSA[58–61]

CASMP Program Overview						
	Week 1	Week 2	Week 3	Week 4	Week 5	Week 6
Overview of Self-management and Chronic Angina	✓					
Making an Action Plan	✓	✓	✓	✓	✓	✓
Relaxation/Cognitive Symptom Management	✓		✓	✓	✓	✓
Feedback/Problem-solving		✓	✓	✓	✓	✓
Common Emotional Responses to Cardiac Pain: Anger/Fear/Frustration		✓				
Staying Active/Fitness		✓	✓			
Better Breathing			✓			
Fatigue/Sleep Management			✓			
Energy Conservation				✓		
Eating for a Healthy Heart				✓		
Monitoring Angina Symptoms and Deciding when to Seek Emergency Help				✓		
Communication				✓		
Angina and Other Common Heart Medications					✓	
Evaluating New/Alternative Treatments					✓	
Cardiac Pain and Depression					✓	
Monitoring Angina Pain Symptoms and Informing the Health Care Team						✓
Communicating with Health Care Professionals About Your Cardiac Pain						✓
Future Self-Management Plans						✓

Figure 1. CASMP overview.

and exceeded 0.8 in this study: PF (0.87), RP (0.86); BP (0.81); RE (0.87); SF (0.83); VT (0.83); MH (0.85); GH (0.83). SF-36 construct, convergent, and discriminant validities have also been well documented.[57–59,62]

Although the SF-36 has discriminated among patient samples with divergent medical, psychiatric, and psychiatric and other serious medical conditions, some evidence suggests that it may inadequately discriminate among those with differing CCS angina functional class.[61] The potential for the SF-36 to be insensitive to changes in angina class necessitated the use of a second disease-specific instrument, the Seattle Angina Questionnaire (SAQ),[61,63] to evaluate HRQL.

The SAQ is a disease-specific measure of HRQL for patients with CAD, consisting of 19 items that quantify five clinically relevant domains of CAD: physical limitation, angina pain stability and frequency, treatment satisfaction, and disease perception.[63] The SAQ is scored by assigning each response an ordinal value and summing across items within each of the five subscales. Subscale scores are transformed (0–100) by subtracting the lowest score, dividing by the range of the scale, and multiplying by 100.[63] Higher scores for each subscale indicate better functioning; no summary score for the five subscales is derived. SAQ reliability, construct validity, and responsiveness to intervention have been demonstrated in a number of studies.[13,14,61,63–65] Internal consistency reliabilities for the SAQ in this study were PL (0.85), AF (0.71), TS (0.73), and DP (0.68).

Secondary Outcomes. *Self-Efficacy and Resourcefulness.* Self-efficacy to manage angina pain and other symptoms was measured with a modified version of the 11-item "Pain and Other Symptom" scale of Lorig et al.'s Self-Efficacy Scale (SES), originally developed for arthritis intervention studies.[66] This scale assesses people's perceived ability to cope with the consequences of chronic arthritis including pain and related symptoms and functioning[66] via a 10-point graphic rating scale ranging from 10 (very certain) to 100 (very uncertain) for each of its 11 items. A total score for perceived self-efficacy is obtained by summing all items and dividing by the number of items completed; a higher score indicates greater perceived self-efficacy.

SES test-retest stability and construct validity have been reported in large samples.[35,36,67] The SES has also performed consistently with theoretical predictions in a prior psychoeducation trial for chronic pain, having negative correlation with pain (−0.35) and disability (−0.61), and strong positive correlation with role functioning (0.62) and life satisfaction (0.48); internal consistency was 0.90.[37] Permission was received from the SES developer to adapt the SES by replacing the word "arthritis" with "angina." The internal consistency of our adapted version of the SES in this study was 0.94.

Resourcefulness was measured by Rosenbaum's Self-Control Schedule (SCS),[68] designed to assess individual tendencies to use a repertoire of complex cognitive and behavioral skills when negotiating stressful circumstances. Thirty-six items are scored using a six-point Likert scale (−3 to +3) to assess individual tendencies to engage in aspects of self-control behaviors including 1) the use of cognitions and positive self-statements to cope with negative situations, 2) application of problem solving strategies, 3) delay of immediate gratification, and 4) maintenance of a general belief in self when dealing with challenging circumstances.[68] Eleven items are reverse scored, and all items are summed to generate a total score for resourcefulness ranging from −108 to 108; higher scores indicate greater resourcefulness.[68] SCS test-retest stability, internal consistency, and validity are well documented.[37,68–73] The internal consistency for the SCS in this study was 0.80.

All instruments were pilot tested prior to the trial on a sample of six CSA patients (aged 46–68 years) to assess their comprehension of items and response burden; no changes were required.

SAMPLE SIZE

Sample size estimation was based on achievement of a moderate effect size in our primary outcome of HRQL. Cardiac patients have reported minimum 10-point improvements in SF-36 scales up to four years postinvasive intervention.[7,11] Prior trials suggested that psychoeducation can achieve comparable minimal levels of short-term change in a number of SF-36 scales for patients with chronic pain via the acquisition of disease self-management skills and the self-attribution of success.[35,37] We specified a 10-point difference in SF-36 scores as being clinically important and the sample size was set to test for this difference. Based on Chronic Pain Self-Management Program (CPSMP) trial data,[37] we used an estimated SD of 18; comparable SDs for five SF-36 scales including physical functioning, bodily pain, general health, social functioning, and mental health have been reported among cardiac patients aged 44–84 years.[7] Larger SDs however were reported for two role functioning scales of the SF-36 including role emotional and role physical functioning, thus requiring estimated sample sizes beyond the allowable time frame for this study.[7,57] We therefore expected potentially inadequate power to detect meaningful change in these two SF-36 scales. Allowing for an alpha of 0.05 and 80% power, the required sample for each group was 52. Telephone reminders and flexibility in CASMP program offerings were expected to help minimize attrition. However, to allow for losses to follow-up, the final sample estimate for each group was 65, or 130 in total. The statistics program nQuery Advisor 4.0 was used to compute this sample size estimate.

DATA ANALYSIS

Analyses were based on intention-to-treat principles.[74] Equivalence of groups on baseline demographic characteristics and pretest scores was examined using Chi-squared analysis for discrete level data and the Student t-test for continuous level data. Change score analyses were conducted to determine the impact of the CASMP on HRQL, self-efficacy, and resourcefulness to manage symptoms. Significant differences in change scores between treatment and control groups were examined via analysis of variance (ANOVA).[75] To guard against Type I error, multivariate analysis of variance (MANOVA) was conducted prior to ANOVA testing on SF-36- and SAQ-related data, due to the multiple subscales involved.[75] We chose a change score approach as opposed to analysis of covariance (ANCOVA) so that observed differences in change scores between treatment and control groups would be accessible to the reader and therefore the magnitude of any intervention effects would be readily apparent.[75,76] For verification, we reanalyzed our data via ANCOVA; the findings supported our change score approach. All data were cleaned and assessed for outliers and departure from normality; assumptions of all parametric analyses were met.

■ Results

DERIVATION OF THE SAMPLE AND ATTRITION

In total, 277 potential participants were assessed for inclusion via telephone during an 18-month period. Of these potential participants, 130 were included and 147 were excluded. Of those excluded, 44% did not meet the inclusion criteria, 30% refused, and 26% missed their initial appointment for consent and completion of baseline questionnaires, despite assiduous follow-up (i.e., three telephone calls and a follow-up letter). Reasons for refusal included: not interested ($n = 18$), too busy to participate ($n = 15$), transportation problems ($n = 6$), and physical limitations precluding travel ($n = 5$). Those who did not arrive for enrollment procedures were also counted as refusals when determining acceptance rate. The acceptance rate for enrollment among those eligible was 61%. Of the 130 consenting participants, 66 were randomized to the CASMP, and 64 were randomized to the wait-list control group.

Thirteen participants (treatment group, $n = 9$; usual care group, $n = 4$) did not complete posttest measures, yielding a 10% loss to follow-up (LTF) rate. Of these, nine participants LTF dropped out of the study without explanation and could not be contacted and four became ineligible to continue due to hospitalization. One hundred seventeen participants (treatment group, $n = 57$; usual care group, $n = 60$) completed pre- and posttest measures that were used for data analyses (see Fig. 2).

PARTICIPANT CHARACTERISTICS AND COMPARABILITY OF GROUPS

Baseline sociodemographic- and angina-related characteristics of the treatment and control groups are presented in Tables 1 and 2, respectively. The mean age of the sample was 68 (SD 11), living with CSA for 7 (SD 7)

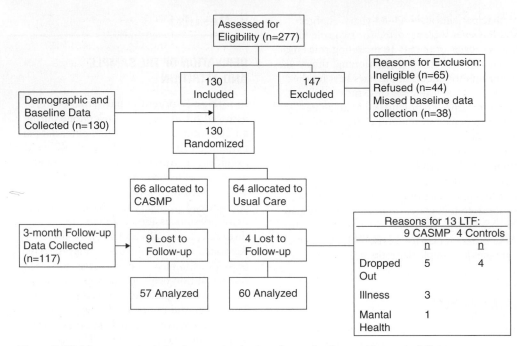

Figure 2. Trial flow: sample derivation, randomization, data collection, and losses to follow-up.

years on average. The majority of the sample was male, married or cohabitating, and Caucasian. Individuals of East Indian and Pakistani origin constituted the second largest racial group enrolled. Most were either retired or working full time. The majority had completed high school and/or had postsecondary education. Approximately half had two prior cardiac revascularization procedures, typically either coronary artery bypass grafting or angioplasty. The majority reported having a comorbid condition, typically a minor medical problem or diabetes. The treatment and control groups were not significantly different on any sociodemographic characteristic, comorbid condition, CCS functional class, number of prior revascularizations, or pretest measure. Comparisons were also made on all sociodemographic characteristics and pretest scores between those LTF ($n = 13$) and those who completed ($n = 117$) the study; no significant differences were found. (All baseline scores available on request from the first author.)

INTERVENTION EFFECTS: BETWEEN-GROUP DIFFERENCES IN CHANGE SCORES

Primary Outcome. *HRQL.* Mean change scores by group, group differences in change scores, and results of MANOVA and ANOVA testing for significant differences in change scores between groups for the SF-36 and SAQ are presented in Tables 3 and 4, respectively. Two omnibus MANOVA tests were performed on the SF-36 data as four subscales reflect mental health aspects of HRQL, and four subscales reflect physical health aspects. MANOVA yielded significantly greater positive change for the treatment group on the overall physical health component of the SF-36 ($F = 4.39$, $P = 0.003$), compared to the usual care group; no significant differences in change were found for the overall mental health component. MANOVA also yielded significantly greater positive change for the treatment group on the SAQ ($F = 3.23$, $P = 0.009$), compared to the usual care group.

Table 1. Sociodemographic Characteristics by Group

Characteristic	Treatment ($n = 66$)	Control ($n = 64$)
Demographics	**n (%)**	**n (%)**
Mean age (years [SD])	67 (11)	70 (11)
Married/ cohabitating	44 (67)	44 (69)
Male	53 (80)	50 (78)
Working full time	16 (24)	15 (23)
Retired	46 (70)	42 (66)
High school	59 (89)	55 (86)
Postsecondary education	42 (64)	44 (69)
Caucasian	48 (73)	54 (84)
Black	3 (5)	0 (0)
Latin American	0 (0)	1 (2)
Asian	2 (3)	1 (2)
East Indian/Pakistani	11 (17)	6 (9)
Middle Eastern	3 (5)	1 (2)
Aboriginal	0 (0)	1 (2)

SD = standard deviation.

Individual-level ANOVA testing on SF-36 subscales indicated significant improvements for the treatment group on physical functioning (PF) [$F = 11.75$ (1,114), $P < 0.001$] and general health (GH) [$F = 10.94$ (1,114), $P = 0.001$]. The Mann-Whitney U test was used to test for significant differences in change between groups for the role physical and role emotional functioning (RP, RE) and bodily pain (BP) subscales, due to their discrete distributions;[75] no significant differences between groups were found. ANOVA also yielded significant improvements for the treatment group on two subscales of the SAQ including angina pain frequency (AF) [$F = 5.57$ (1,115), $P = 0.02$] and stability (AS) [$F = 7.37$ (1,115), $P = 0.001$]. At three

Table 2. Angina and Related Clinical Characteristics by Group

Characteristic	Treatment ($n = 66$)	Control ($n = 64$)
Angina-related history		
Mean (SD) years living with angina	6 (6)	8 (8)
Mean (SD) revascularizations (including CABG, PCI)	2 (1)	2 (1)
Comorbid conditions	**n (%)**	**n (%)**
Heart failure	2 (3)	5 (8)
Asthma	4 (6)	2 (3)
Diabetes	18 (27)	9 (14)
Emphysema	1 (2)	1 (2)
Renal failure	2 (3)	1 (2)
Peptic ulcer	1 (2)	3 (5)
Thyroid problems	3 (5)	7 (11)
Other minor medical problem	34 (52)	27 (42)
Canadian Cardiovascular Society Functional Class		
Class I	23 (35)	19 (30)
Class II	26 (39)	29 (45)
Class III	17 (26)	16 (25)
Medications		
Ace inhibitors	33 (50)	29 (46)
Anti-arrhythmics	3 (5)	2 (3)
Anticoagulants	57 (86)	48 (73)
Beta-blockers	40 (61)	38 (59)
Calcium channel blockers	22 (34)	20 (32)
Cholesterol lowering agents	49 (74)	38 (59)
Diuretics	11 (16)	13 (20)
Insulins	18 (27)	9 (14)

SD = standard deviation; CABG = coronary artery bypass graft; PCI = percutaneous coronary intervention.

months, the CASMP resulted in significantly greater improvements in physical functioning and general health, as measured by the SF-36, and significantly greater improvements in angina pain frequency and stability, as measured by the SAQ, compared to usual care.

Table 3. MANOVA and ANOVA Tests for Significant Differences in SF-36 Change Scores between Groups

SF-36 NBS	Change Treatment	Change Control	Difference in Change between Groups	MANOVA		ANOVA	
Range (0–100)	$\Delta(T_2 - T_1)$ M (SD)	$\Delta(T_2 - T_1)$ M (SD)	$(T_\Delta - C_\Delta)$ M (SD)	F(df)	P	F(df)	P
Physical health-related items							
PF	5.3 (9.4)	−0.68 (9.3)	5.95 (9.3)	4.39 (4,110)	0.003[b]	11.75 (1,114)	<0.001[c]
RP	4.8 (12.7)	3.2 (9.6)	1.66 (11.2)			1.47[a]	ns
BP	4.4 (8.7)	2.1 (9.2)	2.31 (8.95)			1.68[a]	ns
GH	2.27 (7.7)	−1.6 (6.4)	4.33 (7.0)			10.94 (1,114)	0.001[c]
Mental health-related items							
RE	4.9 (12.2)	3.6 (12.2)	1.31 (12.2)	0.47 (4,108)	ns	1.49[a]	ns
SF	2.1 (10.9)	0.1 (9.5)	2.04 (10.2)			0.28 (1,114)	ns
VT	2.3 (8.6)	0.3 (7.3)	1.97 (8.0)			1.77 (1,114)	ns
MH	1.5 (8.8)	0.9 (7.9)	0.58 (8.3)			0.14 (1,114)	ns

NBS = Norm-based scores; T_1 = Time 1; T_2 = Time 2; T = treatment; C = controls; Δ = mean change; T_Δ = mean change, treatment; C_Δ = mean change, controls; PF = physical functioning; RP = role physical functioning; BP = bodily pain; GH = general health; RE = role emotional functioning; SF = social functioning; VT = vitality; MH = mental health.

Note: SD of mean change scores expected to be large as range of scores not bound by zero.

[a]Mann–Whitney U test.

[b]$P < 0.05$.

[c]$P \leq 0.01$.

ns = Nonsignificant ($P > 0.05$).

Table 4. MANOVA and ANOVA Tests for Significant Differences in SAQ Change Scores between Groups

SAQ	Change Treatment	Change Control	Difference in Change between Groups	MANOVA		ANOVA	
Range (0–100)	$\Delta(T_2 - T_1)$ M (SD)	$\Delta(T_2 - T_1)$ M (SD)	$(T_\Delta - C_\Delta)$ M (SD)	F(df)	P	F(df)	P
AF	11.4 (23.7)	2.2 (18.4)	9.23 (21.2)	3.23 (5,109)	0.009[a]	5.57 (1,115)	0.02[a]
AS	18.0 (35.0)	2.9 (24.4)	15.07 (30.0)			7.37 (1,115)	0.001[b]
DP	9.9 (23.5)	3.3 (19.1)	6.61 (21.4)			2.80 (1,115)	ns
PL	7.1 (16.5)	1.6 (15.1)	5.55 (15.8)			3.54 (1,113)	ns
TS	9.7 (24.6)	4.8 (18.7)	4.82 (21.8)			1.43 (1,115)	ns

SAQ = Seattle Angina Questionnaire; T_1 = Time 1; T_2 = Time 2; T = treatment; C = Controls; Δ = mean change; T_Δ = mean change, treatment; C_Δ = mean change, controls; AF = angina frequency; AS = angina stability; DP = disease perception; PL = physical limitation; TS = treatment satisfaction; SD = standard deviation.

Note: SD of change scores expected to be large as range of scores not bound by zero.

[a] $P < 0.05$.

[b] $P \leq 0.01$.

ns = Nonsignificant ($P > 0.05$).

Secondary Outcomes. *Self-Efficacy and Resourcefulness.* Mean change scores by group, group differences in change scores, and results of ANOVA testing for significant differences in change in SES and SCS scores between groups are presented in Table 5. ANOVA yielded significant improvement for the treatment group on the SES [$F = 8.45$ (1,115), $P = 0.004$] compared to controls. No significant group differences in SCS change scores were found. Overall, the CASMP resulted in significantly improved self-efficacy scores at three months, compared to usual care. The CASMP did not impact resourcefulness.

Examination of Intervention Cohort Effects. Because the CASMP was delivered to the treatment group in six small group cohorts of eight to fifteen participants, we examined for significant associations between intervention cohort and differences found in change scores between treatment and control groups. No significant associations between intervention cohort and group differences in change scores were found.

CASMP ATTENDANCE

As a form of process evaluation, an attendance record was kept to track the number of CASMP sessions attended by the treatment group participants. Ninety-three percent of those in the treatment group attended all six program sessions; the remaining 7% attended three or more sessions. The average number of sessions attended overall was 5.8.

■ Discussion

Statistically reliable short-term improvements in HRQL and self-efficacy were found for those who participated in the CASMP as compared to the control group; specific components of HRQL significantly improved included overall physical functioning and general health (SF-36) and frequency and stability of angina pain symptoms (SAQ). As no prior psychoeducation-based trials for CSA have used the SF-36 or the SAQ, direct comparisons of our HRQL-related results were not possible. However, our findings generally compare favorably with those of trials that have used other means to evaluate HRQL. We found four psychoeducation trials that reported significant improvements in symptoms including duration, frequency, and severity of cardiac pain.[40–43] Two of these trials also found significant improvements in physical functioning with respect to exercise tolerance and general

Table 5. ANOVA Tests for Significant Differences in SES and SCS Change Scores between Groups

Variable (Range)	Change Treatment $\Delta(T_2 - T_1)$ M (SD)	Change Control $\Delta(T_2 - T_1)$ M (SD)	Difference in Change between Groups $(T_\Delta - UC_\Delta)$ M (SD)	ANOVA F(df)	P
SES (10–100)	8.4 (17.6)	− 0.2 (14.4)	8.62 (16.1)	8.45 (1,115)	0.004[a]
SCS (0–100)	4.2 (26.5)	−1.6 (19.2)	5.80 (23.0)	1.60 (1,115)	ns

T_1 = Time 1; T_2 = Time 2; T = treatment; C = Controls; Δ = mean change; T_Δ = mean change, treatment; C_Δ = mean change, controls; SES = Self-Efficacy Scale; SCS = Self-Control Schedule; SD = standard deviation.
Note: SD of change scores expected to be large as range of scores not bound by zero.
[a]$P < 0.01$.
ns = Nonsignificant ($P > 0.05$).

disability.[40,42] Although our findings are consistent with these positive trends, comparisons must be viewed with caution due to heterogeneity of methods including design, interventions, timing of outcome measurement, and instrumentation.[39] Nevertheless, sample characteristics across trials are similar to our sample, suggesting that physical functioning and angina symptoms can improve after participation in psychoeducational interventions that target angina pain symptoms, self-management techniques, and physical activity enhancement. Future angina psychoeducation randomized controlled trials (RCT) using robust methods, and standard reliable and valid measures to evaluate HRQL would allow for more direct comparisons to this trial.

Although focused on a different population, LeFort et al.'s CPSMP trial is the only other known study to have used the SF-36 to evaluate the impact of psychoeducation on a persistent pain problem.[37] Comparable to our study with respect to intervention format, design, and sample size, LeFort et al. found that their CPSMP program significantly improved SF-36 role physical functioning, bodily pain, vitality, and mental health for persons with chronic noncancer pain ($P < 0.003$).[37]

LeFort et al.'s significant improvement in a broader array of SF-36 dimensions than those achieved by our program may be attributable to the nature of respective pain problems addressed and participants' corresponding foci for self-management. Participants in LeFort et al.'s study had a number of chronic pain problems, averaging 6.7 somatic locations for pain per participant. Individuals may therefore have focused on a broader range of goals for pain self-management than our sample, leading to improvements across SF-36 physical and mental health components. Participants in our study however were most concerned with reducing their fear of cardiac pain to enhance their physical capacity. Based on pilot data, our program targeted a common misbelief among CSA patients that sedentary behavior will minimize cardiac pain and risks to personal safety.[33] Accordingly, the vast majority of our treatment group identi-

fied their fear of physical activity and subsequent pain as a major contributor to deconditioning, poor overall health, fatigue, and obesity. Enhancement of physical activity was therefore their immediate self-management priority. This concentrated self-management focus may account for our treatment group's narrower, although significant, improvements in SF-36 physical functioning and general health. There is also some evidence to suggest that the SF-36 may inadequately discriminate among those with differing CCS angina functional class.[61] Because our sample included those with CCS Classes I–III angina, some SF-36 subscales may not have been sensitive to improvements in angina-induced disability as a result of our program. Finally, baseline scores on all SF-36 dimensions in this study are below Canadian and U.S. population-adjusted norms.[57,77] Given the deleterious impact of CSA on HRQL, improvement in multiple SF-36 dimensions may be difficult to achieve for CSA patients in the short term.

Prior work has established that a minimum change of 10 points in SAQ subscales reflects clinically meaningful change for angina patients.[13,63,65] In our study, AS and AF scores changed in a positive direction for the treatment group by a mean 18 (35.0) and 11.4 (23.7) points, respectively, and therefore meet this criterion for clinically meaningful change. This finding is consistent with the positive results of recent studies that have tested multifaceted CSA secondary prevention strategies, with some educational components.[65,78] Spertus et al.[65] and Moore et al.[78] reported similar findings resulting from their intervention strategies, featuring combinations of antianginal drug therapy, regional anesthesia, exercise rehabilitation, education sessions, and/or individual counseling. Greater short-term improvement in frequency and stability of angina pain symptoms in our trial as compared to these studies may be due to the self-efficacy enhancing nature of our standardized intervention format. Our significant improvement in treatment group self-efficacy is consistent with LeFort et al.'s CPSMP trial.[37] and Lorig and Holman's psychoeducation trials for arthritis self-management.[35] Consistent with Bandura' self-efficacy theory, health behavior change by instruction—without addressing self-efficacy—has not shown to be as effective as those interventions that target self-efficacy directly.[79]

Other scores not significantly improved at posttest included SAQ-treatment satisfaction, disease perception and physical limitation, and resourcefulness, as measured by the SCS. As with some SF-36 subscales, a longer-term evaluation period may be required to see significant improvement in these scores for CSA patients. In addition, psychometric properties of the SAQ-physical limitation (PL) scale may account for our lack of a significant finding in this disease-specific HRQL dimension. The SAQ-PL scale was adapted by Spertus et al.[63] from Goldman et al.'s Specific Activity Scale,[80] designed to assess CAD patients' capacity for physical stress. Six of nine total SAQ-PL items examine activities known to increase myocardial oxygen demand including climbing a hill or flight of stairs without stopping, gardening, vacuuming or carrying groceries, walking more than a block at a brisk pace, lifting or moving heavy objects, and participating in strenuous sports.[63] However, as our pilot study suggests, most CSA patients will learn to avoid moderate levels of physical activity due to their fear of pain.[33] Therefore, more strenuous activities captured by the SAQ-PL scale may not be relevant to CSA patients. Notably, Spetrus et al.[65] and Moore et al.[78] also found no significant improvements in SAQ-PL for their chronic angina samples. These data suggest that the responsiveness of the SAQ-PL scale to improvements in mild physical activity for CSA patients, such as walking and household activity, warrants further investigation.

The strengths of our study are the robust methods used to minimize biases and random error including a priori power analysis, centrally controlled randomization, valid and reliable measures, blinding of data collectors, intention-to-treat analyses, and examination for possible intervention cohort effects. In addition, assiduous follow-up procedures and the use of a wait-list control condition guarded against attrition bias, ensuring minimal loss to follow up. Treatment integrity was also maximized using a theoretically sound and standardized intervention protocol, verified by an external auditor via audio recording.

Performance bias cannot be ruled out as it is not possible to blind participants or interveners in a socially based intervention study. Social desirability may also be a possibility due to our use of self-report measures.[81] However, randomization should have equally distributed those prone to socially desirable responses.[74] The risk of sample size bias may be further reduced in a future study by obtaining a larger sample to ensure adequate power for the two SF-36 role functioning scales. Also, our follow-up period was limited to three months after baseline. Therefore, the long-term sustainability of the observed intervention effects is not known. In addition, all CASMP sessions were delivered by a single facilitator. Future studies of this intervention should use multiple facilitators to enhance external validity and include longer-term follow-up. Finally, this study was conducted at a university site in central Canada; the clinical utility and knowledge translation potential of future investigations may be enhanced by examining the effectiveness of the CASMP as an adjunctive component to facets of health care with preexisting infrastructure, such as standard cardiac rehabilitation programs (where applicable), or community health-care programs and facilities.

In conclusion, cumulative evidence supports the deleterious impact of CSA on HRQL. The CASMP was found effective for improving physical functioning, perceived general health, angina pain frequency and stability, and self-efficacy to manage angina at three months post-test. Further research is warranted to determine the capacity of the program to improve other dimensions of generic and disease-specific HRQL, and resourcefulness in the longer term. A subsequent long-term evaluation would also allow for examination of the sustainability of the short-term improvements observed in HRQL and self-efficacy for CSA patients.

▪ Acknowledgments

We are grateful to the participants of this trial who generously gave their time and effort. We also thank Dr. Kate Lorig, Stanford University Patient Education Research Center, for permission to adapt the Chronic Disease Self-Management Program; Dr. Ellen Hodnett who supported this trial at the Randomized Controlled Trials Unit, Faculty of Nursing, University of Toronto; and Kim Boswell, Julie Kim, Linda Belford, Linda Brubacher, Peter Neilson, Marion Ryujin, and Viola Webster, expert clinicians and administrators who supported trial recruitment.

Lawrence S. Bloomberg Faculty of Nursing (M.H.M., J.W.-W., B.S.) and Faculty of Medicine (B.S., P.C., A.G.), University of Toronto, Toronto; and School of Nursing (S.M.L.), Memorial University of Newfoundland, St. John's, Newfoundland, Canada

Address correspondence to: Michael Hugh McGillion, RN, PhD, Lawrence S. Bloomberg Faculty of Nursing, University of Toronto, 155 College Street, Suite 130, Toronto, Ontario M5T 1P8, Canada. E-mail: michael.mcgillion@utoronto.ca Accepted for publication: September 26, 2007.

REFERENCES

1. Gibbons RJ, Chatterjee K, Daley J, et al. ACC/AHA-ASIM guidelines for the management of patients with chronic stable angina: executive summary and recommendations [(A report of the American College of Cardiology/American Heart Association Task Force on practice guidelines (Committee on Management of Patients with Chronic Stable Angina)]. *Circulation* 1999;99:2829–2848.

2. Lyons RA, Lo SV, Littlepage BNC. Comparative health status of patients with 11 common illnesses in Wales. *J Epidemiol Community Health* 1994;48:388–390.

3. Pocock SJ, Henderson RA, Seed P, Treasure T, Hampton J. Quality of life, employment status, and anginal symptoms after coronary artery bypass surgery: three-year follow-up in the randomized intervention treatment of angina (RITA) trial. *Circulation* 1996;94:135–142.

4. Erixson G, Jerlock M, Dahlberg K. Experiences of living with angina pectoris. *Nurs Sci Res Nord Countries* 1997;17:34–38.

5. Miklaucich M. Limitations on life: women's lived experiences of angina. *J Adv Nurs* 1998;28:1207–1215.

6. Caine N, Sharples LD, Wallwork J. Prospective study of health related quality of life before and after coronary artery bypass grafting: outcome at 5 years. *Heart* 1999;81:347–351.

7. Brown N, Melville M, Gray D, et al. Quality of life four years after acute myocardial infarction: Short Form 36 scores compared with a normal population. *Heart* 1999;81:352–358.

8. Gardner K, Chapple A. Barriers to referral in patients with angina: qualitative study. *Br Med J* 1999;319:418–421.

9. Wandell PE, Brorsson B, Aberg H. Functioning and well-being of patients with type 2 diabetes or angina pectoris, compared with the general population. *Diabetes Metab (Paris)* 2000;26:465–471.

10. Brorsson B, Bernstein SJ, Brook RH, Werko L. Quality of life of chronic stable angina patients four years after coronary angioplasty or coronary artery bypass surgery. *J Intern Med* 2001;249:47–57.

11. Brorsson B, Bernstein SJ, Brook RH, Werko L. Quality of life of patients with chronic stable angina before and 4 years after coronary artery revascularization compared with a normal population. *Heart* 2002;87:140–145.

12. MacDermott AFN. Living with angina pectoris: a phenomenological study. *Eur J Cardiovasc Nurs* 2002;1:265–272.

13. Spertus JA, Jones P, McDonell M, Fan V, Fihn SD. Health status predicts long-term outcome in outpatients with coronary disease. *Circulation* 2002;106:43 49.

14. Spertus JA, Salisbury AC, Jones PG, Conaway DG, Thompson RC. Predictors of quality of life benefit after percutaneous coronary intervention. *Circulation* 2004;110:3789–3794.

15. Murphy NF, Simpson CR, MacIntyre K, et al. Prevalence, incidence, primary care burden, and medical treatment of angina in Scotland: age, sex and socioeconomic disparities: a population-based study. *Heart* 2006;92:1047–1054.

16. Heart and Stroke Foundation of Canada. The growing burden of heart disease and stroke in Canada 2003. Ottawa: Heart and Stroke Foundation of Canada, 2003.

17. British Cardiac Society, British Hypertension Society, Diabetes UK, et al. JBS 2: Joint British Societies' guidelines on the prevention of cardiovascular disease in clinical practice. *Heart* 2005;91 (Suppl V):v1–v52.

18. Naylor CD. Summary, reflections and recommendations. In: Naylor CD, Slaughter PM, eds. Cardiovascular health and services in Ontario: An ICES atlas. Toronto: Institute for Clinical Evaluative Sciences, 1999:355–377.

19. Stone JA, Arthur HM, Austford L, Blair T. Introduction to cardiac rehabilitation. In: Stone JA, Arthur HM, eds. Canadian guidelines for cardiac rehabilitation and cardiovascular disease prevention, 2nd ed. Winnipeg: Can Assoc Cardiac Rehab, 2004:2–14.

20. Maseri A, Chierchia S, Davies G, Glazier J. Mechanisms of ischemic cardiac pain and silent myocardial ischemia. *Am J Med* 1985;79 (Suppl 3A):7–11.

21. Malliani A. The elusive link between transient myocardial ischemia and pain. *Circulation* 1986; 73:201–204.

22. Aronow WS, Epstein S. Usefulness of silent myocardial ischemia detected by ambulatory electrocardiographic monitoring in predicting new coronary events in elderly patients. *Am J Cardiol* 1988;62:1295–1296.

23. Langer A, Freeman MR, Armstrong PW. ST segment shift in unstable angina: pathophysiology and association with coronary anatomy and hospital outcome. *J Am Coll Cardiol* 1989;13:1495–1502.

24. Tzivoni D, Weisz G, Gavish A, et al. Comparison of mortality and myocardial infarction rates in stable angina pectoris with and without ischemic episodes during daily activities. *Am J Cardiol* 1989;63:273–276.

25. Deedwania PC, Carbajal EV. Silent ischemia during daily life is an independent predictor of mortality in stable angina. *Circulation* 1990;81:748–756.

26. Yeung AC, Barry J, Orav J, et al. Effects of asymptomatic ischemia on long-term prognosis in chronic stable coronary disease. *Circulation* 1991;83: 1598–1604.

27. Sylven C. Mechanisms of pain in angina pectoris: a critical review of the adenosine hypothesis. *Cardiovasc Drugs Ther* 1993;7:745–759.

28. Bugiardini R, Borghi A, Pozzati A, et al. Relation of severity of symptoms to transient myocardial ischemia and prognosis in unstable angina. *J Am Coll Cardiol* 1995;25:597–604.

29. Cannon RO. Cardiac pain. In: Gebhart GF, ed, Progress in pain research and management, Vol. 5. Seattle: IASP Press, 1995:373–389.

30. Malliani A. The conceptualization of cardiac pain as a nonspecific and unreliable alarm system. In: Gebhart GF, ed, Progress in pain research and management, Vol. 5. Seattle: IASP Press, 1995:63–74.

31. Pepine CJ. Does the brain know when the heart is ischemic? *Ann Intern Med* 1996;124(11): 1006–1008.

32. Procacci P, Zoppi M, Maresca M. Heart, vascular and haemopathic pain. In: Wall P, Melzack R, eds. Textbook of pain, 4th ed. Toronto: Churchill Livingstone, 1999:621–659.

33. McGillion MH, Watt-Watson JH, Kim J, Graham A. Learning by heart: a focused groups study to determine the psychoeducational needs of chronic stable angina patients. *Can J Cardiovasc Nurs* 2004;14:12–22.

34. McGillion M, Watt-Watson J, LeFort S, Stevens B. Positive shifts in the perceived meaning of cardiac pain following a psychoeducation for chronic stable angina. *Can J Nurs Res* 2007;39:48–65.

35. Lorig K, Holman HR. Arthritis self-management studies: a twelve year review. *Health Educ Q* 1993; 20:17–28.

36. Lorig K, Mazonson P, Holman HR. Evidence suggesting that health education for self-management in patients with chronic arthritis has maintained health benefits while reducing health care costs. *Arthritis Rheum* 1993;36:439–446.

37. LeFort S, Gray-Donald K, Rowat KM, Jeans ME. Randomised controlled trial of a community based psychoeducation program for the self-management of chronic pain. *Pain* 1998;74:297–306.

38. Barlow JH, Shaw KL, Harrison K. Consulting the "experts:" children and parents' perceptions of psychoeducational interventions in the context of juvenile chronic arthritis. *Health Educ Res* 1999;14:597–610.

39. McGillion MH, Watt-Watson JH, Kim J, Yamada J. A systematic review of psychoeducational interventions for the management of chronic stable angina. *J Nurs Manag* 2004;12:1–9.

40. Bundy C, Carroll D, Wallace L, Nagle R. Psychological treatment of chronic stable angina pectoris. *Psychol Health* 1994;10(1):69–77.

41. Payne TJ, Johnson CA, Penzein DB, et al. Chest pain self-management training for patients with coronary artery disease. *J Psychosom Res* 1994;38:409–418.

42. Lewin B, Cay E, Todd I, et al. The angina management program: a rehabilitation treatment. *Br J Cardiol* 1995;2:221–226.

43. Gallacher JEJ, Hopkinson CA, Bennett ML, Burr ML, Elwood PC. Effect of stress management on angina. *Psychol Health* 1997;12:523–532.

44. Lewin RJP, Furze G, Robinson J, et al. A randomized controlled trial of a self-management plan for patients with newly diagnosed angina. *Br J Gen Pract* 2002;52:194–201.

45. Campeau L. The Canadian Cardiovascular Society grading of angina pectoris revisited 30 years later. *Can J Cardiol* 2002;18:371–379.

46. Lorig K, Lubeck D, Kraines RG, Selenznick M, Holman HR. Outcomes of self-help education for patients with arthritis. *Arthritis Rheum* 1985;28: 680–685.

47. Lorig KR, Sobel DS, Stewart AL, et al. Evidence suggesting that a chronic disease self-management program can improve health status while reducing utilization and costs: a randomized trial. *Med Care* 1999;37:5–14.

48. Lorig K, Gonzalez V, Laurent D. The chronic disease self-management workshop master trainer's guide 1999. Palo Alto, CA: Stanford Patient Education Research Center, 1999.

49. Lorig KR, Ritter P, Stewart AL, et al. Chronic disease self-management program: two-year health status and health care utilization outcomes. *Med Care* 2001;39:1217–1223.

50. Lorig KR, Sobel D, Ritter PL, Laurent D, Hobbs M. One-year health status and health care utilization outcomes for a chronic disease self-management program in a managed care setting. *Eff Clin Pract* 2001;4:256–262.

51. Bandura A. Social foundations of thought and action: A social cognitive theory. Englewood Cliffs: Prentice Hall, 1986.

52. Bandura A. Self-efficacy: The exercise of control. New York: W.H. Freeman, 1977.

53. Braden CJ. A test of the self-help model: learned response to chronic illness experience. *Nurs Res* 1990;39:42–47.

54. Braden CJ. Research program on learned response to chronic illness experience: self-help model. *Holist Nurs Pract* 1993;8:38–44.

55. Rand Corporation, Ware J. The Short-Form-36 Health Survey. In: McDowell I, Newell C, eds. Measuring health: A guide to rating scales and questionnaires, 2nd ed. New York: Oxford University Press, 2006:446–454.

56. Ware JE, Sherbourne CD. The MOS 36-item short-form health survey (SF-36): I Conceptual framework and item selection. *Med Care* 1992;30:473–483.

57. Ware JF, Snow KK, Kosinski M, Gandek B. SF-36® health survey: Manual and interpretation guide. Lincoln: QualityMetric Incorporated, 2005.

58. McHorney CA, Ware JE, Rachel Lu JF, Sherborne CD. The MOS 36-item short-form health survey (SF-36): III. Tests of data quality, scaling assumptions, and reliability across divergent patient groups. *Med Care* 1994;32:40–66.

59. Tsai C, Bayliss MS, Ware JE. SF-36® Health survey annotated bibliography. (1988–1996), 2nd ed. Boston: Health Assessment Lab, New England Medical Center, 1997.

60. Ware JE, Snow KK, Kosinski M, Gandek B. SF-36® health survey: Manual and interpretation guide. Boston, MA: The Health Institute, New England Medical Center, 1993.

61. Dougherty C, Dewhurst T, Nichol P, Spertus J. Comparison of three quality of life instruments in stable angina pectoris: Seattle angina questionnaire, Short Form health survey (SF-36), and quality of life index-cardiac version III. *J Clin Epidemiol* 1998;51(7):569–575.

62. McHorney CA, Ware JE, Raczek AE. The MOS 36-item short-form health survey (SF-36): II. Psychometric and clinical tests of validity in measuring physical and mental health constructs. *Med Care* 1993;31:247–263.

63. Spertus JA, Winder JA, Dewhurst TA, et al. Development and evaluation of the Seattle Angina Questionnaire: a new functional status measure for coronary artery disease. *J Am Coll Cardiol* 1995;25:333–341.

64. Seto TB, Taira DA, Berezin R, et al. Percutaneous coronary revascularization in elderly patients: impact on functional status and quality of life. *Ann Intern Med* 2000;132:955–958.

65. Spertus JA, Dewhurst TA, Dougherty CM, et al. Benefits of an "angina clinic" for patients with coronary artery disease: a demonstration of health status measures as markers of health care quality. *Am Heart J* 2002;143:145–150.

66. Lorig K, Chastain RL, Ung E, Shoor S, Holman H. Development and evaluation of a scale to measure perceived self-efficacy in people with arthritis. *Arthritis Rheum* 1989;32:37–44.

67. Lorig K, Lubeck D, Selznnick M, et al. The beneficial outcomes of the arthritis self-management course are inadequately explained by behaviour change. *Arthritis Rheum* 1989;31:91–95.

68. Rosenbaum M. A schedule for assessing self-control behaviours: preliminary findings. *Behav Ther* 1990;11:109–121.

69. Weisenberg M, Wolf Y, Mittwoch T, Mikulincer M. Learned resourcefulness and perceived control of pain: a preliminary examination of construct validity. *J Res Pers* 1990;24:101–110.

70. Redden EM, Tucker RK, Young L. Psychometric properties of the Rosenbaum schedule for assessing self control. *Psychol Rec* 1983;33:77–86.

71. Rosenbaum M, Palmon N. Helplessness and resourcefulness in coping with epilepsy. *J Consult Clin Psychol* 1984;52:244–253.

72. Richards PS. Construct validation of the self-control schedule. *J Res Pers* 1985;19:208–218.

73. Clanton L, Rude S, Taylor C. Learned resourcefulness as a moderator of burnout in a sample of rehabilitation providers. *Rehabil Psychol* 1992;37: 131–140.

74. Meinart CL. Clinical trials: Design, conduct and analysis. New York: Oxford University Press, 1986.

75. Norman GR, Streiner DL. Biostatistics: The bare essentials, 2nd ed. Hamilton: BC Decker Inc., 2000.

76. Bonate P. Analysis of pretest-posttest designs. Boca Raton: Chapman & Hall/CRC, 2000.

77. Hopman WM, Towheed T, Anastassiades T, et al. Canadian normative data for the SF-36 health survey. *Can Med Assoc J* 2000;163:265–271.

78. Moore RK, Groves D, Bateson S, et al. Health related quality of life of patients with refractory angina before and one year after enrolment onto a refractory angina program. *Eur J Pain* 2005;9: 305–310.

79. Marks R, Allegrante JP, Lorig K. A review and synthesis of research evidence for self-efficacy enhancing interventions for reducing chronic disability: implications for health education practice (Part II). *Health Promot Pract* 2005;6:148–156.

80. Goldman L, Hashimoto B, Cook EF, Loscalzo MS. Comparative reproducibility and validity of systems for assessing cardiovascular functional class: advantages of a new specific activity scale. *Circulation* 1981;22:1227–1234.

81. Sackett DL. Bias in analytic research. *J Chronic Dis* 1979;32:51–63.

CRITIQUE OF McGILLION ET AL.'S STUDY "RANDOMIZED CONTROLLED TRIAL OF A PSYCHOEDUCATION PROGRAM FOR THE SELF-MANAGEMENT OF CHRONIC CARDIAC PAIN"

■ Overall Summary

Overall, this was a well-written report that described a carefully executed study. The research tested a promising intervention to promote better outcomes among patients with chronic stable angina. The researchers used a strong research design and implemented stringent strategies to enhance the study's internal validity. They provided evidence that selection bias, a key threat to internal validity, did not affect their conclusions. They paid careful attention to such issues as blinding data collectors, reducing attrition, standardizing the intervention, and monitoring intervention fidelity. The instruments they used to measure the outcomes demonstrated strong validity and reliability. The study results indicated significant and clinically important improvements for those in the intervention group on many important outcomes (although the nonuse of intention-to-treat principles possibly led to somewhat inflated estimates of effects). The researchers' power analysis led them to recruit a sample sufficiently large to detect moderate intervention effects, but a larger sample likely would have yielded evi-

dence of additional program benefits—the researchers themselves acknowledged this limitation on statistical power. The researchers provided excellent suggestions for further research on the promising psychoeducation intervention that they evaluated.

■ Title

The title of this report was excellent. It communicated the research design (a randomized controlled trial or RCT), the independent variable (participation versus nonparticipation in a special program), the nature of the intervention (psychoeducational program, involving self-management), a dependent variable (self-management of pain), and the study population (patients with chronic pain from cardiac disease). All this information was conveyed succinctly—only 14 words were used. It could be argued that something about health-related quality of life (the primary outcome variable) should have been included in the title, but this would have made the title long. The authors did list health-related quality of life as a keyword for indexing purposes.

▪ Abstract

The abstract, written in the traditional abstract style without subheadings, was excellent, summarizing all major features of the study. The abstract presented a summary of the problem, described the intervention, outlined crucial aspects of the research designs and study methods, described the study sample, summarized major findings, and stated the conclusion that the findings warrant further research on the long-term effects of the intervention. Despite its strength, the abstract could perhaps have been shorter without diminishing its informativeness. For example, statistical details (all of the information about the F statistics and the actual probability values) were not necessary. Names of the specific instruments that measured the outcomes (e.g., the Medical Outcomes Study 36-Item Short Form) could also have been omitted. People review abstracts to decide whether the full article is of interest, and methodologic details are seldom important in making such decisions.

▪ Introduction

The introduction to this study was short—briefer than is typical, in fact. Yet, the introduction covered a lot of ground in a concise and admirable fashion, thus leaving more space in the article for details about the researchers' methods and findings.

The very first sentence, which stated that cardiac pain from chronic stable angina (CSA) is a cardinal symptom of coronary artery disease, introduced the problem. Later sentences indicated that this clinical problem had not been satisfactorily addressed with secondary prevention strategies. Consequences of the problem were summarized (i.e., that CSA has

repercussions for health-related quality of life [HRQL], including pain, poor general health status, impaired role functioning, reduced ability for self-care, and activity restriction). Ample citations supporting these assertions were provided. Next, the researchers presented information about the prevalence of CSA—that is, about the scope of the problem.

McGillion and colleagues then laid the groundwork for the testing of a new intervention. They noted that existing models of secondary prevention are not necessarily accessible to those managing their chronic symptoms in the community. They identified a potential model of self-management for helping patients with CSA—psychoeducation interventions, which they defined as "multimodal, self-help treatment packages that use information and cognitive-behavioral strategies to achieve changes in knowledge and behavior for effective disease management." They described existing evidence about the utility of such interventions for improving outcomes for patients with other types of chronic pain, but stated that the evidence of the effectiveness of psychoeducation for CSA self-management is inconclusive. They briefly noted some of the methodologic problems with existing studies (e.g., inadequate power, lack of a standardized intervention). McGillion and other colleagues themselves undertook a systematic review of this literature, so they were well-poised to critique the existing body of work.[1]

The researchers' argument led logically to the undertaking of this study because it highlighted the need for a well-designed test of a psychoeducation intervention for CSA patients. Their statement of purpose, placed as the last sentence of the introduction, was: "to evaluate the effectiveness of a standardized psychoeducation program, entitled the Chronic Angina Self-Management Program (CASMP) for improving the HRQL, self-efficacy, and resourcefulness of CSA patients." Although the researchers did not explicitly

---

[1]Note that the researchers' presentation of the problem covered all six components we discussed in connection with problem statements in Chapter 4 of the textbook.

state a hypothesis, the clear implication is that the researchers expected that patients who participated in the CASMP intervention would have better outcomes than patients who did not. The introduction to this article indicates that the researchers targeted a problem of clinical significance to the healthcare community.

Overall, the introduction was well-written and clearly organized. It concisely communicated the rationale for the study, and interwove supporting literature nicely. One comment about the literature cited, however, is that many studies were fairly old. Of the 81 citations, 53 were published before the year 2000, and 16 were published before 1990. It is commendable that the researchers were thorough (i.e., they included studies comprehensively, including many older ones). We wonder, however, whether the space devoted to listing so many citations in the reference list could have been better used, given page constraints for journal articles[2] (see below for some suggested additions to the introduction). On a positive note, the researchers did a nice job of citing an interdisciplinary mix of studies from medical, nursing, other healthcare, and psychological journals.

Although the succinctness of the introduction is in many respects laudable, a few additional paragraphs might have better set the stage for readers. Here are some possible supplementary topics that could have strengthened the introduction:

- The authors stated several of the consequences of CSA, but did not document any economic implications (e.g., lost time from work for patients, increased costs from treatment for depression, costs associated with care in emergency departments). Given that psychoeducation programs such as the one tested involve an investment of resources, a more convincing argument for its utility might involve suggesting how

such an intervention might be cost-effective.

- The theoretical basis of the psychoeducation intervention was not alluded to in the introduction (it is briefly mentioned later in the article). It would be useful to have a brief upfront theoretical rationale for why a psychoeducation intervention might translate into improved psychosocial and physical outcomes.

- Relatedly, the introduction did not articulate a rationale for the researchers' selection of intervention outcomes. Several of the consequences of CSA that were mentioned in the first paragraph (e.g., activity restrictions, impaired role functioning) were apparently not specifically viewed as targets for improvement in this study. Also, certain outcomes stated in the purpose statement (self-efficacy, resourcefulness) were not described earlier as being relevant to either the clinical problem or the intervention model. Perhaps if there had been a better description of the theoretical framework in the introduction, the rationale for selecting these outcomes would have been clearer.

- The purpose statement indicated that the study would be testing an existing structured intervention, CASMP. The introduction should perhaps have provided readers with a one- to two-sentence description of what prior research had found concerning the effectiveness of this specific intervention.

■ Method

The method section was well organized, with numerous subheadings so that readers could easily locate specific elements of the design and methods. The method section included useful information about how the researchers designed and implemented their study.

---

[2]We do not know what the limitations of *Journal of Pain and Symptom Management* were when this paper was submitted, but in 2010 the "Guide to Authors" for that journal indicated that articles should be no more than 7500 words, including references. This translates to about 20 pages, double-spaced.

RESEARCH DESIGN

McGillion and colleagues' clinical trial used a strong research design—a pretest–posttest experimental design that involved random assignment of study participants to an experimental (E) group that received the 6-week CASMP program or a control (C) group that received only "usual care" during the study period. Data were collected from all sample members at baseline and then again 3 months later. The researchers chose an ethically strong control group strategy of wait-listing controls for 3 months so that, after the posttest data were collected, control group members could opt to receive the intervention. One of the shortcomings of such a "delay of treatment" design is that it precludes long-term follow-up. That is, once the Cs are allowed to enroll in the intervention, E-C comparisons no longer provide a valid basis for inferring program effects. The researchers were fully aware of this, and noted that their intent in this research was to seek evidence of short-term (3-month) effects as a basis for launching a larger-scale trial with longer follow-up. (The researchers' rationale for collecting posttest data at 3 months—as opposed to, say, 2 months or 4 months, was not stated.)

STUDY POPULATION AND PROCEDURES

The researchers provided a good description of the study population, recruitment strategies, inclusion and exclusion criteria, methods of screening for eligibility, and procedures for obtaining informed consent. This subsection also did an unusually good job of describing the randomization process and methods the researchers used to eliminate certain biases and validity threats. The researchers used a tightly controlled randomization process to ensure proper allocation to treatment, and used "assiduous follow-up procedures" to minimize attrition, which is the single biggest threat to internal validity in experimental studies. As is true for most nonpharmacological interventions, blinding of partici-

pants and interventionists was not possible. Commendably, however, the researchers did take steps to ensure that the research assistant collecting the data was blinded to participants' group status.

The researchers also stated that usual care "consisted of all nursing, medical, and emergency care services as needed" and that Cs did not receive CASMP during the study period. It is noteworthy that the researchers mentioned what *usual care* means—"usual care" is often stated without further elaboration. This section further noted that wait-listed controls were offered entry into the next available CASMP once posttest data were collected. It cannot be ascertained from this article whether there was any possibility of contamination—that is, whether Cs could have been exposed to any part of the intervention during the study period, either through contact with Es being treated at the same hospitals or by the same clinicians, or through more direct contact with intervention agents. Judging from the care the researchers took in implementing the study, contamination likely was not a problem.

INTERVENTION

The CASMP intervention—a psychoeducation program given in 6 weekly sessions of 2 hours in a small classroom-type setting with 8 to 15 patients—was described in this section. The researchers adapted an existing intervention that had been developed at Stanford University and cited four papers by the researchers who developed it. There is no information in the present article about the intervention development process, nor whether early developmental efforts by the original research team involved a mixed methods approach. McGillion, however, had undertaken preliminary research on CSA—a qualitative focus group study—and had used the findings to adapt the CASMP program to their study population.

The researchers selected an intervention that was standardized, meaning that the treatment was presumably the same from one session to the next. Moreover, the nurse who delivered the program used a formal facilitator's manual to ensure consistent delivery. It is noteworthy that the researchers made efforts to assess intervention fidelity: All program sessions were audiotaped and there was an external audit of a random sample of 10% of the tapes. Presumably, these audits provided reassurance to the research team that the intervention was appropriately implemented.

The intervention itself was succinctly but adequately described as an integrated approach using strategies "known to enhance self-efficacy, including skills mastery, modeling, and self-talk." Major strategies included discussion, group problem solving, individual experimentation with self-management techniques, and paired problem solving between sessions to enhance motivation. Figure 1 provided a nice overview of the content covered in the six weekly sessions.

In the description of the intervention, the authors noted that both the content and process aspects of CASMP are "grounded in Bandura's Self-Efficacy Theory," which posits that self-efficacy is critical to improving health-related behaviors. Although space constraints likely limited the researchers' ability to include a well-formulated conceptual map linking program components to mediating effects (such as self-efficacy) and to ultimate outcomes, such a map (or a verbal description of the theoretical pathway) would have been useful in understanding some of the researchers' decisions, including their selection of outcome variables.

MEASURES

The researchers stated that their selection of outcomes was guided by Braden's Self-Help Model of Learned Response to Chronic Illness Experience. According to the authors, this model emphasizes human resilience and people's ability to develop skills to enhance life quality in the face of chronic illness. The rela-

tionship between this model and Bandura's Self-Efficacy Theory and the link between Braden's model and CASMP is not explicated, so the conceptual basis of the study remains a bit cloudy. Again, a conceptual map would be useful. The report stated that the primary outcome was HRLQ and the secondary outcome was enabling skill (patients' self-efficacy and resourcefulness to manage their pain).

HRLQ was measured using the 36-item Medical Outcome Study Short Form (SF-36). The SF-36 has eight subscales used to represent various aspects of health (e.g., physical functioning, bodily pain, vitality) and is a solid, well-respected instrument with strong psychometric properties. The researchers reported that the reliability estimates for the SF-36 in this study (presumably internal consistency estimates as calculated by coefficient alpha) were all respectable, that is, above .80. Commendably, because of some evidence that the SF-36 may not adequately discriminate patients with differing angina function, they administered a supplementary scale, the Seattle Angina Questionnaire (SAQ). This scale has five subscales (e.g., pain stability, physical limitation), and in this study, the reliabilities ranged from .68 to .85.

The secondary outcome of self-efficacy was measured by an adapted 11-item Self-Efficacy Scale (SES), and resourcefulness was measured by Rosenbaum's 36-item Self Control Schedule (SCS). The known psychometric characteristics of these two scales were good, and the researchers found that internal consistency in this study was .94 for the SES and .80 for the SCS.

It is also admirable that the researchers pretested their instrument package with a small sample of patients from the study population. They found that no changes were needed.

Overall, except for some ambiguity about the researchers' rationale for including particular constructs as outcomes (especially resourcefulness) and not including other potential constructs (e.g., ability for self-care, mentioned in the introduction as a documented consequence of CSA), the researchers' data collection plan seems sound and the specific measures they selected had good psychometric characteristics.

The only other comment is that the study might have benefited from a qualitative component. For example, by gathering in-depth information about the participants' program experiences, the researchers could perhaps have gained insight into how the program could be further adapted, which groups are most or least likely to benefit from the intervention, why effects were more modest for some outcomes than for others, or why about 8% of the participants dropped out of the program.

SAMPLE SIZE

The researchers' discussion about their sample size was very good. They assumed a moderate effect size for the effect of the program on their primary outcome, HRQL, and also offered a standard for clinical importance. They provided empirical support from other studies about the viability of their assumption of a moderate effect. Based on their assumption, they projected a need for 52 participants in each study group, to achieve a power of .80 with an alpha of .05. Even though their research plan included methods to keep attrition to a minimum, they built a cushion into their sample size estimates and, therefore, sought to enroll 65 participants in each group. The total number of patients randomized was 130, with 66 being enrolled in CASMP and 64 put in the wait-list control group.

DATA ANALYSIS

The researchers' data analysis strategy was explained in some detail, with information about both analytic strategies and the rationale for analytic decisions.

The first sentence stated that the researchers used an intention-to-treat (ITT) analysis, the approach that is considered the gold standard for analyzing RCT data. A true ITT analysis requires that everyone who is randomized is included in the analysis of outcomes, and that can only happen if there is no loss of study participants or if the missing outcomes for those who withdrew or were lost to follow-up are imputed (estimated). As indicated in the researchers' CONSORT-type flow chart (Figure 2), 130 participants were randomized, but 13 dropped out of the study (9 Es and 4 Cs). Follow-up data were collected from 117. Judging from the degrees of freedom in Tables 3 through 5 (degrees of freedom can be used to determine how many people were in the analysis), the analyses were based on the people who actually provided posttest data, not the full sample of 130 who were randomized. (If the researchers had imputed values for the missing posttest data for the 13 patients who withdrew, they presumably would have explained their method of imputation.) In sum, it does not appear that ITT was actually used.

The data analysis section provided an excellent explanation of the researchers' primary statistical analyses. The results reported in this paper involved comparisons of the *change scores* for the E versus the C group. That is, for every person, the difference between his or her posttest score and baseline score (for all scale and subscale scores) was used as the dependent variable, so that readers could see directly how much improvement had occurred. The report indicated that an alternative analytic method, ANCOVA, was also used and that the results were totally consistent with that reported. (In ANCOVA, posttest scores, rather than change scores were used as the dependent variables, and baseline scores were used as covariates, so that baseline values would be statistically controlled.) Because the researchers had multiple dependent variables—multiple subscale scores for the SF-36, for example—multivariate analysis of variance was used. The tables show results for both ANOVA and MANOVA. The researchers' statistical approach was strong.

■ Results

The results section provided useful information about how many people were recruited and what the flow of participants was in this study. Attrition in this study was fairly low, with follow-up data obtained from 90% of the patients randomized.

An excellent early subsection of the Results was devoted to analyzing potential biases and threats to internal validity. The researchers presented two tables showing the baseline characteristics of the Es and Cs, and reported that none of the baseline group differences were statistically significant at conventional levels. These tables not only demonstrated the initial comparability of the groups (in terms of demographic and clinical variables), but they also communicated vital information about the study population, which is important to readers considering whether the CASMP intervention might be appropriate for their own clients. The researchers also reported their analysis of attrition bias: For all of the demographic and clinical characteristics measured at baseline, people who remained in the study were not significantly different from those who dropped out. (The researchers probably also looked at comparability of the groups in terms of baseline performance on the outcome variables, but these results were not reported.)

Key results were reported in a subsection labeled *Intervention Effects*. The tables summarizing the results were complex, but they were well-organized and clear, with good footnotes to help interpret the symbols and abbreviations used. Text was used judiciously to highlight the main findings. The results indicated that improvements were significantly greater for Es than Cs on several important outcome measures. For the SF-36 outcome measure, group differences in change scores were significantly better for those who were in the program with regard to physical functioning and general health—but not bodily pain, nor any of the mental health subscales. On the Seattle Angina Questionnaire,

significant improvements were observed for both angina frequency and angina stability. In terms of secondary outcomes, the program had significant effects on improving self-efficacy scale scores, but not resourcefulness. One comment is that it would have been desirable to present information about the precision of the change score differences using confidence intervals and (especially) effect size estimates. It is possible, however, that journal page limitations constrained the researchers' ability to include this information.

The researchers also included very valuable information about cohort effects—results that are seldom noted in RCT reports. When an intervention unfolds over time, as many do, it is useful to see if the intervention effects are consistent over time. Changes in the degree of improvement might occur if, for example, sample characteristics changed over time or if program implementation was modified over time (e.g., if it improved as a result of early experiences or declined because of waning enthusiasm of the facilitator). McGillion and colleagues noted that there were six cohorts of patients, and that differences in the amount of improvement among the Es in the six cohorts were not significant.

Finally, the researchers also provided some information about actual program participation using data from their process evaluation. It is reassuring that the vast majority of patients assigned to the intervention group (93%) actually attended all six sessions. This is a very high rate of participation, and shows a strong "dose" of the treatment for almost all participants. Thus, the report indicated that not only was the *delivery* of the independent variable standardized, but its *receipt* was fairly uniform as well.

■ Discussion

McGillion and colleagues offered a thoughtful discussion of their findings. They began by contextualizing their study findings by comparing them to findings from other related studies of psychoeducational interventions. They offered some plausible interpretations of differences and similarities in the results. The results of these studies are broadly consistent, in that positive effects on indicators of quality of life were observed in all studies, though on slightly different dimensions (or measures) of HRQL.

The authors also discussed the clinical significance of their findings. That is, in addition to achieving statistically significant program effects, they argued that the amount of improvement demonstrated by the E group is sufficiently large to be considered clinically significant.

The authors discussed the strengths of their study, which were considerable. They also noted some possible limitations, which included the following: lack of blinding of participants and intervention agents, which could have led to possible performance bias; the possibility that there was inadequate power to detect group differences for some of the outcomes for which program effects were more modest; the short-term follow-up of participants, making it impossible to draw conclusions about the program's longer-term effects; the use of a single facilitator, which could adversely affect the generalizability of the results; and the setting of the study in a university site, which again has implications for external validity. It was admirable and insightful of the investigators to have noted these shortcomings, and they offered suggestions for addressing them in subsequent research.

■ General Comments

PRESENTATION

This report was well written and well organized, and provided an unusually great amount of detail about the researchers' decisions and their rationales. The primary presentational shortcoming concerned the limited elaboration of the conceptual basis of the study. We suspect that the ambiguity about the linkages between the theories/models and the intervention are not conceptual flaws, but rather communication issues. Given the great care that was taken in the design and execution of the study, the researchers likely had a fully developed conceptualization, but opted to abbreviate their presentation.

ETHICAL ASPECTS

The authors did not provide much information about steps they took to ensure that participants were treated ethically. For example, no mention was made of having the study approved by a human subject committee (in Canada, a Research Ethics Board), but that does not mean that such approval was lacking. The only relevant information was a statement about obtaining informed consent. There is no indication in the report that the participants were harmed, deceived, or mistreated in any way. And, indeed, their wait-list design is ethically strong.

VALIDITY ISSUES

McGillion and colleagues undertook an extremely rigorous study. They used a powerful research design and made exemplary efforts to reduce or eliminate many serious validity threats. Many of the limitations of this excellent study were noted by the authors themselves.

The study was quite strong in terms of internal validity: We can be reasonably confident that the CASMP program had beneficial effects on the participants' perceptions of self-efficacy and on aspects of their quality of life. Participants were carefully randomized, and the authors presented evidence that randomization was successful in creating groups that were comparable at the outset of the study. Thus, a key threat to internal validity—selection bias—was adequately addressed. There is no reason to suspect that threats such as history, maturation, or testing played a role in influencing the results. The major plausible internal validity threat in experimental designs is mortality—that is, differential attrition from study groups. Attrition was modestly higher among the Es than the Cs, but overall attrition was low. The authors reported that those who dropped out of the study were not significantly different from those who stayed in the study in terms of baseline characteristics.

In terms of statistical conclusion validity, the fact that the researchers found significant group differences for several outcomes indicates that statistical conclusion validity was good—but it was not excellent, as the authors themselves noted. If one looks at Tables 3 through 5, the differences in change scores favored Es over Cs *for every single outcome*, but not always at statistically significant levels. This suggests that, with a larger sample (i.e., greater statistical power), more E-C differences would likely have been statistically significant.

It might be noted, however, that the positive and significant intervention effects, while likely *real*, might possibly be somewhat inflated, given the fact that an intention-to-treat analysis does not appear to have been done. The people who dropped out of the study might have been patients for whom the CASMP program might not have "worked," for example, because of low motivation, interest, or need. We can do a rough calculation that suggests that even with the dropouts included in the analysis, the group differences favoring Es would have continued to be large and almost certainly significant. For example, the first outcome in Table 3 is for the Physical Functioning subscale of the SF-36. On average, Es improved by 5.3 points on the scale over the 3-month study period, while Cs *deteriorated* by .68 points (mean change = -.68). Based on the degrees of freedom, it appears that the analysis was done with 116 participants; we will assume that the averages shown are for 57 Es and 59 Cs, for a total of 116. The original E group included 66 patients, not 57. So, if we make an extremely

conservative assumption that the average change score for the 9 Es who dropped out of the study was -.68 (i.e., if we imputed the average missing change scores as identical to the average change among the Cs who did not get the intervention), and we compute a new average for all 66 Es, the value would drop from 5.3 to 4.5—still considerably better than −.68 for Cs.[3] In sum, we think that the evidence is persuasive that participation in the program was associated with significant improvement in outcomes.

In terms of construct validity, we have already noted that the researchers could have better communicated information about their conceptualization of the intervention. Performance bias—bias stemming from participants' and researchers' awareness of group status, and having such awareness affect outcomes—is another construct validity issue that the authors acknowledged. It seems more plausible to us, however, that the intervention itself had beneficial effects on angina frequency and physical functioning than that awareness caused these improvements. This is probably more likely to be the case because the posttest outcomes were measured 6 weeks after the end of program sessions, at which point awareness of group status likely would have waned.

Finally, external validity in this study is an issue that needs to be addressed in subsequent research. The researchers noted some of the factors limiting the generalizability of the findings (e.g., the use of a single facilitator, and the setting for the intervention in a university site in Canada). Other limiting factors include the relatively small sample, the exclusion of very high-risk patients, and the refusal of about 20% of eligible patients to participate. As is almost invariably true in clinical trials, the viability of the intervention for broader groups of CSA patients depends on replications.

---

[3]Here is how we arrived at the calculation. First, we multiplied .68 × 9 (the number of Es who dropped out) = 6.12. Then, we multiplied the mean of 5.3 × 57 (the number of Es in the analysis) = 302.1. Next, because the change for the C group was negative, we subtracted 6.12 from 302.1 = 295.98. Finally, this overall sum of change scores was divided by the original number of Es (66), to yield the new average of 4.485, which we rounded to 4.5.

■ Response from the McGillion Team and Further Comments:

Dr. McGillion and his team graciously accepted our invitation to review this critique. Many of their comments confirmed that journal page constraints were the reason that some of the additional details or discussion points were absent from their paper. Here, for example, is their comment about conceptual framing (personal communication, June 23, 2008):

> We appreciate the critical importance of a clear conceptual framing that provides the rationale for outcome selection and related measures. Journal style and limitations imposed on length were again factors in why this particular level of detail was left out of the manuscript. The primary outcome for this trial was HRQOL. Secondary outcomes included self-efficacy and resourcefulness. The conceptual framework that guided examination of these outcomes was Braden's Self-Help Model (*references were provided, but are omitted here*). The effectiveness of the CASMP was tested for improving scores in HRQOL, self-efficacy, and resourcefulness for CSA patients. Braden's Self-Help Model reflects the dynamics of a learned self-management response to chronic illness and was applied in order to link these variables together through the concept of enabling skill. Enabling skill, or one's perceived ability to manage adversity, was the proposed mediating variable by which one learns a self-help capacity, thereby experiencing enhanced life quality.

The authors also commented on the critique of their intention-to-treat analysis. This is what they wrote (personal communication, June 23, 2008):

> Regarding intention to treat (ITT) analysis: We do not agree that an analysis conducted according to ITT principles necessarily involves the imputation of post-test values for those participants lost to attrition. Rather, we would argue that ITT is commonly used as an umbrella term for two separate issues: a) treatment group [i.e. treatment or control] adherence and b) missing data. We state that we have analyzed our data according to ITT because we analyzed the data according to how participants were randomized-control participants remained in the control group and treatment groups participants remained in the treatment group. When data were missing, they were missing;

> we did not use any method to impute or estimate missing data. There are several methods to impute or estimate missing data such as 'last observation carried forward', or propensity scores. We felt that the use of such imputation techniques for an intervention study was inappropriate, as they are all means of estimating what missing outcome data 'might' have been.

We respectfully disagree with parts of this comment. The more appropriate term for the type of analysis that these researchers did is a *per protocol* analysis (analyzing people in groups according to the protocol to which they were randomized). This is the standard analytic approach, not true ITT. Few researchers actually do a classic ITT analysis that maintains all randomized participants in the analysis.

We do agree with the authors, however, that there is a lot of confusion about ITT in the research literature, and outright disagreement about how to (or whether to) impute missing values. The "state of the art" at the moment is to use sophisticated statistical procedures (multiple imputation) to "fill in" missing outcome data, and to then test how different procedures affect the results using a sensitivity analysis.

In the McGillion and colleagues study, we are reasonably confident that if they had performed a true ITT analysis with imputation of outcome data for dropouts, the conclusions that the intervention had positive effects would have remained the same. Our crude demonstration of "imputation" supports this view. Given the low rate of attrition, and the analysis indicating that dropouts were similar to those who remained in the study, it is perhaps understandable that the researchers did not undertake time-consuming and challenging analyses with imputations. The main problem, in our view, is that they used a term that implies a type of analysis they did not pursue.

Despite our disagreement with the authors about this point, the fact remains that this research team took extraordinary steps to ensure the integrity of their study. There is little doubt that their study is extremely high on internal validity—one of the best examples we have seen in the nursing research literature.

DIFFERENCES IN PERCEPTIONS OF THE DIAGNOSIS AND TREATMENT OF OBSTRUCTIVE SLEEP APNEA AND CONTINUOUS POSITIVE AIRWAY PRESSURE THERAPY AMONG ADHERERS AND NONADHERERS

Amy M. Sawyer • Janet A. Deatrick •
Samuel T. Kuna • Terri E. Weaver

▶ **Abstract:** Obstructive sleep apnea (OSA) patients' consistent use of continuous positive airway pressure (CPAP) therapy is critical to realizing improved functional outcomes and reducing untoward health risks associated with OSA. We conducted a mixed methods, concurrent, nested study to explore OSA patients' beliefs and perceptions of the diagnosis and CPAP treatment that differentiate adherent from nonadherent patients prior to and after the first week of treatment, when the pattern of CPAP use is established. Guided by social cognitive theory, themes were derived from 30 interviews conducted postdiagnosis and after 1 week of CPAP use. Directed content analysis, followed by categorization of participants as adherent/nonadherent from objectively measured CPAP use, preceded across-case analysis among 15 participants with severe OSA. Beliefs and perceptions that differed between adherers and nonadherers included OSA risk perception, symptom recognition, self-efficacy, outcome expectations, treatment goals, and treatment facilitators/barriers. Our findings suggest opportunities for developing and testing tailored interventions to promote CPAP use.

▶ **Key Words:** Adherence · compliance · content analysis · decision making · health behavior · mixed methods · sleep disorders · social cognitive theory

Obstructive sleep apnea (OSA), characterized by repetitive nocturnal upper airway collapse resulting in intermittent oxyhemoglobin desaturation and sleep fragmentation, contributes to significant disabling sequelae, including daytime sleepiness, impaired cognitive and executive function, mood disturbances, and increased cardiovascular and metabolic morbidity (Al Lawati, Patel, & Ayas, 2009; Harsch et al., 2004; Nieto, et al.

2000; Peppard, Young, Palta, & Skatrud, 2000). The prevalence of OSA, based on minimal diagnostic criteria (apnea/hypopnea index [AHI] of 5 events/hour), has been estimated at 2% in women and 4% in men in the United States (Young et al., 1993). More recently, large U.S.-cohort studies have provided additional evidence of the prevalence of OSA, estimating that approximately one in five adults with a mean body mass index (BMI) of at least 25 kg/m^2 has at least mild OSA, defined as an apnea-hypopnea index (AHI) $\geq$ 5 events/hour; and one in 15 adults with a mean BMI of at least 25 kg/m^2 has at least moderate OSA (i.e., AHI $\geq$ 15 events/hour; Young, Peppard, & Gottlieb, 2002). Continuous positive airway pressure (CPAP) therapy is the primary medical treatment for adults with OSA, eliminating repetitive, nocturnal airway closures; normalizing oxygen levels; and effectively improving daytime impairments (Gay, Weaver, Loube, & Iber, 2006; Sullivan, Barthon-Jones, Issa, & Eves, 1981; Weaver & Grunstein, 2008).

Nonadherence to CPAP is recognized as a significant limitation in the effective treatment of OSA, with average adherence rates ranging from 30% to 60% (Engleman, Martin, & Douglas, 1994; Kribbs et al., 1993; Krieger, 1992; Reeves-Hoche, Meck, & Zwillich, 1994; Sanders, Gruendl, & Rogers, 1986; Weaver, Kribbs, et al., 1997). Nonadherent users begin skipping nights of CPAP use during the first week of treatment, and their hourly use of CPAP on days used is significantly shorter than those who apply CPAP consistently (Aloia, Arnedt, Stanchina, & Millman, 2007; Weaver, Kribbs, et al., 1997). Patients who are nonadherent during early treatment generally remain nonadherent over the long term (Aloia, Arnedt, Stanchina, et al., 2007; Krieger, 1992; McArdle et al., 1999; Weaver, Kribbs, et al., 1997). The return of symptoms and other manifestations of OSA with even one night of nonuse underscores the critical nature of adherence to CPAP (Grunstein et al., 1996; Kribbs et al., 1993).

Many studies have explored what factors predict adherence to CPAP (Engleman et al., 1996; Engleman, Martin, et al., 1994; Kribbs et al., 1993; Massie, Hart, Peralez, & Richards, 1999; McArdle et al., 1999; Meurice et al., 1994; Reeves-Hoche et al., 1994; Rosenthal et al., 2000; Schweitzer, Chambers, Birkenmeier, & Walsh, 1997; Sin, Mayers, Man, & Pawluk, 2002). Self-reported side effects of CPAP do not distinguish between adherers and nonadherers to CPAP. Subjective sleepiness, severity of OSA as determined by apnea-hypopnea index, and severity of nocturnal hypoxia are inconsistently identified as correlates, albeit weak, of CPAP adherence (Weaver & Grunstein, 2008). The majority of these studies have focused on physiological variables and patient characteristics as predictors of adherence. Over the past 10 years, studies have identified psychological and social factors and cognitive perceptions, such as self efficacy, risk perception, and outcome expectancies, as determinants of CPAP use (Aloia, Arnedt, Stepnowsky, Hecht, & Borrelli, 2005; Lewis, Seale, Bartle, Watkins, & Ebden, 2004; Russo-Magno, O'Brien, Panciera, & Rounds, 2001; Stepnowsky, Bardwell, Moore, Ancoli-Israel, & Dimsdale, 2002; Stepnowsky, Marler, & Ancoli-Israel, 2002; Wild, Engleman, Douglas, & Espie, 2004). Social and situational variables have also been suggested as influential on CPAP adherence, with those who live alone, who have had a recent life event, and who experienced problems with CPAP on the first night of exposure having lower adherence to CPAP therapy (Lewis et al., 2004). Support group attendance has also been identified as contributing to higher CPAP use in older men (Russo- Magno et al., 2001). Findings of both of these studies suggest that social support is an important factor influencing decisions to use CPAP, yet the sociostructural context of accepting and adhering to CPAP treatment has not been described from the perspective of the patient in the extant literature. Other studies have identified that early experiences with CPAP (i.e., during the first week) are an important influence on patients' perceptions and beliefs about the OSA diagnosis and treatment with CPAP (Aloia, Arnedt, Stepnowsky, et al., 2005; Stepnowsky, Bardwell, et al., 2002).

From the collective published evidence, early experiences with CPAP, combined with patients' perceptions and beliefs about OSA and CPAP and the balance of their sociostructural facilitators/barriers, are critical factors that influence patients' decisions to use CPAP. To date, there are relatively few studies that have systematically examined the influence of disease and treatment perceptions and beliefs on CPAP adherence. Because the first week of CPAP treatment is critically influential on OSA patients' decisions to use CPAP, it is imperative that the contextual experiences and underlying beliefs and perceptions of the diagnosis and treatment be described. There are no published studies that have addressed this significant gap in the scientific literature. Furthermore, no study has directly explored patient perspectives, employing qualitative methodology, both at diagnosis and with treatment, to more fully describe contextual factors that differentiate CPAP adherers and nonadherers. Our study addressed several important questions: (a) What are adult OSA patients' beliefs and perceptions about OSA, the associated risks, and treatment with CPAP prior to treatment use? (b) What are the consequences of these beliefs and perceptions on the use of CPAP? (c) What are the beliefs and perceptions of adults with OSA after 1 week of CPAP use, including perceived benefits of treatment, effect of treatment on health, and perceived ability to adapt to CPAP? and (d) Do differences exist between adherers and nonadherers with regard to their beliefs and perceptions at diagnosis and with treatment use that might, in part, explain differences in CPAP adherence outcomes? To our knowledge, our study findings provide the first published description of beliefs of those who adhere and those who choose not to adhere to CPAP treatment. These findings contribute to understanding patient treatment decisions regarding CPAP use, suggest opportunities for identifying those at risk for nonadherence

to CPAP, and contribute toward developing tailored interventions to promote CPAP use.

■ Conceptual Framework

Acceptance and consistent use of CPAP is influenced by a multitude of factors, as is evidenced in previous studies examining predictors of CPAP adherence (Weaver & Grunstein, 2008). It is therefore important to approach the phenomenon of CPAP adherence from a multifactorial perspective that addresses the complex nature of this particular health behavior. The application of social cognitive theory has been widely applied in studies of adoption, initiation, and maintenance of health behaviors (Bandura, 1977, 1992; Schwarzer & Fuchs, 1996). The core determinants of the model include knowledge, perceived self-efficacy, outcome expectations, health goals, and facilitators/barriers. The model posits that health promoting behaviors are primarily influenced by patients' self-efficacy, or their belief in their ability to exercise control over personal health habits, which influences other critical determinants: knowledge, outcome expectations, goals, and perceived facilitators and impediments (Bandura, 2004; see Figure 1). Knowledge of health risks and specific benefits relative to health behaviors is a necessary determinant for health behaviors, but rarely does knowledge alone promote change in behaviors. Outcome expectations, or the expectancies one holds for investing in a particular health behavior, are evaluated by the individual in terms of costs and benefits, including physical, social, and psychological. Individuals who anticipate that the benefits of a health behavior outweigh the costs are more inclined to perceive the health behavior as favorable, and more inclined to set short- and long-term personal goals to guide adoption of that health behavior. This cascade of health behavior determinants does not occur in isolation, but is influenced by barriers and facilitators that derive from personal, social,

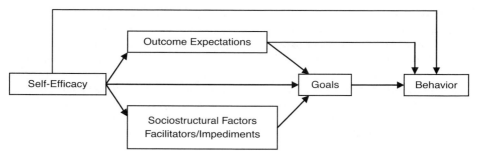

Figure 1. Social cognitive theory health determinants: Pathways of influence of self-efficacy on health behaviors. From Bandura, A. (2004). Health promotion by social cognitive means. *Health Education & Behavior, 31*(2), 146. Copyright 2004 by Sage Publications. Reprinted with permission of the publisher.

and environmental circumstances. As individuals identify facilitators for the health behavior and overcome barriers, their belief in their ability to successfully change or adopt a health behavior (i.e., perceived self-efficacy) increases.

Recognizing that individuals exist within a collective agency or community, the construct of self-efficacy is not confined solely to personal capabilities. Although commonalities in the basic concepts of self-efficacy exist across cultures, the "cultivated identities, values, belief structures, and agentic capabilities are the psychosocial systems through which experiences are filtered" (Bandura, 2002, p. 273). Bandura suggested that the application of social cognitive theory must be situated in context, recognizing that "human behavior is socially situated, richly contextualised, and conditionally expressed" (2002, p. 276). From this conceptual perspective and in a predominantly qualitative research paradigm, we examined patients' perceptions, beliefs, and experiences within their own context to permit an explicit description of salient factors that influenced OSA patients' decisions to use or not use CPAP.

■ Method

DESIGN

Using a concurrent nested, mixed method design, we conducted a longitudinal study extending from initial diagnosis through the first week of home CPAP treatment of newly diagnosed OSA patients. We conducted two individual interviews with participants and collected first-week CPAP adherence data. In contrast to a triangulation design, the concurrent nested study design emphasizes one methodology, and the data are mixed at the analysis phase of the study (Creswell, Plano Clark, Gutmann, & Hanson, 2003). Nesting the less dominant quantitative method within the predominant qualitative method permitted an enriched description of the participants and a more in-depth analysis of the overall phenomenon of interest: CPAP adherence (Creswell et al., 2003).

Sawyer, 2010

PARTICIPANTS

Adults with suspected OSA were recruited from a sleep clinic at an urban Veterans Affairs medical center during a 5-month enrollment period. One sleep specialist referred potential participants who were clinically likely to have OSA to the study. Our purposive sampling strategy was to include patients who (a) provided detailed information during their initial clinical visit and were willing to openly discuss their health and health care; (b) had at least moderate OSA (AHI $\geq$ 15 events/hour; American Academy of Sleep Medicine Task Force, 1999) and were prescribed CPAP treatment; (c) initially accepted CPAP for home use; and (d) were able to speak and understand English. To ensure that participants would be prescribed CPAP treatment based on Veterans Health Administration CPAP prescribing guidelines in place during study enrollment, patients with mild OSA (AHI < 15 events/hour) were excluded. We also excluded participants who had current or historical treatment with CPAP or any other treatment for OSA, a previous diagnosis of OSA, refusal of CPAP treatment by the participant prior to any CPAP exposure (i.e., in-laboratory CPAP titration sleep study), and those who required supplemental oxygen in addition to CPAP and/or bilevel positive airway pressure therapy for treatment of sleep-disordered breathing during their in-laboratory CPAP titration sleep study.

Previous studies have identified that decisions to adhere to CPAP emerge by the second to fourth day of treatment (Aloia, Arnedt, Stanchina, et al., 2007; Weaver, Kribbs, et al., 1997). Therefore, it is possible that patients' beliefs, perceptions, and experiences during the first several experiences with CPAP might significantly influence short- and long-term CPAP adherence patterns. For this reason, we did not include individuals who refused CPAP treatment prior to any CPAP experience, because we sought to describe salient factors preceding and during initial CPAP exposure. The protocol was approved by the research site and the affiliated university's institutional review boards. All participants provided informed consent prior to participating in any study activities.

PROCEDURE

After study enrollment, each participant had two in-laboratory, full-night sleep studies (i.e., polysomnograms). The first sleep study was a diagnostic study and the second sleep study was to determine the therapeutic CPAP pressure necessary to eliminate obstructive sleep apnea events. All sleep studies were performed and scored using standard criteria (American Academy of Sleep Medicine Task Force, 1999; Rechtschaffen & Kales, 1968). The AHI, a

measure of disease severity in OSA, was computed from the diagnostic polysomnogram as the number of apneas and/or hypopneas per hour of sleep. The therapeutic CPAP pressure, the pressure required to eliminate hypopneas and apneas, was determined on a manual CPAP titration polysomnogram performed about 1 week (7.9 ± 6.9 days) after the diagnostic polysomnogram.

Semistructured Interviews. Semistructured interviews, conducted by one study investigator, were scheduled with participants at two intervals: within 1 week following diagnosis but prior to the CPAP titration sleep study, and after the first week of CPAP treatment at home (see Figure 2). All interviews were conducted in an informal, private room at the medical center to ensure privacy, participant comfort, and promote open sharing of information (Streubert Speziale & Carpenter, 2003). To minimize attrition, participants were offered the opportunity to participate in interviews at an alternative location or by telephone if transportation difficulties or ambulatory limitations precluded study participation.

Interview guides, consisting of specific questions and probes (i.e., prompts to encourage focus on the particular issue of interest) were used for each interview to ensure that a consistent sequence and set of questions were addressed across participants. A funnel approach was used in the development and execution of the interview guides. This approach begins with broad questions and gradually progresses to focused questions specific to the phenomenon of interest to promote sharing of experiences by the participants (Tashakkori & Teddlie, 1989). The first interview focused on perceptions of the diagnosis, perceived health effects of the diagnosis, pretreatment perceptions of CPAP, and the social and cultural precedents that led to the participant seeking medical care for their sleep problems (see Table 1). The second interview focused on perceived effects of treatment with CPAP, supportive mechanisms or barriers to using CPAP, and how beliefs and perceptions about the diagnosis, associated risks of

SAWYER

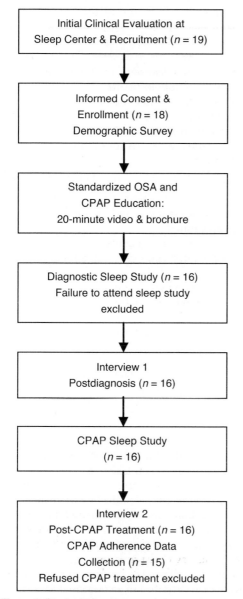

Figure 2. Study design.

after each interview to describe the environment of the interview, describe the participant at the time of the interview, and note any aberrations from the planned interview guide that occurred and a description of such aberrations. The field notes not only served as a descriptive context of the interview, but also served as interviewer reflexivity notations (i.e., interviewer biases, suppositions, and presuppositions of the research topic). The purpose of maintaining reflexivity notations was to ensure that interviewer-imposed assumptions did not take precedent over the participant's described experience.

CPAP Adherence. In accordance with the standard of clinical care at the sleep center, all participants were issued the same model CPAP machine (Respironics Rem- Star Pro®) that records on a data card (SmartCardTM) the time each day that the CPAP circuit is pressurized, an objective measurement of daily CPAP mask-on time. CPAP use was defined as periods when the device was applied for more than 20 minutes at effective pressure. One week of CPAP adherence data were uploaded to a personal computer for software analysis (Respironics EncorePro®) at the time of the second semistructured interview. Graphic adherence data were used as probes to discuss specific occurrences of CPAP nonuse. The objectively measured CPAP adherence data were also used to identify adherent (≥ 6hrs/night CPAP use) and nonadherent participants (< 6hrs/night CPAP use). A cut-off point of 6 hours/night was selected a priori to describe adherers and nonadherers to CPAP treatment, as recent evidence suggests that 6 or more hours of CPAP use per night is necessary to improve both functional and objective sleepiness outcomes (Weaver et al., 2007).

ANALYSIS

A sequential analysis was conducted, with qualitative-directed content analysis of interview data followed by quantitative descriptive

the diagnosis, and the treatment experience might have affected CPAP adherence (see Table 2). Interviews were digitally audio-recorded and transcribed to an electronic format by a professional transcriptionist not affiliated with the study. Field notes were maintained by the interviewer before and

Table 1. Postdiagnosis Interview Guide

Concept	Topic/Question
Perceptions and knowledge of diagnosis	How did you know about sleep disorders and the sleep center before coming to your first appointment? Before being told you have OSA,[a] had you heard of OSA? If so, what did you know about OSA? What do you now understand about OSA? After having your sleep study, what are your thoughts about OSA and what it means to you?
Perceived effects of diagnosis	How do you believe OSA affects you in your daily life?
Sociocultural precedents and influences on health, illness/disease, and care seeking	Do you know anyone else who has been diagnosed with OSA? If so, how did that impact you and your interest in coming to the sleep center? Why did you seek care from the sleep center? Is there anyone who influenced you to seek care for this problem? Is there anyone who has helped you understand what OSA is? If so, how did that information impact your desire to receive treatment? What has you experience with a health care system been to this point? Do sleep, sleeping, and/or the sleep environment have any specific meaning(s) to you? To your family? To your spouse/significant other/bed partner?

[a]OSA = Obstructive sleep apnea

analysis of the CPAP adherence data. By sequentially analyzing the data, the priority of the individual as informant was emphasized and the investigators were blinded to CPAP adherence until the final analysis procedure, a mixed methods analysis, was conducted (see Figure 3). By dividing the participants into categories of adherent (i.e., ≥ 6 hrs/night CPAP use) and nonadherent (i.e., < 6 hrs/night CPAP use), we examined across-case consistencies in subthemes and themes to describe the contextualized experience of adhering or not adhering to CPAP treatment.

Each transcript was read in its entirety, highlighting, extracting, and condensing text from individual interviews that addressed individual beliefs, perceptions, and/or experiences during diagnosis and early treatment with CPAP. This process of text analysis brought forward the manifest content of the qualitative data (Graneheim & Lundman, 2004). These responses were separated from the interview text, identified by participant identification number, and entered into an analysis table. Abstraction, or the process of taking condensed, manifest data and interpreting the underlying meaning (i.e., latent meaning), followed as participant responses were then described in a condensed format and interpreted for meaning within a thematic coding process. Trustworthiness was enhanced as the likelihood of investigator bias was minimized by first highlighting relevant text for coding, extracting relevant text from complete interviews transcripts, and then coding the meaning units for theory-driven categories or themes and then for subthemes (Hsieh & Shannon, 2005).

Table 2. One Week Post-CPAP Use Interview Guide

Concept	Topic/Question
Perceived effects and knowledge of treatment with CPAP	Have you been using CPAP[a] for the treatment of your OSA[b]?
	How would you describe your use of CPAP?
	Are you experiencing any improvement in the way that you feel since you have started using CPAP?
	When did you first learn about CPAP?
	Who first described CPAP to you?
	What did you think when you first learned about CPAP? First saw CPAP? First used CPAP in the sleep laboratory?
	What do you see as the most important reason for using CPAP in the short term? In the long term?
Supportive mechanisms or barriers to incorporating CPAP into daily life	How was the first week of CPAP treatment?
	What kinds of problems are you experiencing using CPAP?
	What has prevented you from regularly using CPAP?
	What has been helpful to you in regularly using CPAP?
Sociocultural perspectives of health-related decisions to use or not use CPAP	Do you believe CPAP treatment is a treatment you can [continue to] use?
	Did this belief change since you first learned about your OSA diagnosis? Since starting CPAP?
	Do you envision yourself using CPAP during the next 3 months? During the next year? During the next 5 years?
	Do you have any concerns about the CPAP unit? About your sleep [ability or quality]? About your sleep environment that might affect your CPAP use?
	How does the diagnosis of OSA and treatment with CPAP affect or been affected by those around you?

[a]CPAP = continuous positive airway pressure.
[b]OSA = obstructive sleep apnea.

The overarching, theory-derived themes were initially determined by applying the broad determinants of health as described in the study's conceptual framework, social cognitive theory (Bandura, 2004). These themes included knowledge, perceived barriers and facilitators, perceived self-efficacy, outcome expectations, and goals. This approach permitted the investigators to examine the applicability of the theoretical framework to the phenomenon of CPAP adherence and elaborate on previous findings suggesting the framework's concepts as measurable predictors of CPAP-related health behaviors (Aloia,

Arnedt, Stepnowsky, et al., 2005; Stepnowsky, Bardwell, et al., 2002; Wild et al., 2004). Emergent subthemes were identified as thematic content analysis progressed. The subthemes were then categorized within the overarching conceptual framework themes (see Table 3). We designed the analysis strategy to be consistent with other recent empirical studies of CPAP adherence while permitting a more robust, narrative description of what these theoretically derived variables mean from the perspective of the OSA patient.

Theme definitions were developed by the investigators and reviewed by an expert

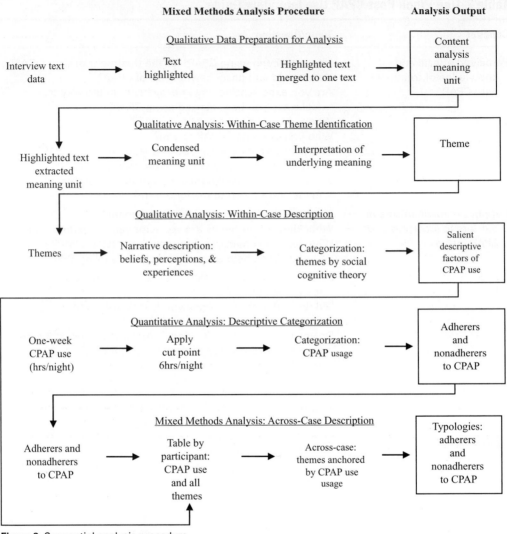

Figure 3. Sequential analysis procedure.

qualitative methodologist and an expert in the research application of theoretical constructs. One study investigator, blinded to CPAP adherence data, coded all interview data for the study. Valid application of the themes was examined by an independent expert coder. Coded interviews were independently recoded by the expert coder to establish validity and reliability of the application of the codes to the interview data. All extracted interview data were eligible for recoding; approximately 15% of the data from each total interview were randomly selected for expert recoding. Agreement of the study coder and the expert coder was 94%, meeting the established criteria of 80% agreement for acceptance of the coded data. When differences in application of codes were identified, code definitions were reviewed by coders, discussion of specific application of the code(s) was held, and

Table 3. Social Cognitive Theory Determinants of Health as Categorizing Framework for Themes From Content Analysis

Determinants of Health Behavior	Themes[a] Derived From Content Analysis
Knowledge	Fear of death
	Gathering information about OSA/CPAP gives rise to determining the importance of getting to treatment and decisions to accept/reject treatment
	Most immediate impact of OSA on daily life [single symptom] as a motivator to pursue diagnosis and treatment
	Justifying symptoms provides explanation for not pursuing diagnosis and/or treatment
	OSA impacts not only health but also quality of life
	Pervasive effects of OSA on life
	Sleepiness plays a limited role in life and can be accommodated
	Perceived health effects of a disorder are important to valuing diagnosis/treatment
	Associating health risks and functional limitations with OSA contributes to recognizing OSA as a health problem with significant effects on overall well-being
	Perception of seriousness of symptoms influenced by perceived effects symptoms have on individual [health risks] and those around individual [social network]
	Perceived health risks of OSA
	Information provided to individual and applicability of information influences individual's assumptions of responsibility for OSA and CPAP treatment
	Symptoms of OSA have impact on social roles, functions, and relationships
Perceived barriers and facilitators	Social influences as motivators to recognize health problem, seek diagnosis/treatment, and use CPAP
	Objective measures of OSA important to health care decision making
	Differences in perception of urgency of treatment between patient and provider influences valuing of diagnosis and treatment by patient
	Social networks contribute to treatment acceptance but not necessarily to treatment use
	Perceived seriousness of symptoms influenced by perceived effects of symptoms on individual [health risks] and those around individual
	Social networks provide support, help problem solve health concerns, and are sources of health-related information commonality of symptoms of OSA promotes perception of normalcy:
	Barrier to seeking diagnosis/treatment

(continued)

Table 3. *(Continued)*

Determinants of Health Behavior	Themes[a] Derived From Content Analysis
	Social influences as motivators to recognize health problem, seek diagnosis and treatment, and use treatment
	Silent symptoms: Fear of what it means if symptoms of OSA are undetectable
	Family and social networks contribute to health beliefs about sleep
	Expectations of health delivery vs. the actual delivery of health care services impact on the importance individual's place on their health and the value they place on their relationship with health care providers
Perceived self-efficacy	Knowledge and information provided to individual and applicability of information influences individual's assumption of responsibility for OSA and CPAP treatment
	Early response to CPAP, consistent or inconsistent with outcome expectations, facilitates or is a barrier to treatment use
	Early experience with CPAP is a source of support or a barrier to belief in own ability to use treatment
	Fitting treatment into life
	Problem-solving difficulties/routinization of CPAP responsibilities contribute to disease management
Outcome expectations	Understanding why symptoms exist and associating specific symptoms with a diagnosis provides hope that treatment will address experienced symptoms and improve overall quality of life
	Expectations of treatment outcomes are facilitators of treatment initiation and use
	Early response to CPAP, consistent or inconsistent with outcome expectations, facilitates or is a barrier to using treatment
Goals	Problem-solving difficulties/routinization of CPAP responsibilities contribute to disease management

[a] Themes derived from participant text data were categorized as a determinant of health behavior from social cognitive theory. Themes are not mutually exclusive. Theme definitions were mutually agreed on by investigators of the study and applied to the directed content analysis procedure by a single investigator acting as the primary coder of text data.

mutual agreement was achieved in all instances of coding differences.

After all interview data were coded for themes, the investigators used the average daily CPAP use during the first week of treatment to separate adherers (≥ 6 hours CPAP use/night) and nonadherers (< 6 hours CPAP use/ night). Descriptive statistics were used in the analysis of 1 week of CPAP adherence data (mean ± standard deviation [SD]).

Across-case analysis of themes and subthemes was then examined from an integrative perspective, using adherent and nonadherent as anchors, or as a unique descriptive qualifier, to identify common perceptions, beliefs, and experiences within the groups of interest. The across-case analysis, including both qualitative and quantitative data sets as complementary within an analysis matrix, gave rise to cases that had common descriptive aspects.

RESULTS

With the recurrence of themes in the content analysis phase, data saturation was reached at 15 participants and the sampling procedure was considered complete. The participants were all veterans, predominantly middleaged (53.9 ± 12.7 years) men (88%; see Table 4). The participants were well educated, with

Table 4. Sample Description

Characteristic	Frequency (%) (*n* = 15)
Gender	
Men	13 (87%)
Women	2 (13%)
Race/ethnicity	
African American	9 (60%)
White	5 (33%)
Other	1 (7%)
Marital status	
Married	7 (47%)
Single	3 (20%)
Divorced	3 (20%)
Widowed	2 (13%)
Highest education	
Middle school	1 (7%)
High school	7 (47%)
2 yr college	4 (27%)
4+ yr college	3 (20%)
Shift work	3 (20%)
Employed	6 (40%)
Retired	6 (40%)

	Mean 6 Standard Deviation
Age, years	53.9 ±12.7
Weight, pounds	248.9 ± 68.7
AHI, events/hour	53.5 ± 26.5
O2 Nadir, %	66.4 ± 13.2
CPAP pressure, cmH_2O	10.7 ± 1.6
1 week CPAP adherence, hours	4.98 ± 0.5

93% (*n* = 14) of the sample achieving a high school education or higher. The sample, on average, had severe OSA (AHI 53.5 ± 26.5 events/hr), with an oxygen nadir of 66.4% (± 13.2%). The average CPAP pressure setting was 10.7 ± 1.6 cmH20. Average CPAP use during the first 7 days of CPAP treatment was 4.98 ± 0.5 hours/night. Sorting on CPAP adherence (i.e. ≥ 6hrs/night CPAP use and < 6 hrs/ night CPAP use), there were six adherers and nine nonadherers. The interview prior to CPAP exposure was conducted after the diagnostic polysomnogram, on average at Day 9 (range 2 to 28 days), and the second interview was conducted following at least 1 week of CPAP treatment (average number of days from Day 1 of CPAP use, 18; range 7 to 47 days).

ADHERERS AND NONADHERERS TO CPAP THERAPY

Knowledge and Perceived Health Risks. Knowledge, or the "knowing" an individual has about the health risks and benefits of health behaviors (Bandura, 2004) was a predominant theme in both interviews for all participants. Saturation on nearly every knowledge theme suggests that participants identified that having an understanding of OSA and CPAP is an important part of the experience of being diagnosed with OSA and treated with CPAP. Adherent participants related their knowledge of risks and benefits of CPAP to their own outcome expectations after being diagnosed with OSA. For some participants, knowledge of OSA being simply more than snoring was a first step in recognizing OSA as a syndrome with health implications. One participant described this, saying, "I knew sleep apnea existed, but it just never dawned on me how serious it was in my case. I just didn't pay any attention to it. I just figured I was going to snore for the rest of my life."

For many participants, "putting the whole picture together" after receiving education about OSA and CPAP treatment helped them understand that they not only were experiencing symptoms of OSA on a daily basis, but their overall health and quality of life was impacted by OSA. During the first interview, participants were provided with a summary of their diagnostic sleep study results. The combination of education about the OSA diagnosis and treatment with CPAP, and relating their own diagnosis to their daily health and functioning, was important to adherent participants' formulation of accurate beliefs and perceptions of OSA and CPAP. These beliefs served to motivate or facilitate adherent participants' determination to pursue CPAP after diagnosis:

> I didn't know anything really, how the CPAP worked or anything like that. I just knew that there was a disease called sleep apnea and that a lot of people have it and people don't realize it. I really still didn't know anything about it til after I went through the test [diagnostic polysomnogram]. . . . Five [breathing events] is normal and thirty is severe and I'm doing ninety an hour. You know that literally scared the hell right out of me because all I could think of is I'm going to die in my sleep.
>
>   [T]hen when you told me about driving, being tired, I remembered that every time we take off on a long trip, the first hour I got to pull over and rest. So it all came together. So I figured maybe I do have it [OSA].

For many adherent participants, knowledge of health risks associated with OSA was limited to "being sluggish" or "having low energy levels." For some, their perception of OSA was only relative to "falling asleep when I sit down." Participants who "put the whole picture together," relating their diagnosis to their own health status, were motivated to accept CPAP treatment from the outset. For example, one participant said, "It's [OSA] got to take a toll in the long run on a lot of things, like high blood pressure. I'm hoping that it helps me to drop my high blood pressure." These perceptions provided hope for adherent participants that expanded beyond the management of their OSA to other disease and health experiences:

> If I have more energy and I'm not so sluggish—because I go to the local high school track and get in five or six laps, walking around the track—I

will have more energy to do those kinds of things that keep you healthy.

Posttreatment, there was less emphasis on knowledge-based themes among adherent participants. This suggested a shift of emphasis among adherers from knowledge of risks and benefits of OSA to perceptions derived from the actual experience of CPAP treatment.

Nonadherent participants' knowledge at diagnosis was not different from adherent participants' knowledge. However, those with knowledge that served as a barrier, rather than a facilitator, to diagnosis were less likely to pursue a diagnostic sleep study in a timely fashion. This was particularly true for those who had inaccurate knowledge and perceptions of OSA, such as OSA being a condition of simple snoring. Even though many acknowledged they probably had OSA, the snoring was the "problem" that defined OSA, not apneic events and resultant untoward health and functional outcomes. As one participant described,

> My brother does it [snores], and he stopped [breathing] all the time in the middle of the night. My father did it, you know, and I do it. I knew I do it so it's been a while, I mean, I don't remember not being a loud snorer. . . . Like I said, my condition is hereditary. I'm sure my oldest son has it and I'm sure my youngest son is going to end up with it. My brother had it and my father had it, you know, my mother probably had it 'cause she's a snorer. I didn't think it was serious of a problem 'cause it's [snoring, stops in breathing] something that I had experienced for so many years.

Furthermore, describing early knowledge of "having to wear a mask" for the treatment of OSA served as a barrier to both seeking diagnosis and treatment for some. This perception was not consistent among only nonadherers though, as many of the participants expressed concerns about the anticipated treatment of their OSA. CPAP adherers and nonadherers described critically important differences in their own ability to reconcile the following: (a) their OSA diagnosis; (b) their experience of symptoms; (c) their goals for treatment use; and (d) their outcome expectations that were met after treatment exposure. These factors, when reconciled by the individual, facilitated overall positive perceptions of the diagnosis and treatment experience.

Goal Setting and Outcome Expectancies.
Outcome expectancies are the expected or anticipated costs and benefits for healthful habits/behaviors that support or deter from an individual's investment in the behavior (Bandura, 2004). Among the participants, postdiagnosis outcome expectancies that were consistently met were highly influential on participants' decisions to use CPAP. For example, after being diagnosed with OSA, one participant brought all his experienced symptoms into perspective, relating them to his OSA. With treatment, he was hopeful that these symptoms would resolve. He stated, "It seems like sleep apnea basically causes all those problems. So I figure if I can get this taken care of [by wearing CPAP], basically the problems will subside." Making sense of symptoms in terms of treatment outcome expectancies helped adherers commit to trying CPAP and believing that CPAP was going to be a positive experience. One participant summarized his perception of symptoms and outcome expectations like this: "But without me even trying it I know that what I'm experiencing and how it's affected me, and that I want to get better if I can and so there's nothing going to keep me away from getting a CPAP."

A particularly important perception described by participants was their early response to CPAP as influential on future/continued use of CPAP. These early, first experiences were helpful to formulating realistic and personally important outcome expectancies for CPAP use. One participant described his response to CPAP after wearing it for the first time in the sleep laboratory during his second sleep study (i.e., CPAP sleep study):

> But being like I got relief the first night I was at the hospital. I drove home that morning after they woke me up, I went down, I got breakfast, and I'm driving home, I'm saying to myself, gee, I feel great and I only got from one o'clock to six, you know. I feel so much better and I felt so much better that whole day. I felt so good after that five hours of sleep with the machine on that it sold me.

For adherent participants, having a positive response to CPAP during the sleep study night with CPAP was highly motivating for continued CPAP use at home. Furthermore, this early response set the stage for participants to develop an early commitment to the treatment, even when faced with barriers. Persistent, positive responses to CPAP throughout the early treatment period (i.e., 1 week) reinforced participants' outcome expectancies and helped them formulate a perception of the treatment that was conducive to long-term use.

Goals for improved health and for achieving certain health behaviors are an important part of being successful with any health behavior. According to Bandura (2004), individuals set goals for their personal health, including establishing concrete plans or strategies for achieving those goals. Goal setting among adherent CPAP users focused on "how best to adapt to using CPAP" or identifying "solutions to difficulties with use of CPAP." These goals were established so that adherent CPAP users were able to achieve their outcome expectations. Goal setting was not specifically discussed by adherent participants before using CPAP. With exposure to and experience with CPAP, adherent participants first identified that using CPAP was important and, thereafter, identified "tricks and techniques" to successfully use CPAP. Whether these strategies originated from the participant or were a collaborative effort between participant and a support source, having a plan that addressed how best to adapt to CPAP promoted continued effort directed at using CPAP, as described by one adherent participant:

> I guess the first night I put it on I sort of got a little feeling of claustrophobia, but I pushed it out of my mind, saying to myself, "Don't let this [bother you], this is a machine that is going to help you, you got to wear it," so I just put it in my mind that I was going to wear it.

As this participant described, it was important for him to devise a way that he could use the treatment so that he might realize his overall health goals. Similarly, one participant found that he could not fall asleep with CPAP at full pressure. He emphasized the importance of using CPAP to treat his OSA, but he equated using CPAP to "a tornado blowing through your nose." He recalled being taught about several features on the CPAP machine that might alleviate this sensation. After testing a few tricks on the CPAP machine, he found that he was able to fall asleep on a lower pressure setting while the pressure increased to full pressure setting after he was asleep (i.e., ramp function). By setting an immediate goal to get to sleep while wearing CPAP, he was able to achieve his longer-term goal to wear CPAP each night. The long-term goal of adherent participants was to feel better or sleep better, but the immediate goal was to be able to wear CPAP.

For nonadherers, a negative experience during their CPAP sleep study led them to have an undesirable outlook on CPAP and the overall treatment of OSA. For example, one participant described experiencing no immediate response to CPAP during the CPAP sleep study; therefore, he didn't expect to experience any response to treatment over a more extended period of time:

> I still had the same kind of sleep, I thought. As a matter of fact I thought it took me longer to get to sleep than it did on the first sleep study [without CPAP]. I believe my sleep was still the same type of sleep that I always get, even though, you know, the machine was supposed to make me sleep better. I still woke up in the same condition that I usually wake up in, is what I'm trying to say. I didn't feel any more vigorous or alert or anything after that first night.

Participants' descriptions of their considerations for using CPAP consistently included the question, "What are the down sides of using CPAP?" Combining early negative perceptions of the treatment and early negative experiences with CPAP, nonadherers tended to see the drawbacks of using the treatment as far outweighing any benefits of using the treatment. One participant described both negative perceptions and negative experiences, which caused him to believe that CPAP treatment outcome expectancies were not worth the torment of using the treatment:

> No, I didn't think I couldn't do it from the beginning. I was believing it was gonna do something more than what it did, and it didn't do anything. I'm not getting sleep, I'm still getting up tired. I guess I expected more from it and I didn't get anything, not anything that I could see anyway. No, just a bunch of botheration and I didn't get any sleep.

Among participants who did not adhere, the goal-oriented theme was not present after diagnosis. Nonadherers did not articulate specific goals for attaining treatment and, furthermore, they did not describe strategies to be able to wear CPAP after 1 week of CPAP treatment. For nonadherers, establishing treatment-related goals for use of CPAP was not a priority.

Facilitators of and Barriers to CPAP use.
Perceived facilitators and barriers can be personal, social, and/or structural. Although perceived facilitators and barriers are influential on health behaviors, this process is mediated by self-efficacy (Bandura, 2004). Therefore, the existence of a barrier, in and of itself, might not be particularly influential on an individual's behavior if their self-efficacy is high. Consistent with this conceptual perspective, some participants identified barriers that were particularly troublesome when using CPAP, but were vigilant users of CPAP despite these barriers. Conversely, those who described numerous facilitators to using CPAP treatment were not necessarily adherent to CPAP.

Adherent participants were less focused on potential or actual facilitators and barriers to using CPAP over time than nonadherers. When adherent participants discussed facilitators and barriers, their overall descriptions were positive, with facilitators being the focus of their experience after using CPAP for 1 week. No adherent participants emphasized barriers to using CPAP after 1 week of treatment. Furthermore, when faced with barriers, adherent participants described perceptions of the treatment as important and identified a belief in their ability to overcome the barrier. For example, one participant experienced a sensation of not being able to breathe during his second night of

CPAP use at home, but his ability to use CPAP was influenced by his commitment to "needing" the treatment:

> Because it was like I couldn't breathe and even though the machine was on, it was like I was paralyzed, and this happened every time when I tried to go back to sleep. How many times? Three more times that very same night until I was getting really anxious because every time I would try to go to sleep, after a while I would get that anxiety again. Finally, I prayed. I got up and I prayed real hard, asked God to really help me with this and I was right to sleep. Ever since then, I pray every night and have no problems.

As this example demonstrates, barriers and facilitators are not independent determinants of health behavior. Participants described situations and experiences that were labeled as either a facilitator or barrier, but the actual behavioral outcome of getting to diagnosis and using CPAP was not necessarily reflective of such experiences being a barrier or facilitator.

The facilitating experiences described by adherent participants centered on social interactions that provided motivation and facilitation of their CPAP use. Facilitating experiences included descriptions of social support, shared experiences of CPAP use with other CPAP users, and recognition that their own improvement as a result of CPAP treatment was an important influence on social relationships. Social relationships and the ability to be fully engaged in social interactions during their first week of CPAP use was described by several adherent participants as a facilitator to ongoing treatment:

> I see the difference. People see the difference. My wife sees the difference. My kids see the difference. That helps. I think that's 50% of it. People telling you that you have changed and things are getting better and you look a lot better and you a sound a lot better and you act a lot better, because when you have feedback like that you know it's [CPAP] helping.
>
> Our relationship [with spouse] is getting better and better. I think since the sleep machine it's even been more because some things that irritate me, I would speak on and it would cause like a little bit of friction, as it happens in couples. But since I've had the sleep machine, I've been letting the minor things go, things that irritate me or I would complain about before. . . . Communication, our rela-

tionship, so we've been able to talk more and enjoy each other even more since then [starting CPAP]. Yeah, I like the machine, I really do, and I like what it's doing.

Adherent participants clearly emphasized the importance of improved social relationships as a result of their CPAP treatment. Many recognized such improvements after a close friend or family member suggested the improvement was obvious.

Nonadherent participants emphasized barriers rather than facilitators to using CPAP after being diagnosed with OSA. However, after using CPAP for 1 week, nonadherers identified few, if any, actual barriers to treatment. Unlike adherent participants, nonadherers did not discuss social interactions as an important part of their post- CPAP treatment experience. Nonadherent participants also identified themselves as single, divorced, or widowed, with the exception of one participant. Nonadherers did not discuss their social networks (i.e., friends, family outside of their residence, coworkers) as important to their experiences of being diagnosed with OSA and starting CPAP treatment.

Perceived Self-Efficacy. Perceived self-efficacy is the belief that one can exercise control over one's own health habits, producing desired effects by one's own health behaviors (Bandura, 2004). This overarching theme was meaningfully described by participants and represented by several subthemes that were important to both adherers and nonadherers in the study. Within these descriptions, participants offered experiences with being diagnosed with OSA and using CPAP that led to their belief in themselves, or lack thereof, to use or not use the treatment.

Adherers in the sample described generally positive perceived self-efficacy regarding future use of CPAP. Adherers had a positive belief in their ability to use CPAP from the outset, which persisted and became increasingly frequent from diagnosis to early CPAP treatment, even if they first doubted their ability to use the treatment. As one participant described, the first thought of wearing a mask during sleep was not appealing, but with a positive first experience with CPAP, the participant was increasingly confident that CPAP was going to be a part of his life:

> I think I seen the masks sitting there and I thought to myself, I hope I don't have to wear one of those things. Then they came in and said, "Now we're going to put the CPAP on you," and I said, "Okay," and they put the CPAP on me and when they came back into the room I felt great when I woke up at six. They had to wake me up at six o'clock because I was sleeping and you know, I think I felt after that, I didn't care what it was if I got that much sleep from one o'clock to six without getting up. I was going to wear or do whatever I had to do to do it [wear CPAP].

Adherent participants also described that they planned to incorporate CPAP into their daily routine, suggesting an underlying positive belief in their ability to accomplish the health behavior of using CPAP. Recognizing that using CPAP would necessitate additional daily "work," adherers had well-defined plans of incorporating the added demands to their daily schedule:

> I have to just add some things that I have to do in order to keep the CPAP machine clean and to make sure that it's dry and each week I have to disinfect it, but once I did it, once I decided I was gonna do it, I just went in the bathroom, did the whole thing, it only took about twenty minutes, twenty-five minutes, and I was all done. And getting up in the morning and doing the daily cleaning, you know, that's not a negative but it's just something I have to make an adjustment to.

Nonadherent participants described having largely negative experiences with CPAP during the first exposure (i.e., CPAP sleep study) or during the early phase of home CPAP use. Few nonadherent participants experienced benefits with treatment and nonadherers described unsuccessful or a lack of problem-solving efforts with CPAP difficulties. These negative experiences were important areas of concern with regard to their perceived ability to use CPAP over the long term (perceived self-efficacy). For example, one participant had such an extremely negative experience during the first week he was exposed to CPAP that he firmly doubted his ability to ever use it:

> I couldn't breathe in [the mask]. This thing, I had to suck in to get a breath out of it. Last night I got a good night's sleep but I woke up, then I was claustrophobic. I felt like I was stuck under a bed someplace and couldn't get out and then I woke up. When I wore it the whole night through I wasn't sleeping so that's one of the reasons [I won't use CPAP], like I didn't sleep with it on; it was too aggravating.

Each participant described getting used to CPAP during the first several nights of treatment. With unsuccessful experiences during this period, participants either identified resources to help improve their experience or made decisions to use CPAP less or not at all. For all participants, early experiences with CPAP contributed to their belief in their own abilities to get used to the therapy.

Individuals who had difficulty fitting CPAP into their lives were challenged to be adherent to the treatment. When CPAP was seen as not fitting into a life routine, participants offered doubts as to their ability to continue to use the treatment. One participant described having a routine of falling asleep with television. With CPAP, she had difficulty watching television and therefore she experienced more difficulty getting to sleep. Although she continued to try to use CPAP, she expressed that using CPAP was generally annoying to her. The complexities presented by using CPAP within the constraints of her normal routine were likely to increasingly influence doubt in her ability to use CPAP.

MARRIED AND UNMARRIED CPAP USERS

With the emerging emphasis placed on social support and social networks by adherers in the study, we explored how the social context of daily life impacted on perceptions of OSA and CPAP treatment by examining married ($n = 7$) and unmarried ($n = 8$) participants' responses. Using married and unmarried status from self-reported demographic characteristics as anchors, or as a unique descriptive qualifier, we sorted the subthemes within an analysis matrix to identify common perceptions, beliefs, and experiences within these qualifier groups. We included all participants who identified themselves as married or common-law married as married; all participants who identified themselves as single, divorced, or widowed were included as unmarried.

These groups described different experiences with both diagnosis and CPAP treatment. Married participants offered descriptions of social support resources within immediate proximity that were positive facilitators of seeking diagnosis and starting/staying on treatment. Married participants expressed positive beliefs in their ability to use CPAP with early treatment use, often described in conjunction with a CPAP problem-solving episode that was collaboratively resolved with their partner/spouse. Married participants described overwhelmingly positive early responses and experiences with CPAP treatment. Their outcome expectations were consistent across time. They generally anticipated positive responses to CPAP prior to exposure and experienced positive responses to treatment after 1 week of use. Married participants also identified success in "fitting CPAP into their lives." These participants were able to identify far more benefits from than difficulties with CPAP, benefits that enhanced their ongoing commitment to use of the treatment. Married participants discussed proximate support sources (i.e., spouse, living partner, family members) as important to providing feedback about their response to treatment, trouble-shooting difficulties, and positive reinforcement for persistent use of CPAP.

Unmarried participants commonly identified friends or coworkers as motivating factors (facilitators) to seek diagnosis but less social influence on/facilitation of treatment use after 1 week of CPAP therapy. Without the presence of immediate social support, unmarried participants did not emphasize important social interactions with actual wearing of CPAP. After 1 week of treatment on CPAP, unmarried participants described less confidence in their ability to use CPAP and described less "response" to CPAP than those participants who were married. Unmarried participants described few facilitators of treatment use during the first week of CPAP therapy. Nearly all unmarried participants identified "self-driven" reasons for pursuing treatment, and there was an absence of social sources of support, or "cheerleaders and helpful problem solvers" while using CPAP during the first week.

TYPOLOGIES OF ADHERENT AND NONADHERENT CPAP USERS

Described differences in beliefs, perceptions, and experiences of being diagnosed with OSA and early treatment with CPAP were explicit between adherers and nonadherers. Adherers perceived health and functional risks of untreated OSA, had positive belief in their ability to use CPAP from early in the diagnostic process, had clearly defined outcome expectations, had more facilitators than barriers as they progressed from diagnosis to treatment, and identified important social influences and support sources for both pursuing diagnosis and persisting with CPAP treatment. Nonadherers described not knowing the risks associated with OSA, perceived fewer symptoms of their diagnosis, did not have clearly defined outcome expectations for treatment, identified fewer improvements with CPAP exposure, placed less emphasis on social support and socially derived feedback with early CPAP treatment, and perceived and experienced more barriers to CPAP treatment. As a result of the across-case analysis in which consistencies and differences emerged among adherers and nonadherers in the described experience of being diagnosed with OSA and treated with CPAP, we suggest typologies, or descriptive profiles, of persons with CPAP-treated OSA (see Table 5). The typologies we propose are consistent with previous empirical studies of CPAP adherence, in that predictive relationships between risk perception, outcome expectancies, perceived self-efficacy, and social support with CPAP use have been identified. Our study findings extend the previous findings by illuminating the importance of contextual meaning persons

Table 5. Typologies of Adherent and Nonadherent CPAP Users

Adherent CPAP Users	Nonadherent CPAP Users
Define risks associated with OSA	Unable to define risks associated with OSA
Identify outcome expectations from outset	Describe few outcomes expectations
Have fewer barriers than facilitators	Do not recognize own symptoms
Facilitators less important later with treatment use	Describe barriers as more influential on CPAP use than facilitators
Develop and define goals and reasons for CPAP use	Facilitators of treatment absent or unrecognized
Describe positive belief in ability to use CPAP even with potential or experienced difficulties	Describe low belief in ability to use CPAP
Proximate social influences prominent in decisions to pursue diagnosis and treatment	Describe early negative experiences with CPAP, reinforcing low belief in ability to use CPAP
	Unable to identify positive responses to CPAP during early treatment

derive from their experiences, beliefs, and perceptions when progressing from diagnosis with OSA to treatment with CPAP. Moreover, the typologies succinctly describe critical differences between these groups of CPAP-treated OSA persons that support the development of patient-centered or -tailored adherence interventions that recognize individual differences.

▪ Discussion

To our knowledge, this is the first study to apply a predominantly qualitative method to describe individuals' beliefs and perceptions of the diagnosis of OSA and treatment with CPAP relative to short-term CPAP adherence. Our findings are consistent with previous, empirical studies with regard to the overall applicability of social cognitive theory to the phenomenon of CPAP adherence. The findings from our study uniquely extend these previous findings by illuminating the importance of the individual experiences, beliefs, and perceptions as influential on decisions to pursue diagnosis and treatment of OSA. The

described differences between adherers and nonadherers in our study suggest critical tailored or patient-centered intervention opportunities that might be developed and tested among patients who are newly diagnosed with OSA and anticipate CPAP treatment. The major findings of the study include the following: (a) adults described and assigned meaning to being diagnosed with OSA and treated with CPAP, which in turn influenced their decisions to accept or reject treatment and the extent of CPAP use; and (b) differences in beliefs and perceptions at diagnosis and with CPAP treatment were identified among CPAP adherers and nonadherers and also described in the social context of married and unmarried CPAP users. The described differences between these groups provide data to support the first published typology, or descriptive profile, of CPAP adherers and nonadherers.

Theoretically derived variables, such as the determinants of health behaviors described in social cognitive theory and applied in our study, are operational concepts that help us understand OSA patients' perceptions and beliefs about OSA and CPAP, and can guide interventions to improve adherence to CPAP.

operational concept (handwritten)

Framed by Bandura's social cognitive theory (1977), differences among adherers and nonadherers to CPAP can be defined across social cognitive theory determinants of health behaviors: (a) knowledge, (b) perceived self-efficacy, (c) outcome expectancies and goals, and (d) facilitators and barriers. As previous studies have demonstrated, psychosocial constructs, such as those consistent with social cognitive theory, provide possibly the most explained variance, to date, among adherers and nonadherers (Aloia, Arnedt, Stepnowsky, et al., 2005; Engleman & Wild, 2003; Stepnowsky, Bardwell, et al., 2002; Weaver et al., 2003). Furthermore, recent intervention studies to promote CPAP adherence have applied similar theoretical constructs with some positive findings (Aloia, Arnedt, Millman, et al., 2007; Richards, Bartlett, Wong, Malouff, & Grunstein, 2007). As our study findings suggest, decisions to use CPAP are individualized and at least in part dependent on the patient's support environment and early experiences with and beliefs about CPAP. Because early commitments to use or not use CPAP predict long-term use (Aloia, Arnedt, Stanchina, et al., 2007; Weaver, Kribbs, et al., 1997), it is critically important to understand and examine opportunities to intervene on factors that influence early commitments to use CPAP. This insight will potentiate the development of patient centered and -tailored interventions to improve CPAP adherence at the individual level while collectively promoting the health outcomes of the OSA population.

Our study confirms that social cognitive theory is applicable to the unique health behavior of using CPAP treatment. Indeed, the interacting determinants of health as described by Albert Bandura (1977) in relationship to decisions to accept and use CPAP were clearly described by our study participants. This affirmation suggests that any one measured domain within the model (i.e., barriers, facilitators, outcome expectancies) is not likely to identify persons at risk for nonadherence to CPAP. Rather, our study findings support the complex and reciprocating nature of the theoretical model as it applies to this

health behavior, and offer clarity to our understanding of CPAP adherence as a multifactorial, iterative decision-making process. It is therefore important to ascertain an understanding of the context of the individual from the initial diagnosis through early treatment use to address the complex nature of the problem of adherence to CPAP and to prospectively identify those likely to be nonadherent to the treatment.

In our study, the experience and perception of symptoms contributed to the participants' motivation to seek diagnosis and treatment and to adhere to CPAP treatment. Although studies that have examined pretreatment symptoms, particularly subjective sleepiness, have produced inconsistent results with regard to subsequent CPAP use, these studies have measured symptoms on quantitative scales that define specific scenarios of "impairment" related to the symptom of interest (i.e., Epworth Sleepiness Scale (Johns, 1993), Functional Outcomes of Sleep Questionnaire (Weaver, Laizner, et al., 1997), Stanford Sleepiness Scale (MacLean, Fekken, Saskin, & Knowles, 1992; Engleman et al., 1996; Hui et al., 2001; Janson, Noges, Svedberg-Randt, & Lindberg, 2000; Kribbs et al., 1993; Lewis et al., 2004; McArdle et al., 1999; Sin et al., 2002; Weaver, Laizner, et al., 1997). Yet, as our study highlights, perceptions of need relative to one's experience of symptoms were highly individual and significantly influenced decisions to pursue both diagnosis and treatment. Consistent with perceptions that influence medicine-taking behavior (Hansen, Holstein, & Hansen, 2009), particular situations necessitated the pursuit of diagnosis and use of the treatment. The experience of symptoms and the impact of symptoms on daily life were highly variable among participants and not readily amenable to discrete categorization. Understanding particular situations is important insight to explaining adherence to CPAP.

Recognizing and acknowledging that perceived symptoms are part of a disease process and logically linked to the diagnosis of OSA was important to the participants of our study, and to their commitment to move forward from diagnosis to treatment, consistent with Engleman and Wild's findings (2003). A recent intervention study to promote CPAP adherence incorporated specific strategies that address "personalization" of OSA symptoms (Aloia, Arnedt, Riggs, Hecht, & Borrelli, 2004; Aloia, Arnedt, Millman, et al., 2007). Results of this randomized controlled trial showed lower CPAP discontinuation rates among those participants who were in the motivational enhancement and education group when compared with "usual care," suggesting the importance of assisting persons diagnosed with OSA to make the connection between the objectively measured disease/diagnosis and their lived experience of the disease (Aloia, Arnedt, Millman, et al., 2007). Personalizing symptoms, recognizing the impact of symptoms on daily function, and identifying the meaning of disease in terms of the perception of one's own health were clearly described by participants in our study. Adherent and nonadherent participants clearly expressed differences in their experiences of having OSA, including the impact of functional impairment on social relationships. From these differing perspectives, participants defined outcome expectations and health risks associated with OSA in different ways, possibly influencing their eventual decision to use or discontinue CPAP.

The described importance of participants' early experiences with CPAP and their initial response to CPAP treatment, both during the CPAP sleep study and during the first week of CPAP use, were influential on participants' interest in continuing to use CPAP. Our study results are consistent with Van de Mortel, Laird, and Jarrett's (2000) findings in which nonadherent, CPAP-treated OSA patients had complaints about their sleep study experience and described "major" problems on the night of their CPAP titration. Similarly, Lewis et al. (2004) found that problems identified on the first night of CPAP use, albeit on autotitrating CPAP, were consistent with lower CPAP use. Not only has the initial experience in terms of difficulties with CPAP been identified as

important to subsequent CPAP adherence, but also the patient's response to the first night of CPAP (i.e., degree of sleep improvement) has been correlated with subsequent CPAP adherence (Drake et al., 2003). The importance of promoting a positive initial experience with CPAP and providing anticipatory guidance about outcome expectations is highlighted by our findings.

The significance of social support, both proximate and within the broader social network, was an important facilitator of CPAP use among adherers in our study. Differences between the experiences of married and unmarried individuals with OSA revealed the described importance of an immediate, proximate source of support for CPAP use. Our finding is consistent with previous findings that those CPAP users who lived alone were significantly less likely to use their CPAP than those who lived with someone (Lewis et al., 2004). Not only are immediate sources of support important for continued use of CPAP, but also shared experiences with CPAP from less-immediate social sources. Participants in our study described social relationships as motivators to seek diagnosis, providing positive reinforcement for persisting with treatment use, and a source for sharing tips on managing OSA and CPAP. Studies exploring reasons for nonadherence to antituberculosis drugs have similarly identified the importance of social influences on seeking treatment and using treatment (Naidoo, Dick, & Cooper, 2009). Among CPAP-treated OSA patients, intervention studies that included feedback to participants, positive reinforcement, inclusion of a support person, and assistance with trouble-shooting difficulties resulted in higher CPAP adherence among participants in the intervention groups as compared with placebo or usual-care groups (Aloia et al., 2001; Chervin, Theut, Bassetti, & Aldrich, 1997; Hoy, Vennelle, Kingshott, Engleman, & Douglas, 1999). Confirming the applicability of these intervention strategies, the described experiences of participants in our study provide empirical support for adherence interventions that include a support person, provide early feedback and positive reinforcement to patients, and assist with trouble-shooting difficulties in the early treatment period.

Barriers to subsequent CPAP use that were identified by participants of our study included the process of having to put a mask on every night, aesthetic issues with mask/headgear use, inconvenience of having to use a machine to sleep, and daily routines that were disrupted by CPAP. Consistent with previous studies (Engleman et al., 1994; Hui et al., 2001; Massie et al., 1999; Sanders et al., 1986), side effects of CPAP were not emphasized by participants as barriers to CPAP use. Although identified barriers did not necessitate nonadherence to CPAP in our study, it was important for individuals who experienced such barriers to identify positive reasons to use CPAP and successfully mitigate barriers, often with the help of others.

This study had several limitations. First, although the sample size of 15 was adequate for a qualitative study, there was limited power to conduct any exploratory quantitative analyses. Although not the objective of this study, quantitative exploration of commonly used measures of subjective sleepiness, functional impairment, and adherence to CPAP correlated with descriptive, quantified typologies of adherent and nonadherent CPAP users would support the findings of the study. Study participants included predominantly male veterans with severe OSA who had relatively high educational preparation. Examining this typology in a larger, more heterogeneous sample of OSA patients is needed. As the relationship of gender, disease severity, symptom perception, and disease- specific literacy with CPAP adherence has not been clearly defined, replicating this study in a more diverse sample and expanding concurrently measured quantitative outcomes would be informative and supportive of typology refinement or expansion. Finally, to reduce the potential confounding effect of clinically delivered psychoeducation, we enrolled participants referred to the study from a single clinical provider with limited participant–provider interaction at the first prediagnostic evaluation. However, participants

may have had telephone contact with the sleep center staff, or had unscheduled visits at the sleep center that were not controlled for in any way in our study.

Our mixed methods, exploratory study, employing a predominantly qualitative methodology, achieved saturation of themes regarding the diagnosis of OSA and nightly CPAP use during the first week of treatment. The study results are consistent with previous studies of CPAP, even when adherence, in many previous studies, was defined as four hours/night of use rather than six hours/night of use, as in our study. With recent evidence suggesting better outcomes with longer nightly CPAP use (Stradling & Davies, 2000; Weaver et al., 2007; Zimmerman, Arnedt, Stanchina, Millman, & Aloia, 2006), applying a definition of CPAP adherence of six hours vs. four hours likely contributed to more robust differences in described beliefs and perceptions among adherers and nonadherers. To our knowledge, the results of our study provide the first published, narrative descriptions of CPAP adherers and nonadherers that support an overall composite of characteristics that might be useful in identifying specific subgroups of patients who are most likely to benefit from tailored interventions to lessen the risk for subsequent CPAP nonadherence. To date, studies have provided adherence promotion interventions to unselected groups, possibly minimizing variation of response between intervention and control groups. Future randomized controlled trials testing CPAP adherence interventions delivered to participants who are selected based on their risk for treatment failure because of nonadherence are necessary to evaluate intervention effectiveness.

■ Acknowledgments

We acknowledge the sleep center staff's commitment to the conduct and completion of the study, and the exemplary transcription services provided by Charlene Hunt at Transcribing4You~Homework4You.

▪ Declaration of Conflicting Interests

The authors declared a potential conflict of interest (e.g., a financial relationship with the commercial organizations or products discussed in this article) as follows: Dr. Kuna has received contractural support and equipment from Phillips Respironics, Inc. Dr. Weaver has a licensing agreement with Phillips Respironics, Inc., for the Functional Outcomes of Sleep Questionnaire.

▪ Funding

The authors disclosed receipt of the following financial support for the research and/authorship of this article: The study was supported by award number F31NR9315 (Sawyer) from the National Institute of Nursing Research. The content is solely the responsibility of the authors and does not necessarily represent the official views of the National Institute of Nursing Research or the National Institutes of Health.

Bios

Amy M. Sawyer, PhD, RN, is a postdoctoral research fellow at the University of Pennsylvania School of Nursing, Philadelphia, Pennsylvania, and a nurse researcher at the Philadelphia Veterans Affairs Medical Center, Philadelphia, Pennsylvania, USA.

Janet A. Deatrick, PhD, RN, FAAN, is an associate professor and associate director, Center for Health Equities Research, at the University of Pennsylvania School of Nursing, Philadelphia, Pennsylvania, USA.

Samuel T. Kuna, MD, is an associate professor of medicine at the University of Pennsylvania School of Medicine and chief, Pulmonary, Critical Care and Sleep Medicine, at the Philadelphia Veterans Affairs Medical Center, Philadelphia, Pennsylvania, USA.

Terri E. Weaver, PhD, RN, FAAN, is the Ellen and Robert Kapito Professor in Nursing Science, chair, Biobehavioral Health Sciences Division, and associate director, Biobehavioral Research Center, at the University of Pennsylvania School of Nursing, Philadelphia, Pennsylvania, USA.

Corresponding Author
Amy M. Sawyer, University of Pennsylvania School of Nursing, Claire
M. Fagin Hall, 307b, 418 Curie Blvd., Philadelphia, PA 19104, USA Email: asawyer@nursing.upenn.edu

REFERENCES

Al Lawati, N. M., Patel, S., & Ayas, N. T. (2009). Epidemiology, risk factors, and consequences of obstructive sleep apnea and short sleep duration. *Progress in Cardiovascular Diseases, 51,* 285–293.

Aloia, M. S., Arndt, J., Riggs, R. L., Hecht, J., & Borrelli, B. (2004). Clinical management of poor adherence to CPAP: Motivational enhancement. *Behavioral Sleep Medicine, 2*(4), 205–222.

Aloia, M. S., Arndt, J. T., Millman, R. P., Stanchina, M., Carlisle, C., Hecht, J., et al. (2007). Brief behavioral therapies reduce early positive airway pressure discontinuation rates in sleep apnea syndrome: Preliminary findings. *Behavioral Sleep Medicine, 5,* 89–104.

Aloia, M. S., Arndt, J. T., Stanchina, M., & Millman, R. P. (2007). How early in treatment is PAP adherence established? Revisiting night-to-night variability. *Behavioral Sleep Medicine, 5,* 229–240.

Aloia, M. S., Arndt, J. T., Stepnowsky, C., Hecht, J., & Borrelli, B. (2005). Predicting treatment adherence in obstructive sleep apnea using principles of behavior change. *Journal of Clinical Sleep Medicine, 1*(4), 346–353.

Aloia, M. S., Di Dio, L., Ilniczky, N., Perlis, M. L., Greenblatt, D. W., & Giles, D. E. (2001). Improving compliance with nasal CPAP and vigilance in older adults with OAHS. *Sleep and Breathing, 5*(1), 13–21.

American Academy of Sleep Medicine Task Force. (1999). Sleep-related breathing disorders in adults: Recommendations for syndrome definitions and measurement techniques in clinical research. *Sleep, 22,* 667–689.

Bandura, A. (1977). Self-efficacy: Toward a unifying theory of behavioral change. *Psychological Reviews, 84,* 191–215.

Bandura, A. (1992). Exercise of personal agency through the self-efficacy mechanism. In R. Schwarzer (Ed.), *Self-efficacy: Thought control of action* (pp. 3–38). Philadelphia: Hemisphere.

Bandura, A. (2002). Social cognitive theory in cultural context. *Applied psychology: An International Review, 51*(2), 269–290.

Bandura, A. (2004). Health promotion by social cognitive means. *Health Education & Behavior, 31*(2), 143–164.

Chervin, R. D., Theut, S., Bassetti, C., & Aldrich, M. S. (1997). Compliance with nasal CPAP can be improved by simple interventions. *Sleep, 20*, 284–289.

Creswell, J. W., Plano Clark, V. L., Gutmann, M. L., & Hanson, W. (2003). Advanced mixed methods research designs. In A. Tashakkori & C. Teddlie (Eds.), *Handbook of mixed methods in social & behavioral research* (pp. 209–240). Thousand Oaks, CA: Sage.

Drake, C. L., Day, R., Hudgel, D., Stefadu, Y., Parks, M., Syron, M. L., et al. (2003). Sleep during titration predicts continuous positive airway pressure compliance. *Sleep, 26*, 308–311.

Engleman, H. M., Asgari-Jirandeh, N., McLeod, A. L., Ramsay, C. F., Deary, I. J., & Douglas, N. J. (1996). Self-reported use of CPAP and benefits of CPAP therapy. *Chest, 109*, 1470–1476.

Engleman, H. M., Martin, S. E., & Douglas, N. J. (1994). Compliance with CPAP therapy in patients with the sleep apnoea/ hypopnoea syndrome. *Thorax, 49*, 263–266.

Engleman, H. M., & Wild, M. (2003). Improving CPAP use by patients with the sleep apnoea/ hypopnoea syndrome (SAHS). *Sleep Medicine Reviews, 7*(1), 81–99.

Gay, P., Weaver, T., Loube, D., & Iber, C. (2006). Evaluation of positive airway pressure treatment for sleep related breathing disorders in adults. *Sleep, 29*, 381–401.

Graneheim, U. H., & Lundman, B. (2004). Qualitative content analysis in nursing research: Concepts, procedures and measures to achieve trustworthiness. *Nursing Education Today, 24*, 105–112.

Grunstein, R. R., Stewart, D. A., Lloyd, H., Akinci, M., Cheng, N., & Sullivan, C. E. (1996). Acute withdrawal of nasal CPAP in obstructive sleep apnea does not cause a rise in stress hormones. *Sleep, 19*, 774–782.

Hansen, D. L., Holstein, B. E., & Hansen, E. H. (2009). "I'd rather not take it, but · · ·": Young women's perceptions of medicines. *Qualitative Health Research, 19*, 829–839.

Harsch, I., Schahin, S., Radespiel-Troger, M., Weintz, O., Jahrei, H., Fuchs, S., et al. (2004). Continuous positive airway pressure treatment rapidly improves insulin sensitivity in patients with obstructive sleep apnea syndrome. *American Journal of Respiratory & Critical Care Medicine, 169*, 156–162.

Hoy, C. J., Vennelle, M., Kingshott, R. N., Engleman, H. M., & Douglas, N. J. (1999). Can intensive support improve continuous positive airway pressure use in patients with the sleep apnea/hypopnea syndrome? *American Journal of Respiratory & Critical Care Medicine, 159*, 1096–1100.

Hsieh, H., & Shannon, S. (2005). Three approaches to qualitative content analysis. *Qualitative Health Research, 15*,1277–1288.

Hui, D., Choy, D., Li, T., Ko, F., Wong, K., Chan, J., et al. (2001). Determinants of continuous positive airway pressure compliance in a group of Chinese patients with obstructive sleep apnea. *Chest, 120*, 170–176.

Janson, C., Noges, E., Svedberg-Randt, S., & Lindberg, E. (2000). What characterizes patients who are unable to tolerate continuous positive airway pressure (CPAP) treatment? *Respiratory Medicine, 94*, 145–149.

Johns, M. (1993). Daytime sleepiness, snoring, and obstructive sleep apnea. The Epworth Sleepiness Scale. *Chest, 103*, 30–36.

Kribbs, N. B., Pack, A. I., Kline, L. R., Smith, P. L., Schwartz, A. R., Schubert, N. M., et al. (1993). Objective measurement of patterns of nasal CPAP use by patients with obstructive sleep apnea. *American Review of Respiratory Diseases, 147*, 887–895.

Krieger, J. (1992). Long-term compliance with nasal continuous positive airway pressure (CPAP) in obstructive sleep apnea patients and nonapneic snorers. *Sleep, 15*, S42–S46.

Lewis, K., Seale, L., Bartle, I. E., Watkins, A. J., & Ebden, P. (2004). Early predictors of CPAP use for the treatment of obstructive sleep apnea. *Sleep, 27*, 134–138.

MacLean, A. W., Fekken, G. C., Saskin, P., & Knowles, J. B. (1992). Psychometric evaluation of the Stanford Sleepiness Scale. *Journal of Sleep Research 1*, 35–39.

Massie, C., Hart, R., Peralez, K., & Richards, G. (1999). Effects of humidification on nasal symptoms and compliance in sleep apnea patients using continuous positive airway pressure. *Chest, 116*, 403–408.

McArdle, N., Devereux, G., Heidarnejad, H., Engleman, H. M., Mackay, T., & Douglas, N. J. (1999). Long-term use of CPAP therapy for sleep apnea/hypopnea syndrome. *American Journal of Respiratory and Critical Care Medicine, 159*, 1108–1114.

Meurice, J. C., Dore, P., Paquereau, J., Neau, J. P., Ingrand, P., Chavagnat, J. J., et al. (1994). Predictive factors of long-term compliance with nasal continuous positive airway pressure treatment in sleep apnea syndrome. *Chest, 105*, 429–434.

Naidoo, P., Dick, J., & Cooper, D. (2009). Exploring tuberculosis patients' adherence to treatment regimens and prevention programs at a public health site. *Qualitative Health Research 19*, 55–70.

Nieto, F., Young, T., Lind, B., Shahar, E., Samet, J., Redline, S., et al. (2000). Association of sleep-disordered breathing, sleep apnea, and hypertension in a large community-based study. *Journal of the American Medical Association, 283*, 1829–1836.

Peppard, P., Young, T., Palta, M., & Skatrud, J. (2000). Prospective study of the association between sleep-disordered breathing and hypertension. *New England Journal of Medicine, 342*, 1378–1384.

Rechtschaffen, A., & Kales, A. (Eds.). (1968). *A manual of standardized terminology, techniques and scoring system for sleep stages in human subjects.* Los Angeles: BIS/BRI. Reeves-Hoche, M. K., Meck, R., & Zwillich, C. W. (1994). Nasal CPAP: An objective evaluation of patient compliance. *American Journal of Respiratory & Critical Care Medicine, 149*, 149–154.

Richards, D., Bartlett, D. J., Wong, K., Malouff, J., & Grunstein, R. R. (2007). Increased adherence to CPAP with a group cognitive behavioral treatment intervention: A randomized trial. *Sleep, 30,* 635–640.

Rosenthal, L., Gerhardstein, R., Lumley, A., Guido, P., Day, R., Syron, M. L., et al. (2000). CPAP therapy in patients with mild OSA: Implementation and treatment outcome. *Sleep Medicine, 1,* 215–220.

Russo-Magno, P., O'Brien, A., Panciera, T., & Rounds, S. (2001). Compliance with CPAP therapy in older men with obstructive sleep apnea. *Journal of American Geriatric Society, 49,* 1205–1211.

Sanders, M. H., Gruendl, C. A., & Rogers, R. M. (1986). Patient compliance with nasal CPAP therapy for sleep apnea. *Chest, 90,* 330–333.

Schwarzer, R., & Fuchs, R. (1996). Self-efficacy and health behaviours. In M. Conner & P. Norman (Eds.), *Predicting health behaviour: Research and practice with social cognition models* (pp. 163–196). Philadelphia: Open Press.

Schweitzer, P., Chambers, G., Birkenmeier, N., & Walsh, J. (1997). Nasal continuous positive airway pressure (CPAP) compliance at six, twelve, and eighteen months. *Sleep Research, 16,* 186.

Sin, D., Mayers, I., Man, G., & Pawluk, L. (2002). Long-term compliance rates to continuous positive airway pressure in obstructive sleep apnea: A population-based study. *Chest, 121,* 430–435.

Stepnowsky, C., Bardwell, W. A., Moore, P. J., Ancoli-Israel, S., & Dimsdale, J. E. (2002). Psychologic correlates of compliance with continuous positive airway pressure. *Sleep, 25,* 758–762.

Stepnowsky, C., Marler, M. R., & Ancoli-Israel, S. (2002). Determinants of nasal CPAP compliance. *Sleep Medicine,3,* 239–247.

Stradling, J., & Davies, R. (2000). Is more NCPAP better? *Sleep, 23,* S150–S153.

Streubert Speziale, H., & Carpenter, D. (2003). *Qualitative research in nursing* (3rd ed.). Philadelphia: Lippincott Williams & Wilkins.

Sullivan, C., Barthon-Jones, M., Issa, F., & Eves, L. (1981). Reversal of obstructive sleep apnea by continuous positive airway pressure applied through the nares. *Lancet, 1,* 862–865.

Tashakkori, A., & Teddlie, C. (1989). *Mixed methodology: Combining qualitative and quantitative approaches.* London: Sage.

Van de Mortel, T. F., Laird, P., & Jarrett, C. (2000). Client perceptions of the polysomnography experience and compliance with therapy. *Contemporary Nurse, 9,* 161–168.

Weaver, T. E., & Grunstein, R. R. (2008). Adherence to continuous positive airway pressure therapy: The challenges to effective treatment. *Proceedings of the American Thoracic Society, 5,* 173–178.

Weaver, T. E., Kribbs, N. B., Pack, A. I., Kline, L. R., Chugh, D. K., Maislin, G., et al. (1997). Night-to-night variability in CPAP use over first three months of treatment. *Sleep, 20,* 278–283.

Weaver, T. E., Laizner, A. M., Evans, L. K., Maislin, G., Chugh, D. K., Lyon, K., et al. (1997). An instrument to measure functional status outcomes for disorders of excessive sleepiness. *Sleep, 20,* 835–843.

Weaver, T. E., Maislin, G., Dinges, D. F., Bloxham, T., George, C. F. P., Greenberg, H., et al. (2007). Relationship between hours of CPAP use and achieving normal levels of sleepiness and daily functioning. *Sleep, 30,* 711–719.

Weaver, T. E., Maislin, G., Dinges, D. F., Younger, J., Cantor, C., McCloskey, S., et al. (2003). Self-efficacy in sleep apnea: Instrument development and patient perceptions of obstructive sleep apnea risk, treatment benefit, and volition to use continuous positive airway pressure. *Sleep, 26,* 727–732.

Wild, M., Engleman, H. M., Douglas, N. J., & Espie, C. A. (2004). Can psychological factors help us to determine adherence to CPAP? A prospective study. *European Respiratory Journal, 24,* 461–465.

Young, T., Palta, M., Dempsey, J., Skatrud, J., Weber, S., & Badr, S. (1993). The occurrence of sleep-disordered breathing among middle-aged adults. *New England Journal of Medicine, 328,* 1230–1235.

Young, T., Peppard, P., & Gottlieb, D. (2002). Epidemiology of obstructive sleep apnea: A population health perspective. *American Journal of Respiratory & Critical Care Medicine, 165,* 1217–1239.

Zimmerman, M. E., Arndt, T., Stanchina, M., Millman, R. P., & Aloia, M. S. (2006). Normalization of memory performance and positive airway pressure adherence in memory-impaired patients with obstructive sleep apnea. *Chest, 130,* 1772–1778.

CRITIQUE OF SAWYER ET AL.'S STUDY "DIFFERENCES IN PERCEPTIONS OF DIAGNOSIS AND TREATMENT OF OBSTRUCTIVE SLEEP APNEA AND CONTINUOUS POSITIVE AIRWAY PRESSURE THERAPY AMONG ADHERERS AND NON-ADHERERS"

■ Overall Summary

This was a very well-written, interesting report of a study on a significant topic. The mixed methods QUAL(quan) approach that was used was ideal for combining rich narrative interview data with objective, quantitative measures of adherence to continuous positive airway pressure treatment. The use of a longitudinal design enabled the researchers to gain insights into changes in patients' perceptions from diagnosis to treatment. The study design and methods were described in commendable detail, and the methods themselves were of exceptionally high quality. The authors provided considerable information about how the trustworthiness of the study was enhanced. The results were nicely elaborated, and the researchers incorporated numerous excerpts from the interviews. This was, overall, an excellent paper about a very strong study.

■ Title

The title of this report was long and perhaps a few words could have been omitted (e.g., "differences in" could be removed without affecting readers' understanding of the study). Nevertheless, the title did describe key aspects of the research. The title conveyed the central topic (perceptions about obstructive sleep apnea [OSA] and continuous positive airway pressure [CPAP] therapy). It also communicated the nature of the analysis, which compared perceptions of adherers and nonadherers to CPAP. If this paper had been published in a different journal, it probably would have been desirable to communicate in the title that the study was primarily qualitative, but inasmuch as it was published in *Qualitative Health Research*, that was not necessary. (However, "qualitative" was not used as a keyword for retrieving this study, either. The keywords included "content analysis" and "mixed methods," but in a search for qualitative studies on OSA or CPAP, this paper might be missed.)

■ Abstract

As required by *Qualitative Health Research* (QHR), the abstract was written in the traditional abstract style without subheadings. The abstract was brief, also in accordance with QHR's specifications for abstracts of 150 words or fewer. Yet, the abstract clearly described major aspects of the study so that readers could quickly learn whether the entire paper might be of interest. The abstract described the significance of the topic in the first sentence. The methods were succinctly presented, covering the overall mixed methods design, the longitudinal nature of the study (two rounds of interviews), the sample (15 OSA patients), the basic type of analysis (content analysis), and the focus on comparing adherent and nonadherent patients using objectively measured CPAP use. The use of social cognitive theory to guide the inquiry was noted. Although specific results were not described, the abstract indicated areas in which differences between adherers and nonadherers were observed. Finally, the last sentence suggests some possible applications for the results in terms of developing tailored interventions to promote CPAP use.

■ Introduction

The introduction to this study was concise but well organized and well written. It began with a paragraph about OSA as an important chronic health problem, describing its prevalence, its effects, and its primary medical treatment, that is, CPAP. This first paragraph helps readers understand the significance of the topic.

Much of the rest of the introduction discussed adherence to CPAP, which has consis-

tently been found to be low. The researchers nicely set the stage for their study by summarizing evidence about rates of adherence and factors predicting adherence. They also described prior research that affected some of their design decisions, such as studies that have found that early experiences with CPAP—that is, in the first week of use—influence patients' perceptions. The studies cited in the introduction include both older studies and ones written very recently, suggesting that the authors were summarizing state-of-the-art knowledge.

The introduction then further set the stage for the new study by describing knowledge gaps: "To date, there are relatively few studies that have systematically examined the influence of disease and treatment perceptions and beliefs on CPAP adherence." The report clearly stated four interrelated research questions for the new study. The questions were well suited to an in-depth qualitative approach.

■ Conceptual Framework

The article devoted a section to a description of the conceptual framework that underpinned the research. The authors justified the need for such a framework: "Acceptance and consistent use of CPAP is influenced by a multitude of factors . . . It is therefore important to approach the phenomenon of CPAP adherence from a multifactorial perspective that addresses the complex nature of this particular health behavior."

Sawyer and colleagues used a conceptual framework that is widely used in health behavior research, Bandura's social cognitive theory. The authors presented a nice summary of the theory and included a useful conceptual map (Figure 1). They also noted that Bandura's model is relevant within a qualitative inquiry because of explicit recognition of the role of context: "Bandura suggested that the application of social cognitive theory must be situated in context, recognizing that 'human behavior is socially situated, richly contextualized, and conditionally expressed.'"

One puzzling thing, however, is that both in this section and in the first subsection of the Results, considerable attention is paid to the role of *knowledge* in influencing health behaviors. Yet, knowledge is not a component of the theory as depicted in Figure 1.

▪ Method

The Method section was well organized into four subsections, and was unusually thorough in providing detail about how the researchers conducted this study.

DESIGN

Sawyer and colleagues used a mixed methods design to study patients' perceptions and beliefs about OSA and CPAP, and to explore differences among adherers and nonadherers. The researchers used terminology that was slightly different than that used in the textbook, which is not unusual because the field of mixed methods research methodology is a new one that is evolving. They described their design as a concurrent nested mixed methods design and provided a citation for their terminology. The citation was to a paper (2003) written by Creswell and Plano Clark, the two authors whose more recent terminology was used in this textbook. (The 2003 paper was probably a recent publication when the Sawyer et al. study was being planned.) Using the terminology presented in the textbook, the design would best be described as an embedded QUAL(quan) design. Had Sawyer and colleagues used Morse's notation system, they might have characterized the study as QUAL + quan, which indicates that the data for the two strands were collected concurrently, and that the qualitative component was dominant.

The design section also noted that the design was longitudinal, with data collected both at initial OSA diagnosis through the first week of CPAP treatment. Such a longitudinal design is an excellent way to track patients' perceptions and beliefs from diagnosis to the early treatment phase. The decision about *when* to collect the two rounds of data was well supported by earlier research. An excellent graphic (Figure 2) illustrated the study design and the timing of key events in the conduct of the study, such as enrollment and collection of demographic data, receipt of treatment education, conduct of the diagnostic sleep study and the CPAP sleep study, and the two interviews.

PARTICIPANTS

The researchers clearly defined the group of interest and described how participants were recruited into the study. Participants were adults with suspected OSA who were recruited from a Veterans Affairs sleep clinic. To be eligible, patients had to meet various clinical criteria (e.g., had at least moderate OSA, defined as at least 15 apnea or hypopnea events per hour in a sleep study) and practical criteria (had to speak and understand English). Patients were excluded if their responses could have been confounded by prior CPAP experiences, because the researchers were interested in understanding the perceptions and beliefs early in the diagnosis and CPAP treatment transition.

The researchers also excluded individuals who refused CPAP treatment prior to the actual treatment, and Figure 1 suggests that one such person was dropped from the study. That is, 16 patients were interviewed for the pretreatment interview, but only 15 were interviewed a second time, and the analysis was based on responses from 15 patients. (Sample size issues were discussed in a later section.)

One comment about this section is that we would have described the sampling approach more as convenience sampling than as purposive sampling. Many qualitative researchers say that their sampling was purposive when they purposefully select people with the characteristic or experience that is the focus of the research. However, we think of these more as eligibility criteria, which need to be identified to ensure that those in the study can provide "expert testimony" about the experience of interest. It would appear that the participants were a convenience sample of those meeting the eligibility criteria, and who were referred by a sleep specialist in one particular clinic. In our view, the term *purposive* connotes conscious and deliberate efforts to sample *particular* examplars from those who are eligible and who can best meet the conceptual needs of the study. For example, maximum variation sampling is a purposive strategy that involves a deliberate attempt to select participants who not only meet the eligibility criteria, but who vary along dimensions thought to be important in understanding the full range of the phenomenon of interest. In this study, the researchers could (for example) have deliberately sampled people with varying degrees of social support, to ensure that this important dimension would have adequate representation. As it turns out, there was variation in social support (marital status) among the study participants, but this does not appear to have been the result of a purposive strategy. With a small sample, and with a goal of looking at differences between adherers and nonadherers, a purposive strategy of sampling patients on dimensions known to differentiate these groups would have increased the likelihood that both groups would be adequately represented—although this was fortunately not an issue.

Few mixed methods studies discuss their approach to sampling within the mixed methods framework. In terms of the designs discussed in the textbook, the sampling approach for this study would be described as identical sampling. All study participants provided both qualitative and quantitative data.

PROCEDURES

The section on "Procedures" presented considerable information, focusing primarily on data collection. The section began by describing the two sleep studies that all study participants underwent. In both sleep studies, the patient's Apnea-Hypopnea Index (AHI) was computed via a polysomnogram. The initial AHI provided information that helped to determine study eligibility.

Next, the researchers described the major forms of data collection, which included semi-structured interviews and instrumentation to assess CPAP adherence objectively. In the subsection on the in-depth interviews, the article specified that the data were collected by a single investigator at two points in time: within a week following OSA diagnosis but before treatment, and then after the first week of treatment. The authors noted that participants were given choices about where the interviews would take place, in an effort to minimize attrition. And, in fact, there was no attrition in this study.

The interview guides were described in admirable detail. Table 1 listed the questions that guided the initial interview, and Table 2 listed questions for the post-treatment interview. These tables were an excellent way to communicate the nature of the interviews to readers, and the text provided even more detail. For example, a rationale for using a topic guide was provided ("to ensure that a consistent sequence and set of questions were addressed across participants"). Consistency was also enhanced by having a single interviewer responsible for conducting all interviews. To maximize data quality, the interviews were digitally recorded and transcribed by a professional transcriptionist.

The interviewer also maintained field notes before and after each interview. Commendably, these field notes were not only descriptive (i.e., describing participants and the interview environments), but also "served as interviewer reflexivity notations (i.e., interviewer biases, suppositions, and presuppositions of the research topic").

An important feature of this study was that CPAP adherence was not assessed by self-report. Rather, adherence was objectively determined based on quantitative data from the CPAP machine. A standard definition of "CPAP use" was provided, and a criterion of

6 hours or more per night of CPAP use was established for adherence. The researchers provided a convincing rationale for using the 6-hour limit as the cutoff point for adherence versus nonadherence.

One further note is that the researchers might have considered administering a self-efficacy scale during the course of their study, to anchor their discussion of self-efficacy, which is a key construct in their conceptual model. Although many of the major constructs in the model were ones that merited qualitative exploration, self-efficacy is one that perhaps could have been examined from both a qualitative and quantitative perspective, especially in a study that is explicitly mixed methods in design.

DATA ANALYSIS

The authors are to be congratulated for their detailed description of their data analysis methods. Not only did they carefully explain data analytic procedures in the text, but they also provided a wonderful flow chart (Figure 3) illustrating the sequence of steps they followed. It is extremely rare to find such rich information about data analysis in a qualitative or mixed methods study.

The qualitative data were content analyzed, an approach that is appropriate, given that the study was primarily descriptive. That is, this study was not designed to shed light on the lived experience of the patients (phenomenology), nor on their process of adapting to CPAP treatment (e.g., in a grounded theory study). The purpose was to obtain descriptive information at two points in time about participants' perceptions and beliefs relevant to OSA and CPAP. The researchers explained the procedures used in the content analysis, and provided citations for the approach used (although the two references cited [Hsieh & Shannon, and Graneheim & Lundman] are secondary sources rather than classic content analysis references).

The data analysis section explained how theory-driven themes were extracted in a manner consistent with the broad conceptualization of health behavior articulated in Bandura's theory. The authors offered specific illustrations in Table 3, which listed broad theoretical determinants of health behavior in the first column, and then relevant themes for each determinant as derived from the content analysis. For example, for the broad construct "Perceived self-efficacy," there were five relevant themes, such as "Fitting treatment into life" and "Problem-solving difficulties."

The section on data analysis also included important information about methods the researchers used to enhance trustworthiness—and these methods were strong. For example, one investigator coded all the interview data. Then, an independent expert recoded a randomly selected 15% of the data from each interview. Overall agreement between the study coder and the expert coder was a high 94%. For any differences of opinion about coding, the discrepancy was resolved by consensus. The theme definitions used in the coding, which were developed by the investigative team, were reviewed by two experts, a qualitative methodologist and an expert in the application of the theoretical constructs.

Importantly, the qualitative data were coded and content analyzed for themes by an investigator who was blinded to whether the participant was classified as adherent or nonadherent based on the quantitative data. Only after coding was complete was the adherence status of participants revealed. At that point, across-case analysis was examined "from an integrative perspective, using adherent and nonadherent as anchors . . . to identify common perceptions, beliefs, and experiences within the groups of interest." A meta-matrix was used to integrate the qualitative and quantitative data.

▪ Results

The results section began with a description of the study sample, all of whom were military veterans. Table 4 showed basic descriptive statistics on the demographics of the 15 participants, including their gender, race/ethnicity, marital and employment status, educational background, and age. Clinical information (e.g., mean weight, AHI events/hour, and CPAP adherence in terms of hours per night) was also presented. The text stated that the sample included six adherers and nine nonadherers.

The introductory paragraph of the Results section also noted that data saturation was reached at 15 participants and that sampling stopped at that point. From the point of view of providing readers with the details needed to evaluate the study methods, information about the approach to sampling and sample size might have been more usefully presented in the subsection labeled "Participants" in the method section.

Much of the results section was organized according to differences between adherers and nonadherers to CPAP therapy. The differences were nicely organized into major thematic categories, such as "Knowledge and perceived health status," "Goal setting and outcome expectancies," "Facilitators of and barriers to CPAP use," and "Perceived self-efficacy." Key differences between the two groups (and a few areas of overlap) within these major groupings were described and supported with rich excerpts from the interview transcripts.

Social support emerged as an important issue in CPAP adherence, consistent with previous studies. Thus, the researchers performed a useful supplementary analysis in which they examined differences between married and unmarried patients.

The analysis section concluded with a typology (descriptive profiles) of adherent and nonadherent CPAP users, based on an integration of the data across themes. Table 5 nicely summarized their typology.

■ Discussion

Sawyer and colleagues offered a thoughtful discussion of their findings. Their discussion highlighted ways in which their findings complement and extend the existing body of evidence on CPAP adherence. The discussion nicely wove together findings from the current study and previous studies. It also discussed the findings within the context of the theoretical framework.

The authors also noted some of the study's limitations. They pointed out, for example, that study participants were all veterans with fairly high levels of education, and thus exploration with a more diverse population of OSA patients would be desirable. The researchers also pointed out that the small sample size of 15 provided limited power for conducting quantitative analyses of numerical data they had at their disposal, such as measures of subjective sleepiness and functional impairment. They noted that with a larger sample, they could have explored correlations between such quantitative measures and the thematic typology.

Although the discussion is reasonably lengthy, relatively little space was devoted to the implications of the study findings. The researchers noted that "the described differences between adherers and nonadherers in our study suggest critical tailored or patient-centered intervention opportunities . . . " Indeed, they mentioned the opportunity for tailored interventions several times in connection with their discussion of their theoretically derived themes. However, perhaps a bit more elaboration of how the findings could be used in an intervention would have been helpful.

■ General Comments

PRESENTATION

This report was clearly written, well organized, and offered an exemplary amount of detail about the research methods. The inclusion of several tables and figures provided readers with explicit and concrete information about aspects of the study that are often ignored or described in a single sentence. We applaud the authors, and we also applaud the journal, *Qualitative Health Research*, for not having strict page limits.[1] The need for page limits is understandable given the explosion of research that is being undertaken. However, the ability for readers to judge the quality of research evidence is also crucial, and this is sometimes hampered by constraints on researchers' ability to provide thorough information about how the research was conducted.

ETHICAL ASPECTS

The authors briefly stated steps they took to ensure ethical treatment of participants in the subsection labeled "Participants." All participants provided informed consent, and the study protocols were approved by the Institutional Review Boards of the affiliated university and the research site.

■ Response from the Sawyer Team:

Dr. Sawyer and her colleagues were asked if they wished to comment on this critique. Dr. Sawyer remarked that she was "in near 100% agreement with the draft critique that you provided" and that there was nothing she felt she needed to rebut (personal communication, July 13, 2010). Given the generally positive nature of the critique, Dr. Sawyer noted, "I don't know that I have much in the way of response to offer—however, the suggestion to include a self-efficacy instrument is "'spot on.'"

Her email concluded with the following statement: "My study colleagues and I are very pleased with the published paper in QHR and firmly believe the paper is an excellent teaching resource for mixed methods research in health and disease." We agree.

---

[1] The QHR guidelines to authors that were in effect in 2010 state the journal's page limit policy as follows: "There is no predetermined word or page limit. Provided they are 'tight' and concise, without unnecessary repetition and/or irrelevant data, manuscripts should be as long as they need to be."

THE DEVELOPMENT AND TESTING OF THE NURSING TEAMWORK SURVEY

Beatrice J. Kalisch • Hyunhwa Lee • Eduardo Salas

Editor's Note

A copy of the Nursing Teamwork Survey instrument can be obtained by emailing bkalisch@umich.edu

▶ **Background:** There is a lack of an acceptable, reliable, and valid survey instruments to differentiate levels of nursing teamwork on inpatient units in acute care facilities.

▶ **Objective:** The aim of this study was to test the psychometric soundness of the Nursing Teamwork Survey (NTS).

▶ **Methods:** The survey was administered to 1,758 inpatient nursing staff members using the NTS (return rate = 56.9%), and measures of content, predictive (concurrent), and construct (factorial, contrast, and convergent) validity were completed.

▶ **Results:** Content validity was established by a panel of experts. Concurrent validity showed a significant correlation between teamwork scores and an imbedded question related to overall satisfaction with teamwork ($r = .633$, $p < .001$). The exploratory factor analysis on a random half of the sample predicted a 33-item five-factor solution, whereas the confirmatory factor analysis on the remaining half of the sample confirmed the factor structure (comparative fit index = .884, root mean square error of approximation = 0.055, standardized root mean square residual = 0.045). Contrast validity showed that staff in a non-inpatient unit did not answer the questions in the same way ($r_{WG(J)} = .25$) as the inpatient unit staff ($r_{WG(J)} > .90$). Convergent validity of the teamwork tool was measured by correlating the Teamwork subscale of the Safety Attitudes Questionnaire with the NTS ($r = .76$, $p < .01$). The NTS had good test–retest reliability ($r = .92$ for overall 33 items; $r = .77$ to .87 for the five subscales) and internal consistency ($\alpha = .94$ for overall items; $\alpha = .74$ to .85 for the subscales). Aggregation of individual-level responses to the unit level was supported by intraclass correlation coefficient 1 = .16 ($p < .001$), intraclass correlation coefficient 2 = .9 ($p < .001$), and mean $r_{WG(J)} = .98$.

▶ **Discussion:** The NTS was demonstrated to have good psychometric properties. Further NTS research should include testing the tool in hospitals with varying characteristics and exploring the links to clinical and operational outcomes.

▶ **Key Words:** nursing · patient safety · scale · survey · teamwork · psychometrics · work environment

The impact of teamwork on patient safety and quality of care has been well documented in healthcare (Leonard, Graham, & Bonacum, 2004; Salas, Rosen, & King, 2007; Shortell & Singer, 2008). Leonard et al. (2004) emphasized the importance of effective communication and teamwork for the delivery of high-quality and safe patient care. They pointed out that communication failures are common causes of inadvertent patient harm. Salas et al. (2007) showed the close association of patient safety with team effectiveness and shared mindset. Shortell and Singer (2008) suggested that we need to emphasize safety over productivity and teamwork over individual autonomy to reduce errors and mistakes and to improve patient safety.

Most of the research on healthcare teamwork has been focused on emergency and perioperative departments (Mills, Neily, & Dunn, 2008; Morey et al., 2002; Salas et al., 2007; Silen-Lipponen, Tossavainen, Turunen, & Smith, 2005). Although a large proportion of healthcare is delivered by nursing work teams in acute care hospitals, there has been very little research about teamwork in this setting. One of the barriers to studying these work groups has been the lack of acceptable, reliable, and valid instruments to differentiate levels of nursing teamwork in these settings. Such a tool is needed to study the status and the characteristics of nursing teamwork and to test teamwork-enhancing interventions.

A team is made of two or more people who work interdependently with a common purpose. The definition of a nursing work group for the purposes of this study is the staff members—registered nurses (RNs), licensed practical nurses (LPNs), nursing assistive personnel (NAs), and unit secretaries (USs)—who work together on a given patient care unit in an acute care hospital setting. This inpatient nursing work team provides the care and related administrative tasks for a group of patients. The nursing staff work in shifts of 4, 8, or 12 hours. They hand off to one another when they change shifts or take a break, and two or more of these team members engage in the care of each patient during a work shift. Moreover, the total care of any patient in a hospitalized setting requires numerous nursing staff members around the clock. The complexity and the high demands for specialized nursing knowledge and skill also require nursing staff to consult with one another on a regular basis.

Although the teamwork between nursing unit-based staff and other individuals who visit the team, such as physicians, physical therapists, respiratory therapists, and dietitians, is of equal importance, this study is targeted on the permanent acute care nursing teams. Unless these work teams can achieve a high level of teamwork, they will not be able to work effectively with others outside their unit (Heinemann, Schmitt, Farrell, & Brallier, 1999; Lichtenstein, Alexander, Jinnett, & Ullman, 1997). The tool developed in this study is the Nursing Teamwork Survey (NTS).

TEAMWORK MEASUREMENT TOOLS

Many survey tools have been developed to measure teamwork in general, yet a review of these instruments uncovered several problems. In addition to structure issues (e.g., item redundancy from one subscale to the next, no counterbalance of positive and negative items, unclear answer choices, labels, and items that do not match), many of these measurement instruments were developed with the purpose of education or consultation, not research (Dimock, 1991; Glaser & Glaser, 1995; Phillips & Elledge, 1994; Wheelan, 1994). Others had a very specific use such as measuring the development of new groups or teams (Campbell & Hallan, 1997; Dimock, 1991; Farrell, Heinemann, & Schmitt, 1992; Weisbond, 1991) or formal meeting situations (Burns & Gragg, 1981; Harper & Harper, 1993). A number of these tools are proprietary and thus require payment for each use (Glaser & Glaser, 1995). A few require that the researcher send the results to a company for analysis (Sexton et al., 2006). The most important barrier to using a substantial number of existing tools is that they have not been tested for their psychometric properties (Burns & Gragg, 1981; Chartier, 1991; Francis & Young, 1992; Hall, 1988; Pfeiffer & Jones, 1974; Phillips & Elledge, 1994; Schein, 1988; Varney, 1991).

Looking specifically at existing teamwork measurement tools within healthcare, Heinemann and Zeiss (2004) reported that 12 survey tools were designed or adapted to teams in healthcare. Of these, several centered on teams that care for specific types of patients such as geriatric (Farrell et al., 1992; Heinemann et al., 1999; Hepburn, Tsukuda, & Fasser, 1998), psychiatric (Lichtenstein et al., 1997), and rehabilitation (Heinemann & Zeiss, 2004). Although Attitudes Toward Health Care Teams Scale (Heinemann et al., 1999) has excellent psychometric properties, it is used to measure attitudes toward teams such as whether the physician should be the director of the team as opposed to the actual functioning of the team. Others are designed to measure collaboration between nurses and physicians (Baggs, 1994; Shortell, Rousseau, Gillies, Devers, & Simons, 1991). Using the cognitive-motivational model, Millward and Jeffries (2001) developed and tested the Team Survey with 10 healthcare teams and 124 professionals in the United Kingdoms' National Health Trust (Millward & Jeffries, 2001). Although initially promising, this tool was used with inpatient nursing work groups and was found to not demonstrate the ability to differentiate among teams. Thus, it was concluded that a new instrument is needed to be able to measure levels of nursing teamwork in acute care settings.

PSYCHOMETRIC TESTING PROCESS

Assessment of the psychometric properties of a new instrument involves tests of acceptability, validity, and reliability (Nunnally & Bernstein, 1994; Vogus & Sutcliffe, 2007; Waltz, Strickland, & Lenz, 2005). Acceptability, or ease of use, is judged by the number of respondents who completed the scale without omitting items and the length of time required to complete the survey.

Validity of an instrument refers to the extent the scale provides data relative to commonly accepted meanings of the concept (or whether it actually measures what it claims to measure). Validity has been given three major meanings: (a) content validity—sampling from a pool of required content; (b) predictive validity—establishing a statistical relationship with a particular criterion; and (c) construct validity—measuring psychometric attributes (Nunnally & Bernstein, 1994, p. 83). Content validity focuses on the content of the meas-

urement instrument, assessing whether it is reflective of the relevant content domain being measured. Predictive validity focuses on the correlation of the instrument being validated with some well-respected outside measure of the same construct (Bagozzi, Yi, & Phillips, 1991). Predictive validity is measured through concurrent validity, which refers to the extent to which a measure may be used to estimate an individual's present standing on the criterion. For construct validity, two major scientific aspects are (a) developing measures of individual constructs and (b) finding functional relations between measures of different constructs (Nunnally & Bernstein, 1994, p. 85). Exploratory and confirmatory factor analyses provide constructs. Contrast and convergent validity testing measures the relationships between (a) two groups who are known to be different in the characteristic being measured by the instrument and (b) different measures of the same construct (Waltz et al., 2005).

Reliability refers to consistency or repeatability of a set of measurements. Reliability is tested by the test–retest method and measures of internal consistency. Test–retest reliability refers to the likelihood that a given measure will yield the same description of a given phenomenon if that measure is repeated. In concept, it allows the direct measurement of consistency from administration to administration (Pallant, 2005). Internal consistency estimates the extent to which factors made up of survey questions within a scale are assessing a single construct and is measured by the Cronbach's alpha. Internal consistency is scored from 0 to 1, where the coefficient of .7 is considered acceptable for newly developed scales, and .8 or higher indicates good reliability as evidence that the items may be used interchangeably (Waltz et al., 2005). Intraclass correlations are another measure of internal consistency. Factors that evolved from a tool are tested by computing the F statistic from a one-way analysis of variance (ANOVA), an intraclass correlation coefficient (ICC1 and ICC2), and an $r_{WG(J)}$ (within-group agreement). ICC1 and ICC2 are statistical measures used to determine two important aspects of the reliability of a survey instrument: (a) that the members of each unit report similar scores on a given measure, and (b) that the units have significant between-unit variance for a given measure (Vogus & Sutcliffe, 2007). The ICC1 can be interpreted as the proportion of total variance that is explained by unit membership with values ranging from -1 to $+1$ and values between .05 and .30 being the most typical. The ICC2 provides an overall estimate of the reliability of unit means as it becomes closer to 1, with .70 being acceptable. The $r_{WG(J)}$ is a measure of the variance that determines the agreement of responses within a group. The closer the value is to 1.0, the more interchangeable the responses are among the individuals in a group.

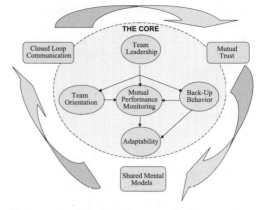

Figure 1. The "Big Five" framework of teamwork. Reprinted with permission from Salas, Sims, & Burke (2005).

CONCEPTUAL FRAMEWORK

Although there are many theories of teamwork, the Salas theory (Salas, Sims, & Burke, 2005) was selected as a framework for the NTS because it is based on teamwork behaviors and offers a practical explanation of the dynamics of teamwork. This framework (Figure 1) includes five core elements of teamwork—(a) team orientation (cohesiveness and the group's awareness of itself as a team), (b) team leadership (structure, direction, and support provided by the formal leader and on the part of team members), (c) mutual performance monitoring (observation and awareness of team members of one another while completing their own work), (d) backup (team members helping one another with their tasks and responsibilities), and (e) adaptability (adjusting work as the environment changes)—and three coordinating mechanisms—(a) communication (active exchange of information between two or more team members), (b) shared mental models (collective mindset), and (c) mutual trust (belief that team members will act in ways that promote the aims of the team). Team leadership and team orientation are required for mutual performance monitoring and backup behavior. Backup behavior is mediated by adaptability and

affects team effectiveness directly by making sure that all team tasks are completed. Mutual performance monitoring impacts team effectiveness through backup behavior. Mutual performance monitoring and communication require both shared mental models and trust. Effective backup behavior and adaptability requires shared mental models to achieve team effectiveness. Adaptability has a direct impact on team effectiveness by the quality of mutual performance monitoring and backup behavior.

PURPOSE

The aim of this study was to develop and to test the NTS, designed to measure nursing teamwork in acute care hospital settings at the patient unit level.

▪ Methods

SETTING AND PARTICIPANTS

The participants for this methodological study were nursing team members on 38 acute care patient care units in an academic healthcare center (936 beds) and a community hospital (120 beds). The total number of participants was 1,758. These included the nurses (RNs and LPNs), the NAs, and the USs who base their work on a given patient care unit. In addition, a survival team (*n* = 11) was administered the survey for contrast validity testing purposes.

INSTRUMENT

Items for the NTS were generated on theoretical grounds, informed by the Salas teamwork model (Salas et al., 2005). In addition, qualitative data from 34 focus groups with 116 RNs, 7 LPNs, 28 NAs, and 19 USs (mean age = 42 years, 97% female) were used (Kalisch, Weaver, & Salas, 2009). From these data, 74 potential items were generated with seven categories for the NTS.

Experts in nursing teamwork (staff nurses, nurse managers, and teamwork experts) were asked to make judgments about the degree to which the survey content matched a detailed description of what constitutes the content domain. There were 10 different versions of the survey. Starting with a 74-question survey and proceeding to the final version of 45 questions, each version was reviewed, and suggestions were made for modification by expert panels. Items not clear or not relevant were eliminated. The content validity index was 91.2%(on the final version of the NTS) based on the review of the expert panels' assessment of the relevance and clarity of the NTS (Lynn, 1986).

The 45-question NTS uses a 5-point Likert-type scale (1 = *rarely,* 2 = 25% *of the time,* 3 = 50% *of the time,* 4 = 75% *of the time,* and 5 = *always*). The tool is designed to be self-administered and focuses on the within-team performance. The survey also contains questions about the demographic characteristics of the respondents, satisfaction, and number of patients cared for during their last shift.

PROCEDURES

After acquiring institutional review board approvals, the study was initiated with a presentation to the directors and managers of

nursing at the facilities used in the study. The NTS and a cover letter detailing procedures for maintenance of confidentiality were placed in a 9 × 11-inch envelope along with a candy bar as a token of appreciation. These were distributed to the staff members' mailboxes on each participating unit. In the instructions, staff members were asked to complete the survey, to place it in a provided letter-size envelope, to seal it, and to drop it in the lockbox placed on each unit. Those units that completed at least a 50% return rate were given a pizza party as an incentive to participate in the research. The same procedures were made for the nursing survival flight team, which served as a contrasting group for validity testing.

DATA ANALYSIS

Analyses were completed using the Statistical Package for the Social Sciences (version 16.0; SPSS Inc., Chicago, IL). Before proceeding with any analyses, the negatively worded items were reversed coded. To increase the total number of cases for the factor analysis, we carried out imputations to fill in missing values using the SAS version 9.1 implementation Imputation and Variation Estimation Software. The Imputation and Variation Estimation Software imputation process allowed specific explicit replacement models for variables with missing data and conditioning of the resulting imputed values on values in fully observed variables.

Concurrent validity was tested by comparing answers to a question imbedded in the demographic section of the survey that asked respondents to complete an overall rating of their satisfaction with teamwork on their unit with the total score on the NTS.

A series of exploratory factor analyses (EFA) were conducted with the 45-question NTS. The EFA was run on a random half of the imputed data set (*n* = 879). The EFA was examined using principal components factor analysis as the extraction technique and Varimax as the orthogonal rotation method to obtain a distinct and maximally interpretable solution (Thompson & Daniel, 1996). As suggested by various experts, the following five commonly used decision rules were applied: (a) the use of a simple factor structure, (b) a minimum eigenvalue of 1 as a cutoff value for extraction, (c) the point of discontinuity of the scree plot, (d) the deletion of items with factor loadings less than .35 or items cross-loaded on more than two factors, and (e) the exclusion of single-item factors from the standpoint of parsimony (Hair, Tatham, Anderson, & Black, 1998; Price & Mueller, 1986; Straub, 1989). In addition, some items with relatively lower means or more variations compared with the others were detected from descriptive statistics of all initial 45 teamwork items. Also looking at the correlation matrix, any items with correlation coefficients less than .30 were identified. As in the correlation matrix, there were some commonalities less than .60, which reflect that variables are not related to each other. The concordance of conceptual meaning with each factor was also examined.

The next step was to run confirmatory factor analysis (CFA) models on the remaining half of the data set using AMOS version 16. The results of the EFA, intended to inform factor structures, were then tested using the CFA. To establish a model with the closest fit to the data, we performed CFA on the other random half ($n = 879$) of the data set. The root mean square error of approximation (RMSEA) and the standardized root mean square residual (SRMR) fit indices were used following the two-index presentation strategy recommended by Hu and Bentler (1999). The two-index presentation strategy reflects the fact that several fit indices have been shown to be correlated highly and thus provide somewhat redundant information. To compensate for this, we chose two indices, RMSEA and SRMR, because they have been shown to be dissimilar under various sample sizes, distributional violations, and model misspecifications. Using the combinatorial cutoff of RMSEA <.06 and SRMR <.09 minimizes Type I and Type II error rates and was thus selected for evaluating all models. A good fit is indicated by RMSEA values of less than .06 (Hu & Bentler, 1999). A value of .90 for the compar-

ative fit index (CFI) and incremental fit index has served as a lower limit rule-of-thumb cutoff for acceptable fit (Byrne, 1994).

Contrast validity was tested using the responses of a nursing survival flight team ($n = 11$). It was hypothesized that a group that practiced in a different type of nursing practice environment would score lower than the inpatient nursing teams.

For convergent validity, the NTS scores were correlated with the Teamwork Climate subscale (six questions) of the Safety Attitudes Questionnaire (SAQ; Sexton et al., 2006). The SAQ was designed to measure various provider attitudes about patient safety. Reliability of the SAQ is reported to be .9. The instrument is made up of six subscales; only the Teamwork Climate subscale was used, and it was compared with the overall score on the NTS. The hypothesis was that the results of the NTS would correlate with the SAQ Teamwork subscale. To test this hypothesis, we administered both the NTS and the SAQ on 82 staff nurses on one patient care unit. A measure of convergent validity for the NTS was performed by generating a Pearson correlation coefficient test between the NTS and the SAQ subscales.

For the test–retest reliability, identical forms of the instrument were administered to the same 49 nurses 2 weeks apart. Simple additive scores were computed for the survey to examine test–retest reliability. By conducting a one-way ANOVA using the factors as the dependent variable and the units as the independent variable, the F statistic values were evaluated with a $p < .05$ level of significance. Then, using the between-group mean square and the within-group mean square calculated from the one-way ANOVA, the ICCs (ICC1 and ICC2) were computed.

■ Results

PARTICIPANTS

Data were collected in 2008 from 1,802 RNs, LPNs, NAs, and USs. Once cases were removed that could not be used (e.g., staff did not spend most time on the unit, too much missing data), the sample size was 1,758. The ratio of sample size to number of survey items was 40:1, which exceeds the minimum 10:1 ratio recommended by Kerlinger (1978). The return rate was 56.9%.

Nursing staff survey respondents worked on a variety of types of units: 30.3% (n = 532) intensive care units (ICUs), of which 17.2% (n = 302) were adult ICUs and 13.1% (n = 230) were pediatric ICUs; 11.7% (n = 205) adult intermediate-level units; 28.7% (n = 505) adult medical-surgical units; 13% (n = 228) pediatric units; 6.8% (n = 119) emergency

departments and related units; 5.7% (n = 101) maternity units; and 3.8% (n = 67) other units.

Of these 1,758 participants, 68.1% (n = 1,198) were female, 77.4% (n = 1,360) reported their job title as nurse (e.g., RN, LPN, clinical nurse specialist), most worked full time (80.2%, n = 1,397), and approximately half held a baccalaureate degree (48.2%, n = 848). Two thirds of the staff members were 26 to 44 years of age. The average number of years of work experience in nursing was 10 years. The study participant characteristics are shown in Table 1. Of 11 survival team nurses, used for contrast validity, all worked full time, 27.3% (n = 3) were female, 54.5% (n = 6) held a

Table 1. Sample Characteristics (N = 1,758)

		Frequency (%)
Gender	Male	156 (9.2)
	Female	1533 (90.8)
Age	Under 25 years old	193 (11.0)
	26 to 34 years old	518 (29.6)
	35 to 44 years old	475 (27.2)
	45 to 54 years old	412 (23.6)
	55 to 64 years old	148 (8.5)
	Over 65 years old	3 (0.2)
Years of experience (mean ± *SD*)	9.84 ± 9.38	
Highest nursing degree	Grade/high school and GED	220 (12.5)
	Associate degree	576 (32.8)
	Bachelors degree	848 (48.2)
	Graduate degree	96 (5.5)
Employment status	>30 hours/week	1397 (80.2)
	<30 hours/week	344 (19.8)
Unit	Adult ICU	302 (17.2)
	Pediatric ICU	230 (13.1)
	Adult intermediate	205 (11.7)
	Adult medical-surgical/ rehabilitation	505 (28.7)
	Pediatric	228 (13.0)
	Maternity	101 (5.7)
	ER-SWAT-SVF	119 (6.8)
	Other	67 (3.8)

Note. GED = General Educational Development; ER-SWAT-SVF = Emergency Department/ Transport team.

baccalaureate degree, half of them ($n = 5$) were 45 to 54 years of age, and the average number of years of work experience in nursing was 14.4 years ($SD = 6.8$ years). These groups are similar except there were more males in the survival team sample.

ACCEPTABILITY

The percentage of respondents completing the instrument without omitting any items was 80.4%. Another 11.5% omitted only one item, 2.9% omitted two items, and 5.2% omitted more than two items. Most respondents completed the questionnaire in 10 minutes or less.

VALIDITY

Factor Analysis and Subscale Development. The results from EFA and CFA determined that 12 items should be excluded from the original 45 items, leaving 33 questions in the final instrument (Table 2). A five-factor solution evolved from the modified 33-item NTS scale: (a) Trust, (b) Team Orientation, (c) Backup, (d) Shared Mental Model, and (e) Team Leadership. The large value calculated by the Bartlett's test of sphericity indicated that the correlation matrix is not an identity matrix ($\chi^2 = 12,860.195$, $df = 528$, $p < .001$), and the Kaiser–Meyer–Olkin measure showed that sampling adequacy was excellent (.961). The five factors explained 53.11% of the variance. The Trust factor was composed of 7 items with loadings greater than .40, the Team Orientation factor was composed of 9 items with loadings greater than .45, the Backup factor was composed of 6 items with loadings greater than .40, the Shared Mental Model factor was composed of 7 items with loadings greater than .45, and the Team Leadership factor was composed of 4 items with loadings greater than .40 (Table 2). The minimum possible score is 0 for each subscale, and the maximum possible scores are 35 for Trust, 35

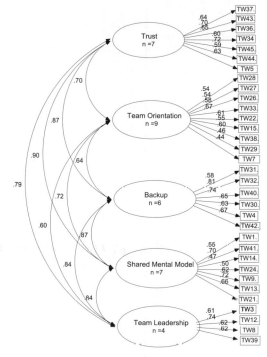

Figure 2. Standardized confirmatory factor analysis (CFA) path diagram for five-factor teamwork model.

for Team Orientation, 30 for Backup, 35 for Shared Mental Model, and 20 for Team Leadership. Higher scores indicate higher levels of trust among team members, more cohesive team orientation, more backup behaviors, more shared mental models, and better team leadership.

The CFA yielded a 33-item five-factor model that fit the data from the NTS very well (CFI = .884, RMSEA = .055, SRMR = .045; Figure 2). The analysis resulted in a chi-square value of 1,745.30 ($df = 485$, $p < .001$). A CFI that is close to the .9 criteria level indicates a close fit. Therefore, using this rule, the five-factor structure suggested by the earlier EFA was confirmed and resulted in a good model fit, thereby contributing to the stability of the tool. The model fit statistics from the CFA are displayed in Table 3.

Table 2. Five-Factor Principal Component Analysis of the Nursing Teamwork Items

Factor	Eigenvalue	% of Variance	Cronbach's Alpha	Item	Factor Loadings				
					1	2	3	4	5
1. Trust	11.854	35.92	.847	Clarifying the intended message with one another	.695				
				Constructive feedback	.670				
				Sharing ideas and information	.647				
				Engaging in changes to make improvements	.627				
				Trust	.569				
				Fair reallocation of responsibilities	.461				
				Communication of expectation	.407				
2. Team Orientation	2.262	6.85	.831	Conflict avoidance	.659				
				Dominated by staff members with strong personalities		.654			
				Complaint by oncoming shift staff about incomplete work		.645			
				Judgmental feedback		.633			
				Defensive response		.594			
				Extra break time		.585			
				Focusing on their own work than working together		.567			
				Nursing assistants and nurses not working well together		.554			
				Ignoring mistakes and annoying behavior		.462			

Factor				Item	Loading
3. Backup	1.223	3.71	.841	Noticing a member falling behind	.688
				Pitching in together to get the work done	.631
				Keeping an eye out for each other without falling behind	.608
				Charge nurses or team leaders assist team members	.564
				Knowing when assistance is needed before being asked	.555
				Response to other team members' patients	.551
4. Shared Mental Model	1.145	3.47	.834	Understanding of own responsibilities throughout the shift	.699
				Understanding of others' role and responsibilities	.559
				The shift change reports contain necessary information	.550
				Awareness of the strengths and weaknesses of other team members	.521
				Following through on commitment	.508
				Working together for a quality job	.506
				Respect	.469
5. Team Leadership	1.043	3.16	.744	Charge nurses or team leaders monitoring the progress of the team	.629
				Charge nurses or team leaders balance team workload	.486
				Extended plan to deal with changes in the workload	.485
				Charge nurses or team leaders give clear and relevant directions	.410

Table 3. Model Fit Statistics From CFA for the Five-Factor Teamwork Model

CFI	.884
RMSEA	.055
SRMR	.045
NFI	.846
RFI	.833
IFI	.884
TLI	.873

Note. CFA = confirmatory factor analysis; CFI = comparative fit index;
RMSEA = root mean square error of approximation; SRMR = standardized root mean square residual; NFI = normed fit index; RFI = relative fit index; IFI = incremental fit index; TLI = Tucker–Lewis index.

Concurrent Validity. As the result of concurrent validity, a one-way ANOVA showed that nursing staff who were very satisfied and satisfied with the level of teamwork on their unit had a significantly higher NTS score overall (4.10 and 3.70, respectively) than the nursing staff who were dissatisfied (2.95; $p < .001$). As predicted, the overall unit teamwork score correlated significantly with the responses to this item ($r = .633$, $p < .001$).

Contrast and Convergent Validities. An examination of contrasting group validity showed that the items on the NTS were focused on inpatient nursing teams and their work. The responses of inpatient teams, contrasted with a survival flight team, showed that every unit except the survival flight unit had an $r_{WG(J)}$ value of .90 and higher, indicating that the individuals on the survival flight unit did not respond to the survey in the same way as the nursing staff on the other units. As hypothesized, the survival flight unit had a low $r_{WG(J)}$ value of .25. Between the SAQ Teamwork Climate scale and the total score on the NTS, a correlation of .76 was found to be significant at a .01 level.

RELIABILITY

Test–Retest Reliability. The overall test–retest coefficient with 33 items was .92, and each subscale had the test–retest reliability coefficients ranging from .77 to .87.

Internal Consistency. The alpha coefficient for the overall 33 items was .94, and the alpha coefficients for the subscales ranged from .74 to .85. From the analyses of intraclass correlations, significant F statistic values inferred that the responses between nursing staff on different units were not similar at $p < .001$. The ICC1 and the ICC2 reflect the homogeneity of the staff responses on a unit level for each of five factors (described below). Table 4 contains the F statistic, ICC1, and ICC2 values for the five factors and teamwork total for the 38 units. The ICC1 values all remained in the range, indicating the reliability of an individual's assessment of the unit's teamwork. The ICC2 values were all above .84, indicating that the response of the unit as a whole was reliable.

The computation of $r_{WG(J)}$ revealed that the aggregation of the data on the unit level was feasible because the degree of congruence between individual nursing staff survey responses was shown to be correlated by unit. Every unit had an $r_{WG(J)}$ value of .90 and higher, with a median of .98, indicating that all the individuals responded to the questions in the same direction.

▪ Discussion

The aim of this study was to develop and to test the psychometric properties of the NTS. It was administered to 1,758 nursing staff in 38 patient care units in a large academic health sciences center and a community hospital.

Although there is not an exact match with Salas's teamwork theory (Salas et al., 2005), the results from the NTS demonstrate a relatively strong fit. Salas's model of teamwork includes five elements of teamwork (team orientation,

Table 4. Teamwork Reliability Measures ($N = 1,758$); 38 Units

		Sum of Squares	df	Mean Square	F	Significance	ICC1	ICC2
Trust	Between groups	103.043	37	2.785	6.247	.00	.10	.84
	Within groups	765.497	1717	0.446				
	Total	868.540	1754					
Team Orientation	Between groups	112.097	37	3.030	6.788	.00	.11	.85
	Within groups	766.829	1718	0.446				
	Total	878.926	1755					
Backup	Between groups	138.770	37	3.751	8.777	.00	.15	.89
	Within groups	734.165	1718	0.427				
	Total	872.935	1755					
Shared Mental Model	Between groups	78.929	37	2.133	7.317	.00	.12	.86
	Within groups	501.194	1719	0.292				
	Total	580.123	1756					
Team Leadership	Between groups	124.116	37	3.354	6.938	.00	.12	.86
	Within groups	829.183	1715	0.483				
	Total	953.299	1752					
Teamwork total	Between groups	98.894	37	2.673	9.717	.00	.16	.90
	Within groups	472.848	1719	0.275				
	Total	571.742	1756					

Note. ICC1 = (MSB − MSW) / (MSB + [(k−1) × MSW]); ICC2 = (MSB − MSW) / MSB.
ICC = intraclass correlation coefficient; MSB = between-group mean square; MSW = within-group mean square; k = average sample size in each unit.

team leadership, mutual performance monitoring, backup, and adaptability) and three coordinating mechanisms (communication, shared mental models, and trust). Five factors or subscales emerged for the NTS. These are Trust, Team Orientation, Backup, Shared Mental Model, and Team Leadership. Mutual performance monitoring, adaptability, and communication were not represented in the NTS. It is possible that these are embedded in the Backup and Trust factors.

The seven items in the Trust factor measure whether team members trust each other enough to communicate ideas and information and to value, to seek, and to give each other constructive feedback; the nine items in the Team Orientation factor measure whether the team works together in improving each others weaknesses efficiently and effectively;

the six items in the Backup factor measure if team members willingly aid and help one other when they recognize someone is busy or overloaded with work; the seven items in the Shared Mental Model factor are used to measure whether all team members understand their role and responsibilities and thus respectively work together to achieve a quality work outcome; and the four items in the Team Leadership factor are used to measure whether the nurses who serve as charge nurses or managers adequately monitor, distribute, balance, and willingly assist the workload of the nurses.

The analyses of acceptability, reliability, and validity demonstrated strong psychometric properties. The results showed that the NTS is easy to use, as indicated by the relatively low proportion of omitted survey items. It was also demonstrated that the NTS can be used as a unit-level variable, as indicated by the intraclass correlation results. This finding makes it possible to compare nursing teams by team functioning. The use of the NTS with groups of nursing staff could potentially provide benchmark data, allowing healthcare organizations to judge the performance of various nursing teams.

Limitations of this study include the fact that the sample came from only two hospitals, and therefore the findings may not be generalizable to other settings. Nevertheless, the two study hospitals fell within similar score ranges, demonstrating stability of the distribution of scores. The NTS has not been used yet to measure teamwork interventions, so it is not known whether the tool is sensitive to changes designed to increase teamwork. Further research using the NTS should test the tool in hospitals with varying characteristics and explore the links to clinical and operational outcomes.

Beatrice J. Kalisch, PhD, RN, FAAN, is Titus Distinguished Professor of Nursing and Director, Nursing Business and Health Systems, School of Nursing, University of Michigan, Ann Arbor.
Hyunhwa Lee, MS, RN, is Doctoral Candidate, School of Nursing, University of Michigan, Ann Arbor.
Eduardo Salas, PhD, is Professor and Trustee Chair, Department of Psychology and Director, Institute for Simulation and Training, University of Central Florida, Orlando.

Accepted for publication September 2, 2009.
This project was funded by The Michigan Center for Health Intervention, University of Michigan School of Nursing, National Institutes of Health, National Institute of Nursing Research (P30 NR009000). The authors thank Laura Shakarjian, Susan Wright, and Julie Juno for data collection and Unmesh Lal and Anne Shin for their contributions to data analysis.
Corresponding author: Beatrice J. Kalisch, PhD, RN, FAAN, Nursing Business and Health Systems, School of Nursing, University of Michigan, 400 N. Ingalls Street, Ann Arbor, MI 48103 (e-mail: bkalisch@umich.edu).

REFERENCES

Baggs, J. G. (1994). Development of an instrument to measure collaboration and satisfaction about care decisions. *Journal of Advanced Nursing, 20*(1), 176–182.
Bagozzi, R. P., Yi, Y., & Phillips, L. W. (1991). Assessing construct validity in organizational research. *Administrative Science Quarterly, 36*(3), 421–458.
Burns, F., & Gragg, R. (1981). Brief diagnostic instruments. In J. E. Jones & J. W. Pfeiffer (Eds.), *The annual handbook for group facilitators* (pp. 87–93). San Diego, CA: Pfeiffer & Company.
Byrne, B. M. (1994). *Structural equation modeling with EQS and EQS/WINDOWS: Basic concepts, applications, and programming.* Thousand Oaks, CA: Sage.
Campbell, D., & Hallan, G. L. (1997). *Team development survey.* Rosemont, IL: National Computer Systems, Inc.
Chartier, M. R. (1991). Trust-orientation profile. In W. J. Pfeiffer (Ed.), *Annual, developing human resources* (pp. 136–148). San Diego, CA: Pfeiffer & Company.
Dimock, H. G. (1991). Survey of team development. In J. W. Pfeiffer (Ed.), *Encyclopedia of team-development activities* (pp. 243–246). San Diego, CA: Pfeiffer & Company.
Farrell, M. P., Heinemann, G. D., & Schmitt, M. H. (1992). A measure of anomie in health care teams. In J. R. Snyder (Ed.), *Interdisciplinary health care teams: Proceedings of the Fourteenth Annual Conference in Chicago* (pp. 186–197). Indianapolis, IN: School of Allied Health Sciences, Indiana University School of Medicine, Indiana University Medical Center.
Francis, D., & Young, D. (1992). *The team review survey.* San Diego, CA: Pfeiffer & Company.
Glaser, R., & Glaser, C. (1995). *Team effectiveness profile.* King of Prussia, PA: Organization Design and Development, Inc.
Hair, J. F., Tatham, R. L., Anderson, R. E., & Black, W. (1998). *Multivariate data analysis* (5th ed.). Upper Saddle River, NJ: Prentice Hall.
Hall, J. (1988). *Teamness index: An assessment of your team's readiness for effective team work.* The Woodlands, TX: Teleometrics International.
Harper, A., & Harper, B. (1993). In A. Harper & B. Harper, *Skill-building for self-directed team members* (pp. 88–90). Yorktown, NY: MW Co.
Heinemann, G. D., Schmitt, M. H., Farrell, M. P., & Brallier, S. A. (1999). Development of an Attitudes Toward Health Care Teams Scale. *Evaluation & the Health Professions, 22*(1), 123–142.
Heinemann, G. D., & Zeiss, A. M. (Eds.). (2004). *Team performance in health care: Assessment and development.* New York: Kluwer Academic/Plenum.
Hepburn, K., Tsukuda, R. A., & Fasser, C. (1998). Teams skills scale. In E. L. Siegler, K. Myer, T. Fulmer, & M. Mazey (Eds.), *Geriatric interdisciplinary team training* (pp. 264–265). New York: Springer.

Hu, L.-T., & Bentler, P. M. (1999). Cutoff criteria for fit indexes in covariance structure analysis: Conventional criteria versus new alternatives. *Structural Equation Modeling, 6*(1), 1–55.

Kalisch, B. J., Weaver, S. J., & Salas, E. (2009). What does nursing teamwork look like? A qualitative study. *Journal of Nursing Care Quality, 24*(4), 298–307.

Kerlinger, F. N. (1978). *Foundations of behavioral research*. New York: McGraw-Hill.

Leonard, M., Graham, S., & Bonacum, D. (2004). The human factor: The critical importance of effective teamwork and communication in providing safe care. *Quality & Safety in Health Care, 13* (Suppl. 1), i85–i90.

Lichtenstein, R., Alexander, J. A., Jinnett, K., & Ullman, E. (1997). Embedded intergroup relations in interdisciplinary teams: Effects on perceptions of level of team integration. *Journal of Applied Behavioral Science, 33*(4), 413–434.

Lynn, M. R. (1986). Determination and quantification of content validity. *Nursing Research, 35*(6), 382–385.

Mills, P., Neily, J., & Dunn, E. (2008). Teamwork and communication in surgical teams: Implications for patient safety. *Journal of the American College of Surgeons, 206*(1), 107–112.

Millward, L. J., & Jeffries, N. (2001). The Team Survey: A tool for health care team development. *Journal of Advanced Nursing, 35*(2), 276–287.

Morey, J. C., Simon, R., Jay, G. D., Wears, R. L., Salisbury, M., Dukes, K. A., et al. (2002). Error reduction and performance improvement in the emergency department through formal teamwork training: Evaluation results of the MedTeams project. *Health Services Research, 37*(6), 1553–1581.

Nunnally, J. C., & Bernstein, I. H. (1994). *Psychometric theory* (3rd ed.). New York: McGraw-Hill Inc.

Pallant, J. (2005). In J. Pallant, *SPSS survival manual* (2nd ed., pp. 6). New York: Open University Press.

Pfeiffer, J. W., & Jones, J. E. (1974). Post meeting reaction form. In J. W. Pfeiffer (Ed.), *A handbook of structured experiences for human relations training* (Vol. 3, p. 30). San Diego, CA: Pfeiffer & Company.

Phillips, S. L., & Elledge, R. L. (1994). In S. L. Phillips & R. L. Elledge, *Team building for the future: Beyond the basics* (pp. 10–31). San Diego, CA: Pfeiffer & Company.

Price, J. L., & Mueller, C. W. (1986). *Handbook of organizational measurement*. Marshfield, MA: Pitman.

Salas, E., Rosen, M. A., & King, H. (2007). Managing teams managing crises: Principles of teamwork to improve patient safety in the emergency room and beyond. *Theoretical Issues in Ergonomics, 8*(5), 381–394.

Salas, E., Sims, D. E., & Burke, C. S. (2005). Is there a "Big Five" in Teamwork? *Small Group Research, 36*(5), 555–599.

Schein, E. H. (1988). In E. H. Schein, *Process consultation: Its role in organization development* (2nd ed., Vol. 1, pp. 76–83). Reading, MA: Addison Wesley Publishing Company.

Sexton, J. B., Helmreich, R. L., Neilands, T. B., Rowan, K., Vella, K., Boyden, J., et al. (2006). The Safety Attitudes Questionnaire: Psychometric properties, benchmarking data, and emerging research. *BMC Health Services Research, 6*, 44.

Shortell, S. M., Rousseau, D. M., Gillies, R. R., Devers, K. J., & Simons, T. L. (1991). Organizational assessment in intensive care units (ICUs): Construct development, reliability, and validity of the ICU nurse-physician questionnaire. *Medical Care, 29*(8), 709–726.

Shortell, S. M., & Singer, S. J. (2008). Improving patient safety by taking systems seriously. *JAMA, 299*(4), 445–447.

Silen-Lipponen, M., Tossavainen, K., Turunen, H., & Smith, A. (2005). Potential errors and their prevention in operating room teamwork as experienced by Finnish, British and American nurses. *International Journal of Nursing Practice, 11*(1), 21–32.

Straub, D. W. (1989). Validating instruments in MIS research. *MIS Quarterly, 13*(2), 147–169.

Thompson, B., & Daniel, G. (1996). Factor analytic evidence for the construct validity of scores : A historical overview and some guidelines. *Educational and Psychological Measurement, 56*(2), 197–208.

Varney, G. H. (1991). In G. H. Varney, *Building productive teams* (pp. 29–30). San Francisco: Jossey-Bass.

Vogus, T. J., & Sutcliffe, K. M. (2007). The Safety Organizing Scale: Development and validation of a behavioral measure of safety culture in hospital nursing units. *Medical Care, 45*(1),46–54.

Waltz, C. F., Strickland, O. L., & Lenz, E. R. (2005). In C. F. Waltz, O. L. Strickland, & Lenz, E. R. *Measurement in nursing and health research* (3rd ed., pp. 137–214). New York: Springer.

Weisbond, M. R. (1991). Team development rating form. In J. W. Pfeiffer (Ed.), *Encyclopedia of team-development activities* (pp. 249–250). San Diego, CA: Pfeiffer & Company.

Wheelan, S. A. (1994). *The group development questionnaire: A manual for professionals*. Provincetown, MA: GDQ Associates.

A META-ANALYSIS OF INTERVENTIONS TO PROMOTE MAMMOGRAPHY AMONG ETHNIC MINORITY WOMEN

Hae-Ra Han • Jong-Eun Lee • Jiyun Kim • Haley K. Hedlin • Heejung Song • Miyong T. Kim

how Search for relevant art

Editor's Note

Additional information provided by the authors expanding this article is on the Editor's Web site at http://www.nursing-research-editor.com.

▶ **Background:** Although many studies have been focused on interventions designed to promote mammography screening among ethnic minority women, few summaries of the effectiveness of the interventions are available.

▶ **Objective:** The aim of this study was to determine the effectiveness of the interventions for improving mammography screening among asymptomatic ethnic minority women.

▶ **Methods:** A meta-analysis was performed on intervention studies designed to promote mammography use in samples of ethnic minority women. Random-effects estimates were calculated for interventions by measuring differences in intervention and control group screening rates postintervention.

▶ **Results:** The overall mean weighted effect size for the 23 studies was 0.078 ($Z = 4.414$, $p < .001$), indicating that the interventions were effective in improving mammography use among ethnic minority women. For mammography intervention types, access-enhancing strategies had the biggest mean weighted effect size of 0.155 ($Z = 4.488$, $p < .001$), followed by 0.099 ($Z = 6.552$, $p < .001$) for individually directed approaches such as individ-ual counseling or education. Tailored, theory-based interventions resulted in a bigger effect size compared with nontailored interventions (effect sizes = 0.101 vs. 0.076, respectively; $p < .05$ for all models). Of cultural strategies, ethnically matched intervention deliveries and offering culturally matched intervention materials had effect sizes of 0.067 ($Z = 2.516$, $p = .012$) and 0.051 ($Z = 2.365$, $p = .018$), respectively.

▶ **Discussion:** Uniform improvement in mammography screening is a goal to address breast cancer disparities in ethnic minority communities in this country. The results of this meta-analysis suggest a need for increased use of a theory-based, tailored approach with enhancement of access.

▶ **Key Words:** ethnic minority women · mammography · meta-analysis

Despite considerable progress in breast cancer control in the United States over the past 20 years, ethnic minority women continue to face an unequal burden of cancer (Chu, Miller, & Springfield, 2007; Lantz et al.,

2006). For example, African American and Hispanic women are more likely to be diagnosed at an advanced stage of breast cancer (American Cancer Society, 2008; Lantz et al., 2006) and have worse stage-for-stage survival than do White women (Carey et al., 2006; Shavers, Harlan, & Stevens, 2003). Traditionally, Asian American women have had lower breast cancer incidence rates than White women had (American Cancer Society, 2008). Over the past decade, however, the incidence of breast cancer in Asian women has been increasing at a much higher rate than that of White women (annual increase of 6.3% vs. <1.5%; Deapen, Liu, Perkins, Bernstein, & Ross, 2002). In addition, similar to Black and Hispanic women, Asian American women are significantly more likely than White women to discover breast cancer at a later stage (Miller, Hankey, & Thomas, 2002).

Researchers have ascribed a large portion of this disparity in the late-stage diagnosis and poor survival of breast cancer to racial and ethnic differences in the utilization of mammography screening, which is a critical strategy in early detection and timely treatment of breast cancer (Smith-Bindman et al., 2006). The U.S. Preventive Services Task Force (2002) recommends that women have a mammogram every 1–2 years beginning at age 40 years. Although differences in mammography rates between White and African American women have narrowed during the past decade (Smigal et al., 2006), ethnic differences in screening do persist in some groups. The American Cancer Society's most recent annual report of cancer statistics revealed that regular use of mammography was especially low among Hispanic and Asian women relative to the national level (Cokkinides, Bandi, Siegel, Ward, & Thun, 2007). According to a recent report on national surveys (Town, Wholey, Feldman, & Burns, 2007), ethnic minority women are less likely than their White counterparts to have health insurance (69.7% vs. 87%). Minority women who lack health insurance or have lived in the United States for less than 10 years have been found particularly vulnerable to insufficient mammography screening

(Cokkinides et al., 2007; Purc-Stephenson & Gorey, 2008; Rakowski et al., 2006).

Many studies have been focused on promoting mammography screening among ethnic minority women using a variety of intervention strategies. For example, *promotora* (lay health advisor) interventions have been generally well received by ethnic minority women, positively affecting their use of preventive health services, including mammography (Erwin et al., 2003; Mock et al., 2007; Navarro et al., 1998; Taylor et al., 2002). Without a sufficient amount of monitoring, support, and opportunities for advancement, however, the utility of the *promotora* approach is uncertain because the content and frequency of interactions between the *promotora* and the study participant may change by the discretion of the *promotora* (Suarez et al., 1997; Wasserman, Bender, & Lee, 2007). Well-validated theories can be used to guide an intervention effectively by specifying the ingredients and correct implementation of the intervention, making replication of the intervention easier (Sidani & Braden, 1998). Theory-guided tailored interventions (i.e., providing intervention materials adjusted to the characteristics of an individual) have been effective in promoting various forms of health behavior such as healthy diet (Park et al., 2008; Resnicow et al., 2008) and smoking cessation (Schumann et al., 2008). Likewise, recent strategies to promote breast cancer screening include theory-based tailored interventions (Allen & Bazargan-Hejazi, 2005; Champion et al., 2006, 2007; Jibaja-Weiss, Volk, Kingery, Smith, & Holcomb, 2003), although no systematic evaluation of this intervention approach across studies has been done.

The purpose of this meta-analysis was to determine the effects of intervention programs on mammography screening among ethnic minority women. Identification of the determinants of mammography use can facilitate more effective strategies to reduce barriers to breast cancer screening. Meta-analyses of mammography interventions (Denhaerynck et al., 2003; Edwards et al., 2006; Legler et al., 2002; Sohl & Moyer, 2007; Yabroff & Mandelblatt, 1999) found that combined approaches enhancing access—in addition to individual strategies such as reminder letters, telephone calls, or personal contact—can increase mammography use. Specifically, in the Legler et al. (2002) meta-analysis, access-enhancing strategies were the strongest intervention approach, resulting in an increase in mammography use by 18.9% (95% confidence interval [CI] = 10.4–27.4), followed by individually directed interventions in a healthcare setting (17.6%; 95% CI = 11.6–24.0). Yabroff and Mandelblatt (1999) included two studies that used access-enhancing strategies (financial incentives) in their meta-analysis but did not perform meta-analysis with two interventions. They found that patient-targeted behavioral interventions improved mammography utilization by 13.2% (95% CI = 4.7–21.2). Effect sizes of interventions using social networks were revealed to be in the range of 5.8% (Legler et al., 2002) to 12.6% (Yabroff & Mandelblatt, 1999).

However, most previous meta-analyses have not been focused specifically on ethnic minority women, nor have culturally tailored or recent intervention approaches most effective for these groups of women with traditionally lower use of mammography been discussed. The goal of this study was to fill this gap by conducting analyses on more recent studies (published since September 2000, where the review by Legler et al., 2002, left off) that were targeted specifically to ethnic minority women. Specifically, the objective of the meta-analysis was to describe mammography intervention approaches used for ethnic minority (Asian American, African American, and Hispanic) women in the United States.

■ Methods

STUDY SELECTION

Literature for this review was identified using electronic searches of databases and hand searches from reference collections. The literature search was limited to articles published

in the English language from 2000 onwards. Two authors independently searched Medline, CINAHL, PsycINFO, and Web of Science using combinations of the key word phrases *Asian, African American, Hispanic or Latino, breast cancer screening, mammography, experimental studies, interventions, and intervention studies.*

The electronic and hand searches generated a combined total of 749 titles and abstracts for assessment. Screening of relevant studies for inclusion was conducted using titles and abstracts based on the following criteria: (a) the study aimed to increase use of mammography screening among asymptomatic women, either exclusively or in addition to other health behaviors; (b) the study included more than 40% of women with ethnic minority background (i.e., Asian American, Black, or Hispanic) in the sample; (c) outcomes were based on a woman's adherence to mammography screening, documented either by self-report or in a clinical database or medical record; (d) an experimental or quasi-experimental design was used in the study; and (e) the study was reported between September 2000 and August 2008. Not included were international studies because the focus was on intervention strategies to improve breast cancer screening among ethnic minority women in the United States.

The titles and abstracts of all identified studies were reviewed by two study team members. Of these 749 studies, 607 were excluded. A total of 142 full-text articles were reviewed systematically to confirm eligibility for this study. Of the 142 articles examined, 43 did not include more than 40% of ethnic minority women, or ethnicity was unclear; 23 did not have a control group; 2 were only system directed; and 6 did not specify an intervention component clearly. In addition, 13 did not include enough information to calculate an effect size; 18 did not include a woman's adherence to mammography screening as an outcome; and 14 had an international study setting or reported on the same sample as another that was already included. As a result, a total of 23 studies were included in the meta-analysis (Figure 1).

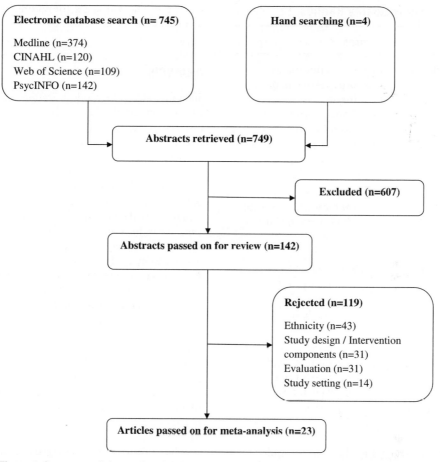

Figure 1. Summary of the study selection process.

STUDY CODING

The specific outcome of interest in this analysis was the difference in the proportion of mammography screening in the intervention group versus the control group. A number of variables were selected for inclusion in the database of articles. The following were coded: first author, year, study design, setting, sample (percentage of ethnic minority women), unit of assignment, type of intervention, intervention period, time to outcome measure (months), method of outcome ascertainment, number of participants in the study groups, mean age of the study sample, proportion of mammogra-

phy screening for the treatment and control groups, theory, control group (no intervention, minimal intervention or usual care, or other non-breast-cancer intervention), any cultural strategies used, and study quality. Following the typology used in previous reviews (Legler et al., 2002; Rimer, 1994), interventions were categorized as follows: (a) individual directed (e.g., one-on-one counseling, tailored and nontailored letters and reminders, and telephone counseling), (b) system directed (e.g., provider prompts), (c) access enhancing (e.g., mobile vans and reduced-cost mammograms), (d) social network (e.g., peer educators and lay health advisors), (e) community

Table 1. Study Quality Ratings

Items	Scores
Study design	0 = Nonrandomized prospective experiment 1 = Randomized experiment
Outcome measure	0 = Subjective measure of mammogram receipt (self-reports) 1 = Objective measure of mammogram receipt (claims data, chart review)
Clarity of outcome definition	0 = No definition of study outcome (mammogram adherence) 1 = Clearly defined mammogram adherence
Information on withdrawal	0 = Not clearly discussed 1 = The number and the reasons for withdrawals in each group are stated

education, (f) mass media, and (g) multiple strategies (combinations of the intervention approaches listed above). As in a prior review (Legler et al., 2002), in five studies comparing two or more intervention groups to one control group, the intervention with the most components (i.e., highest dose group) was considered. To rate study quality, four items were used from relevant literature (Jadad et al., 1996; Soeken, Lee, Bausell, Agelli, & Berman, 2002). The range of total quality scores was 0 to 4 (Table 1). For the purpose of this analysis, studies with scores of 1–2 were considered to be *low quality* and those with scores of 3–4 were considered to be *high quality*. Using Microsoft Excel, two raters independently coded the variables. Every discrepancy was identified and resolved by discussion among team members. The average κ for coding agreement was sufficient, 0.86.

ANALYSIS

Stata (StataCorp LP, College Station, TX) was used to conduct the data analysis. An effect size (d) was calculated for each study using the difference in the postintervention adherence rates between the intervention and control groups (p_i and p_c, respectively). An overall mean weighted effect size (MWES) for the 23 studies was computed using the *meta* command in Stata, which weights d by the inverse of the estimated study variance in fixed-effects models. For the effect size of $d = p_i - p_c$, the study variance was defined to be $p_i (1 - p_i)/n_i + p_c (1 - p_c)/n_c$, where n_i and n_c are the number of participants in the intervention and control groups, respectively (DerSimonian & Laird, 1986).

A test for heterogeneity of the intervention effects was performed using the DerSimonian and Laird (1986) Q statistic. When significant, a random-effects model was used to accommodate this heterogeneity (DerSimonian & Laird, 1986). This process was repeated to calculate MWES for various subgroups of the 23 studies. In addition, 95% CIs were estimated for each MWES.

The sensitivity analyses consisted of refitting the meta-analysis for the overall MWES to determine whether the results varied by potentially influential studies (i.e., extreme effect size, large sample size) or study quality. A leave-one-out approach was taken and the overall MWES was reestimated by removing the influential studies one at a time. Also conducted were meta-analyses restricted to high- and low-quality studies to compare to the overall MWES. Finally, additional analyses using funnel plot and fail-safe N were performed to examine publication bias. In the absence of publication bias, the plot should be symmetric, resembling an inverted funnel (Light & Pillemer, 1984). Because visual inspection of the funnel plot involves subjective interpretation, Rosenthal's (1984) fail-safe N was calculated also. This calculation is an estimate of the number of studies having no effect (i.e., zero effect size) that is needed to reduce the overall effect size in the meta-analysis from significant to nonsignificant. If the estimated fail-safe N is greater than a cutoff value (formula $= 5k + 10$, where k is the number of studies in the meta-analysis; Rosenthal, 1984), it is suggested that there is no evidence of publication bias.

■ Results

STUDY CHARACTERISTICS

Of the 23 studies, 6 studies included predominantly African Americans; 2 studies, Hispanics; 5 studies, Asians; and 10 studies, combined ethnic samples. Randomized experimental study design (61%), group-level assignment (57%), and community setting (83%) were common features of the studies. Sample sizes varied; smaller studies included <100 participants in the sample, whereas the biggest study was done on >5,000 women, totaling 22,849 women. (See Table, Supplemental Digital Content 1, which summarizes the characteristics of studies included in this meta-analysis, http://links.lww.com/A1244.) This table is also included on the Editor's Web site at http://www.nursing-research-editor.com.

The studies used single or multiple intervention strategies, with individually directed print materials being the most frequently used approach, followed by peer or lay health worker education or support and telephone counseling. Access-enhancing strategies such as low- or no-cost mammograms, making appointments, mobile vans, or vouchers were included in 6 studies. For the comparison group, 15 studies (65%) provided no intervention or usual care; 6 studies, minimal intervention; and 2 studies, other active non breast intervention (e.g., education on cholesterol or physical activity). Self-report rather than medical records was more frequently used as a method of outcome measurement (74% vs. 26%). The Health Belief Model was the

most popular theory and was used in 6 studies alone or in combination with other theories such as Transtheoretical Model of Change and Social Learning theory, although in 9 studies, the theoretical approach was unspecified. These theories offered a basis for targets of individualized tailoring (e.g., providing intervention materials attuned to the characteristics of a person) in 4 studies. Most interventions involved some form of cultural strategies except for 2 (both conducted in a healthcare setting). Culturally matched intervention materials and ethnically matched intervention deliveries were equally common, whereas 5 studies indicated participation of members of the target ethnic community as a way of increasing cultural sensitivity of their intervention. Nine (39%) of the studies received a high quality rating, whereas 14 (61%) were rated as low quality.

POOLED RESULTS

The estimated intervention effect and 95% CI for each study are presented in Table 2. As shown in Table 2, the overall MWES for the 23 studies was 0.078 ($Z = 4.414$, $p < .001$) with a 95% CI of 0.043 to 0.113, indicating that the interventions were effective in improving mammography screening among ethnic minority women. This effect size was computed using a random effects model to account for significant heterogeneity among interventions as indicated by a significant Q statistic ($Q = 92.95$, $df = 22$, $p < .001$).

SUBGROUP ANALYSES

Also shown in Table 2 is the effectiveness of the different intervention methods. Access-enhancing interventions had the biggest MWES of 0.155 ($n = 6$, $Z = 4.488$, $p < .001$), followed by individually directed interventions ($n = 19$, MWES $= 0.099$, $Z = 6.552$, $p < .001$). Estimated effect sizes for other intervention approaches involving mass media ($n = 4$, MWES $= 0.065$, $Z = 1.759$, $p = .079$), community education ($n = 4$, MWES $= 0.013$,

Table 2. Estimated Effect Sizes With 95% Confidence Intervals (CIs)

Element	Category	No. of Studies	Effect Size (95% CI)
Overall		23	0.078 (0.043 to 0.113)
Intervention type[a,b]	Individual directed	19	0.099 (0.073 to 0.110)
	Access enhancing	6	0.155 (0.087 to 0.223)
	Social network	6	−0.023 (−0.078 to 0.032)
	Community education	4	0.013 (−0.067 to 0.094)
	Mass media	4	0.065 (−0.007 to 0.138)
Theory	Theory based	14	0.090 (0.042 to 0.137)
	Nontheory based	9	0.062 (0.009 to 0.116)
Tailored	Yes[c]	4	0.101 (0.057 to 0.145)
	No	19	0.076 (0.035 to 0.116)
Cultural strategies[b]	Involved target community members	5	0.074 (−0.055 to 0.203)
	Culturally matched materials	15	0.051 (0.009 to 0.092)
	Matched intervention deliveries	14	0.067 (0.015 to 0.120)
Setting	Healthcare[c]	4	0.113 (0.081 to 0.114)
	Community	19	0.067 (0.027 to 0.107)
Ethnic groups[d]	African American	9	0.098 (0.023 to 0.174)
	Asian Pacific Islanders	5	0.094 (0.000 to 0.189)
	Hispanic	5	0.036 (−0.034 to 0.106)
Quality	High (3 or 4)[c]	9	0.099 (0.076 to 0.122)
	Low (1 or 2)	14	0.061 (0.008 to 0.114)

[a]Type of intervention: individual directed = counseling (in person, telephone), letters, reminders; access enhancing = facilitated scheduling, mobile vans, vouchers, reduced-cost or free mammograms; social network = peer leaders or lay health advisors; community education = community workshops, seminars.
[b]Studies may be classified as using more than one type of intervention or cultural strategies.
[c]Fitted with a fixed-effects model (p for Q statistic > .05).
[d]Included studies with samples >40% of specified ethnic groups.

$Z = 0.324$, $p = .746$), or social networks ($n = 6$, MWES = −0.023, $Z = −0.817$, $p = .414$) were not statistically significant.

Tailoring an intervention according to the individual's characteristics based on valid behavioral theory was more effective than not doing so, with the MWES being 0.101 ($n = 4$, $Z = 4.476$, $p < .001$) and 0.076 ($n = 19$, $Z = 3.677$, $p < .001$), respectively. Theory-based interventions ($n = 14$) resulted in a bigger effect size compared with nontheory-based interventions ($n = 9$; effect sizes = 0.090 vs. 0.062, respectively; $p < .05$ for all tests). Of

cultural strategies, ethnically matched intervention deliveries ($n = 14$, MWES = 0.067, $Z = 2.516$, $p = .012$) and culturally matched intervention materials ($n = 15$, MWES = 0.051, $Z = 2.365$, $p = .018$) significantly improved mammography screening. Interventions involving members of the target community were a cultural strategy, with the biggest effect size of 0.074 ($n = 5$, $Z = 1.124$, $p = .261$), but the result was not significant. Interventions delivered in healthcare settings ($n = 4$) were associated with a bigger effect size compared with interventions done in community settings

(n = 19; MWES = 0.113 vs. 0.067; p < .01 for all models). When combined intervention effects were examined for each ethnic group (included studies with samples >40% of specified ethnic groups), the estimated intervention effect was significant for African American women with a MWES of 0.098 (n = 9, Z = 2.550, p = .011). Studies with other ethnic minority women yielded no significant findings with a MWES of 0.094 for Asian and Pacific Islanders (n = 5, Z = 1.955, p = .051) and 0.036 for Hispanic women (n = 5, Z = 1.004, p = .315).

SENSITIVITY ANALYSES

Sensitivity analyses were conducted using potentially influential studies such as Kim and Sarna (2004), Sauaia et al. (2007), and Welsh, Sauaia, Jacobellis, Min, and Byers (2005) to gauge the impact on the variability of effect sizes. When the Kim and Sarna study was removed, the MWES for remaining studies was 0.069 (Z = 4.153, p < .001). Removing Sauaia et al. resulted in a MWES of 0.082 (Z − 4.292, p < .001) for the remaining studies. Without Welsh et al., the MWES for the other 22 studies was 0.085 (Z − 5.198, p < .001). Also performed were analyses with studies of high versus low quality ratings (quality rating 3–4 vs. 1–2). The MWES for the high-quality studies (n = 9) was 0.099 (Z = 8.452, p < .001), whereas the MWES for the low-quality studies (n = 14) was 0.061 (Z = 2.239, p = .025).

PUBLICATION BIAS

The likelihood of publication bias was examined by first plotting the standard error by the natural logarithm of the logged odds ratio for the estimated effect sizes. The funnel plot appeared slightly asymmetrical. The fail-safe N, however, indicated that 411 nonsignificant studies would be necessary (cutoff = 125) to show that these interventions used to promote mammography screening among traditionally nonadherent ethnic minority women have no effect on mammography adherence, making the aggregate result from this analysis fairly robust.

■ Discussion

The results indicate that there was an average of 7.8% increase in the rate of mammography use for minority women in the treatment groups receiving a variety of interventions. Access-enhancing interventions yielded the biggest increase in mammography use (15.5%), followed by individually directed interventions (9.9%). Even though the result cannot be compared directly with those of other meta-analyses due to different study selection criteria and intervention typology, this finding is similar to that of Legler et al. (2002) and Yabroff and Mandelblatt (1999).

Interventions using social networks such as *promotoras* or lay health advisors were associated with a small and negative effect size (i.e., reduced mammography screening rates after intervention). The finding of the negative effect size associated with *promotora* interventions might have been a result of study design. Specifically, the six *promotora* interventions included in the meta-analysis (Earp et al., 2002; Fernandez-Esquer, Espinoza, Torres, Ramirez, & McAlister, 2003; Nguyen, Vo, McPhee, & Jenkins, 2001; Powell et al., 2005; Sauaia et al., 2007; Welsh et al., 2005) were all nonrandomized, community-based trials with mostly large sample sizes (mean sample size = about 2,299) and low quality ratings; five studies received a quality rating of 2 and one study received a quality rating of 1. Our finding indicates that *promotora* interventions may be better suited for smaller community applications. When a large-scale community-based intervention trial is planned, interventions using *promotoras* may need to be considered as an alternative with well-prepared *promotora* training and a rigorous monitoring plan.

In analyzing effect sizes by the use of theory, the results indicated that theory-based interventions were more effective than nontheory-based interventions. Tailored interventions guided by theory also resulted in a greater effect size than did nontailored interventions. Indeed, tailored interventions included in this meta-analysis used single or multiple theories to structure the content of the intervention messages. Considering the few tailored interventions with larger improvement in mammography screening, more tailored intervention studies based on valid theories are warranted.

Interventions involving target community members as a way to enhance cultural sensitivity yielded a bigger effect size as compared with interventions using other cultural strategies (e.g., providing culturally matched materials or matching intervention deliveries), although the random-effects model for testing of its effect was not statistically significant. We cannot compare the result with those of other meta-analyses because no previous meta-analyses specifically examined cultural strategies as part of intervention typology. The nonsignificance might be attributable to the small number of studies in this category ($n = 5$). Although the finding offers some implications in designing mammography-enhancing interventions for ethnic minority women, future meta-analysis is needed as more empirical evidence becomes available.

Consistent with previous meta-analysis (Legler et al., 2002), it was found that the intervention effect was bigger for studies conducted in a healthcare setting (e.g., health maintenance organizations and community health centers) than for the community-based studies. Healthcare settings naturally offer increased contact with medical providers. It is likely that women in the healthcare setting might have had fewer barriers to screening, with more support for obtaining mammograms through individualized letters or counseling (Champion et al., 2007; Young, Waller, & Smitherman, 2002), scheduling of screening appointments (Beach et al., 2007), or case management (Beach et al., 2007; Dietrich et al., 2006). As Legler et al. (2002) pointed out, additional support or cues are necessary to facilitate mammography use

even when access may no longer be a problem.

Effect sizes for studies including more than 40% African American and more than 40% Asian or Pacific Islander women were similar (9.8% and 9.4%, respectively), although the effect size for Asian or Pacific Islander women was marginally significant ($p = .051$); however, the MWES (3.6%) was not statistically significant for comparisons consisting of more than 40% Hispanic women. The estimated effect for intervention groups with more than 40% African American women in the Legler et al. (2002) meta-analysis was 11.6% (95% CI = 6.4−16.7), slightly bigger than that in this study. Although no published analysis of intervention effects for Asian or Pacific Islanders or Hispanic women were found, the nonsignificant result might have been due, in part, to the small number of studies available for these subgroup analyses (five studies each for Asian or Pacific Islander and Hispanic women). A careful examination of the characteristics of each individual study included in the ethnic subgroup analyses also revealed some design issues—particularly for studies involving Hispanic women—that are worth pointing out: three out of five studies with more than 40% Hispanic women (Fernandez-Esquer et al., 2003; Sauaia et al., 2007; Welsh et al., 2005) used a nonrandomized experimental design with a large sample size ($N >$ 5,000 for Sauaia et al., 2007, and Welsh et al., 2005). A large-scale community trial is likely to put researchers in a less controlled situation. Diffusion might occur between groups or control communities may receive interventions with substantial amount through other mechanisms (e.g., the Breast and Cervical Cancer Program for free mammograms). A traditional randomized controlled trial could pose ethical and logistical dilemmas in community research because control groups do not benefit from study participation, which is often perceived as *unfair* (Learmonth, 2000). Nevertheless, this analysis suggests that more tightly controlled trials may be necessary to improve mammography screening among minority groups, particularly

Hispanic women. Researchers may need to consider and engage more actively in alternative research designs (e.g., waiting list design and attention control design) to ensure that the benefits of the research are made available to all ethnic minority communities (Corbie-Smith et al., 2003).

Several limitations of this meta-analysis should be noted. One limitation is the reliance of this review on published sources in Medline, CINAHL, PsycINFO, and Web of Science databases. This might have led to an overestimation or underestimation of effect sizes by excluding unpublished sources (e.g., dissertations) or government documents that might not be readily available, although researchers have found no differences related to inclusion or exclusion of unpublished literature (Conn, Valentine, Cooper, & Rantz, 2003). Second, due to the focus of interest in ethnic minority women in the United States who face unique cultural and linguistic challenges, this review was limited to articles of samples in the United States; thus, the findings may not be generalizable to studies that have been conducted in other countries. Third, as is common in meta-analyses, the uneven quality and quantity of studies are also limitations. An attempt was made to address this issue by offering estimates for high- versus low-quality studies. Several analyses included only four to six studies with nonsignificant MWES. Findings from the analyses with only a small number of studies should be considered as preliminary evidence and not definitive estimates of the effectiveness of the studies. It will be important to conduct additional analyses when results from more studies become available. Finally, most studies included in this meta-analysis used multiple intervention components. One problem in interventions with multiple components is that it is difficult to tease out the effect of each individual component. Some researchers suggest conducting factorial design studies to address this issue (Legler et al., 2002), although the cost to conduct such studies would likely be higher.

In conclusion, uniform improvement in cancer screening is a national goal to address cancer disparities among ethnic minority communities in the United States. The results of this meta-analysis suggest important directions for the design of future interventions to promote mammography screening among ethnic minority women. Access-enhancing strategies are an important intervention component for minority women who are likely to lack the resources to obtain mammography screening readily. Also highlighted in this analysis is a need for increased use of a theory-based, tailored approach. More active engagement of community partners in the research process should be considered also to improve screening outcomes. Finally, based on the pooled MWES estimated in this meta-analysis, well-controlled studies are needed to improve the effectiveness of mammography intervention programs among ethnic minority women, particularly among Hispanic women. Consistent use of the rate difference of mammography screening as an outcome measure is important for additional meta-analyses and promotion of further knowledge development in this important area.

Hae-Ra Han, PhD, RN, is Associate Professor, School of Nursing; Jong-Eun Lee, PhD, RN, is Postdoctoral Fellow, School of Nursing; Jiyun Kim, PhD, RN, is Postdoctoral Fellow, School of Nursing; Haley K. Hedlin, BA, is Doctoral Student, Bloomberg School of Public Health; Heejung Song, PhD, is Research Associate, Bloomberg School of Public Health; and Miyong T. Kim, PhD, RN, FAAN, is Professor, School of Nursing, Bloomberg School of Public Health, and School of Medicine, The Johns Hopkins University, Baltimore, Maryland.

Supplemental digital content is available for this article. Direct URL citations appear in the printed text and are provided in the HTML and PDF versions of this article on the journal's Web site (www.nursingresearchonline.com).

Accepted for publication March 12, 2009.
This study was supported by a grant from the National Cancer Institute (R01 CA129060). Editorial support was provided by the Johns Hopkins University School of Nursing Center for Collaborative Intervention Research. Funding for the Center is provided by the National Institute of Nursing Research (P30

NRO 8995). The content is solely the responsibility of the authors and does not necessarily represent the official views of the National Institute of Nursing Research or the National Institutes of Health.

Corresponding author: Hae-Ra Han, PhD, RN, School of Nursing, The Johns Hopkins University, 525 North Wolfe Street, Room 448, Baltimore, MD 21205-2110 (e-mail: hhan@son.jhmi.edu).

REFERENCES

*Allen, B. Jr., & Bazargan-Hejazi, S. (2005). Evaluating a tailored intervention to increase screening mammography in an urban area. *Journal of the National Medical Association, 97*(10), 1350–1360.

American Cancer Society. (2008). *Cancer facts and figures* 2008. Atlanta, GA: Author.

*Avis, N. E., Smith, K. W., Link, C. L., & Goldman, M. B. (2004). Increasing mammography screening among women over age 50 with a videotape intervention. *Preventive Medicine, 39*(3), 498–506.

*Beach, M. L., Flood, A. B., Robinson, C. M., Cassells, A. N., Tobin, J. N., Greene, M. A., et al. (2007). Can language-concordant prevention care managers improve cancer screening rates? *Cancer Epidemiology, Biomarkers & Prevention, 16*(10), 2058–2064.

Carey, L. A., Perou, C. M., Livasy, C. A., Dressler, L. G., Cowan, D., Conway, K., et al. (2006). Race, breast cancer subtypes, and survival in the Carolina Breast Cancer Study. *JAMA, 295*(21), 2492–2502.

*Champion, V. L., Springston, J. K., Zollinger, T. W., Saywell, R. M. Jr., Monahan, P. O., Zhao, Q., et al. (2006). Comparison of three interventions to increase mammography screening in low income African American women. *Cancer Detection and Prevention, 30*(6), 535–544.

*Champion, V., Skinner, C. S., Hui, S., Monahan, P., Juliar, B., Daggy, J., et al. (2007). The effect of telephone versus print tailoring for mammography adherence. *Patient Education and Counseling, 65*(3), 416–423.

Chu, K. C., Miller, B. A., & Springfield, S. A. (2007). Measures of racial/ethnic health disparities in cancer mortality rates and the influence of socioeconomic status. *Journal of the National Medical Association, 99*(10), 1092–1100, 1102–1104.

Cokkinides, V., Bandi, P., Siegel, R., Ward, E. M., & Thun, M. J. (2007). *Cancer prevention & early detection facts & figures 2008.* Atlanta, GA: American Cancer Society.

Conn, V. S., Valentine, J. C., Cooper, H. M., & Rantz, M. J. (2003). Grey literature in meta-analyses. *Nursing Research, 52*(4), 256–261.

Corbie-Smith, G., Ammerman, A. S., Katz, M. L., St. George, D. M., Blumenthal, C., Washington, C., et al. (2003). Trust, benefit, satisfaction, and burden:

A randomized controlled trial to reduce cancer risk through African-American churches. *Journal of General Internal Medicine, 18*(7), 531–541.

*Danigelis, N. L., Worden, J. K., Flynn, B. S., Skelly, J. M., & Vacek, P. M. (2005). Increasing mammography screening among low-income African American women with limited access to health information. *Preventive Medicine, 40*(6), 880–887.

Deapen, D., Liu, L., Perkins, C., Bernstein, L., & Ross, R. K. (2002). Rapidly rising breast cancer incidence rates among Asian-American women. *International Journal of Cancer, 99*(5), 747–750.

Denhaerynck, K., Lesaffre, E., Baele, J., Cortebeeck, K., Van Overstraete, E., & Buntinx, F. (2003). Mammography screening attendance: Meta-analysis of the effect of direct-contact invitation. *American Journal of Preventive Medicine, 25*(3), 195–203.

DerSimonian, R., & Laird, N. (1986). Meta-analysis in clinical trials. *Controlled Clinical Trials, 7*(3), 177–188.

*Dietrich, A. J., Tobin, J. N., Cassells, A., Robinson, C. M., Greene, M. A., Sox, C. H., et al. (2006). Telephone care management to improve cancer screening among low-income women: A randomized, controlled trial. *Annals of Internal Medicine, 144*(8), 563–571.

*Duan, N., Fox, S. A., Derose, K. P., & Carson, S. (2000). Maintaining mammography adherence through telephone counseling in a church-based trial. *American Journal of Public Health, 90*(9), 1468–1471.

*Earp, J. A., Eng, E., O'Malley, M. S., Altpeter, M., Rauscher, G., Mayne, L., et al. (2002). Increasing use of mammography among older, rural African American women: Results from a community trial. *American Journal of Public Health, 92*(4), 646–654.

Edwards, A. G., Evans, R., Dundon, J., Haigh, S., Hood, K., & Elwyn, G. J. (2006). Personalised risk communication for informed decision making about taking screening tests. *Cochrane Database of Systematic Reviews,* (4), CD001865.

Erwin, D. O., Ivory, J., Stayton, C., Willis, M., Jandorf, L., Thompson, H., et al. (2003). Replication and dissemination of a cancer education model for African American women. *Cancer Control, 10*(5 Suppl.), 13–21.

*Fernandez-Esquer, M. E., Espinoza, P., Torres, I., Ramirez, A. G., & McAlister, A. L. (2003). A su salud: A quasi-experimental study among Mexican American women. *American Journal of Health Behavior, 27*(5), 536–545.

*Husaini, B. A., Sherkat, D. E., Levine, R., Bragg, R., Van, C. A., Emerson, J. S., et al. (2002). The effect of a church-based breast cancer screening education program on mammography rates among African-American women. *Journal of the National Medical Association, 94*(2), 100–106.

Jadad, A. R., Moore, R. A., Carroll, D., Jenkinson, C., Reynolds, D. J., Gavaghan, D. J., et al. (1996). Assessing the quality of reports of randomized clinical trials: Is blinding necessary? *Controlled Clinical Trials, 17*(1), 1–12.

*Jibaja-Weiss, M. L., Volk, R. J., Kingery, P., Smith, Q. W., & Holcomb, J. D. (2003). Tailored messages for breast and cervical cancer screening of low-income and minority women using medical records data. *Patient Education and Counseling, 50*(2), 123–132.

*Kim, Y. H., & Sarna, L. (2004). An intervention to increase mammography use by Korean American women. *Oncology Nursing Forum, 31*(1), 105–110.

Lantz, P. M., Mujahid, M., Schwartz, K., Janz, N. K., Fagerlin, A., Salem, B., et al. (2006). The influence of race, ethnicity, and individual socioeconomic factors on breast cancer stage at diagnosis. *American Journal of Public Health, 96*(12), 2173–2178.

Learmonth, A. M. (2000). Utilizing research in practice and generating evidence from practice. *Health Education Research, 15*(6), 743–756.

Legler, J., Meissner, H. I., Coyne, C., Breen, N., Chollette, V., & Rimer, B. K. (2002). The effectiveness of interventions to promote mammography among women with historically lower rates of screening. *Cancer Epidemiology, Biomarkers & Prevention, 11*(1), 59–71.

Light, R. J., & Pillemer, D. B. (1984). *Summing up: The science of reviewing research.* Cambridge, MA: Harvard University Press.

*Maxwell, A. E., Bastani, R., Vida, P., & Warda, U. S. (2003). Results of a randomized trial to increase breast and cervical cancer screening among Filipino American women. *Preventive Medicine, 37*(2), 102–109.

Miller, B. A., Hankey, B. F., & Thomas, T. L. (2002). Impact of sociodemographic factors, hormone receptor status, and tumor grade on ethnic differences in tumor stage and size for breast cancer in US women. *American Journal of Epidemiology, 155*(6), 534–545.

*Mishra, S. I., Bastani, R., Crespi, C. M., Chang, L. C., Luce, P. H., & Baquet, C. R. (2007). Results of a randomized trial to increase mammogram usage among Samoan women. *Cancer Epidemiology, Biomarkers & Prevention, 16*(12), 2594–2604.

Mock, J., McPhee, S. J., Nguyen, T., Wong, C., Doan, H., Lai, K. Q., et al. (2007). Effective lay health worker outreach and media-based education for promoting cervical cancer screening among Vietnamese American women. *American Journal of Public Health, 97*(9), 1693–1700.

*Moskowitz, J. M., Kazinets, G., Wong, J. M., & Tager, I. B. (2007). "Health is strength": A community health education program to improve breast and cervical cancer screening among Korean American women in Alameda County, California. *Cancer Detection and Prevention, 31*(2), 173–183.

Navarro, A. M., Senn, K. L., McNicholas, L. J., Kaplan, R. M., Roppe, B., & Campo, M. C. (1998). Por La Vida model intervention enhances use of cancer screening tests among Latinas. *American Journal of Preventive Medicine, 15*(1), 32–41.

*Nguyen, T., Vo, P. H., McPhee, S. J., & Jenkins, C. N. (2001). Promoting early detection of breast cancer among Vietnamese- American women. Results of a controlled trial. *Cancer, 91*(1 Suppl.), 267–273.

Park, A., Nitzke, S., Kritsch, K., Kattelmann, K., White, A., Boeckner, L., et al. (2008). Internet-based interventions have potential to affect short-term mediators and indicators of dietary behavior of young adults. *Journal of Nutrition Education and Behavior, 40*(5), 288–297.

*Powell, M. E., Carter, V., Bonsi, E., Johnson, G., Williams, L., Taylor-Smith, L., et al. (2005). Increasing mammography screening among African American women in rural areas. *Journal of Health Care for the Poor and Underserved, 16*(4 Suppl. A), 11–21.

Purc-Stephenson, R. J., & Gorey, K. M. (2008). Lower adherence to screening mammography guidelines among ethnic minority women in America: A meta-analytic review. *Preventive Medicine, 46*(6), 479–488.

Rakowski, W., Meissner, H., Vernon, S. W., Breen, N., Rimer, B., & Clark, M. A. (2006). Correlates of repeat and recent mammography for women ages 45 to 75 in the 2002 to 2003 Health Information National Trends Survey (HINTS 2003). *Cancer Epidemiology, Biomarkers & Prevention, 15*(11), 2093–2101.

Resnicow, K., Davis, R. E., Zhang, G., Konkel, J., Strecher, V. J., Shaikh, A. R., et al. (2008). Tailoring a fruit and vegetable intervention on novel motivational constructs: Results of a randomized study. *Annals of Behavioral Medicine, 35*(2), 159–169.

*Reuben, D. B., Bassett, L. W., Hirsch, S. H., Jackson, C. A., & Bastani, R. (2002). A randomized clinical trial to assess the benefit of offering on-site mobile mammography in addition to health education for older women. *American Journal of Roentgenology, 179*(6), 1509–1514.

Rimer, B. K. (1994). Mammography use in the U.S.: Trends and the impact of interventions. *Annals of Behavioral Medicine, 16*(4), 317–326.

Rosenthal, R. (1984). *Meta-analysis procedures for social research.* Beverly Hills, CA: Sage.

*Sauaia, A., Min, S. J., Lack, D., Apodaca, C., Osuna, D., Stowe, A., et al. (2007). Church-based breast cancer screening education: Impact of two approaches on Latinas enrolled in public and private health insurance plans. *Preventing Chronic Disease, 4*(4), A99.

Schumann, A., John, U., Ulbricht, S., Ruge, J., Bischof, G., & Meyer, C. (2008). Computer-generated tailored feedback letters for smoking cessation: Theoretical and empirical variability of tailoring. *International Journal of Medical Informatics, 77*(11), 715–722.

Shavers, V. L., Harlan, L. C., & Stevens, J. L. (2003). Racial/ethnic variation in clinical presentation, treatment, and survival among breast cancer patients under age 35. *Cancer, 97*(1), 134–147.

Sidani, S., & Braden, C. J. (1998). *Evaluating nursing interventions: A theory-driven approach.* Thousand Oaks, CA: Sage.

Smigal, C., Jemal, A., Ward, E., Cokkinides, V., Smith, R., Howe, H. L., et al. (2006). Trends in breast cancer by race and ethnicity: Update 2006. *CA: A Cancer Journal for Clinicians, 56*(3), 168–183.

Smith-Bindman, R., Miglioretti, D. L., Lurie, N., Abraham, L., Barbash, R. B., Strzelczyk, J., et al. (2006). Does utilization of screening mammography explain racial and ethnic differences in breast cancer? *Annals of Internal Medicine, 144*(8), 541–553.

Soeken, K. L., Lee, W. L., Bausell, R. B., Agelli, M., & Berman, B. M. (2002). Safety and efficacy of S-adenosylmethionine (SAMe) for osteoarthritis. *Journal of Family Practice, 51*(5), 425–430.

Sohl, S. J., & Moyer, A. (2007). Tailored interventions to promote mammography screening: A meta-analytic review. *Preventive Medicine, 45*(4), 252–261.

StataCorp. (2005). *Stata statistical software: Release 9.* College Station, TX: Author.

Suarez, L., Roche, R. A., Pulley, L. V., Weiss, N. S., Goldman, D., & Simpson, D. M. (1997). Why a peer intervention program for Mexican-American women failed to modify the secular trend in cancer screening. *American Journal of Preventive Medicine, 13*(6), 411–417.

Taylor, V. M., Jackson, J. C., Yasui, Y., Kuniyuki, A., Acorda, E., Marchand, A., et al. (2002). Evaluation of an outreach intervention to promote cervical cancer screening among Cambodian American women. *Cancer Detection and Prevention, 26*(4), 320–327.

Town, R. J., Wholey, D. R., Feldman, R. D., & Burns, L. R. (2007). Hospital consolidation and racial/income disparities in health insurance coverage. *Health Affairs, 26*(4), 1170–1180.

U.S. Preventive Services Task Force. (2002). *Screening for breast cancer: Recommendations and rationale.* Retrieved May 8, 2008, from http://www.ahcpr.gov/clinic/3rduspstf/breastcancer/brcanrr.htm

Wasserman, M., Bender, D., & Lee, S. Y. (2007). Use of preventive maternal and child health services by Latina women: A review of published intervention studies. *Medical Care Research and Review, 64*(1), 4–45.

*Welsh, A. L., Sauaia, A., Jacobellis, J., Min, S. J., & Byers, T. (2005). The effect of two church-based interventions on breast cancer screening rates among Medicaid-insured Latinas. *Preventing Chronic Disease, 2*(4), A07.

*Wood, R. Y., & Duffy, M. E. (2004). Video breast health kits: Testing a cancer education innovation in older high-risk populations. *Journal of Cancer Education, 19*(2), 98–104.

Yabroff, K. R., & Mandelblatt, J. S. (1999). Interventions targeted toward patients to increase mammography use. *Cancer Epidemiology, Biomarkers & Prevention, 8*(9), 749–757.

*Young, R. F., Waller, J. B. Jr., & Smitherman, H. (2002). A breast cancer education and on-site screening intervention for unscreened African American women. *Journal of Cancer Education, 17*(4), 231–236.

*Indicates studies included in this meta-analysis.

STRANGERS IN STRANGE LANDS

A Metasynthesis of Lived Experiences of Immigrant Asian Nurses Working in Western Countries

Yu Xu

▶ Nurses from Asian countries make up the majority of immigrant nurses globally. Although there are a limited number of studies on the lived experiences of Asian nurses working in Western countries, the development of nursing science will be impeded if the rich understanding gleaned from these studies is not synthesized. Using Noblit and Hare's (*Metaethnography: Synthesizing Qualitative Studies*. Newbury Park, Calif: Sage; 1988) procedures, a metasynthesis was conducted on 14 studies that met preset selection criteria. Four overarching themes emerged: (*a*) communication as a daunting challenge; (*b*) differences in nursing practice; (*c*) marginalization, discrimination, and exploitation; and (*d*) cultural differences. Based on the metasynthesis, a large narrative and expanded interpretation was constructed and implications for nursing knowledge development, clinical practice, and policy making are elaborated.

▶ *Key Words: adaptation · Asian nurses · foreign nurses · lived experiences · metasynthesis*

Nurse Shortage is a global issue.[1,2] Asian nurses from the Philippines and India have been the major targets of international recruitment.[3] For instance, internationally educated nurses made up 3.5% of the estimated 2.9 million US nurse workforce in 2004 and among them 50.2% were from the Philippines alone.[4] Buchan reported that India and the Philippines were the top 2 source countries for internationally recruited nurses (IRNs) in the United Kingdom during 2004–2005.[5]

Both published literature and anecdotal evidence suggest that Asian nurses working in Western countries encounter unique challenges that profoundly affect their relationships with their patients, coworkers, physicians, supervisors, employers, and the host country at large. In addition, these challenges impact their relationships with peers from their home countries, their own immediate and extended families, and most importantly, their inner most selves. Because these challenges and associated issues are intertwined with gender, race, and culture, the dynamics of the interactions among these factors significantly affect the work and life experiences of Asian nurses and deserve a serious and rigorous examination.

As early as the 1970s, researchers started documenting and examining the experiences of Asian nurses working in the United States.[6–9] Most of the early studies were concentrated on Filipino nurses in the United States, primarily because they were the predominant subgroup of international nurses. In the last decade and particularly in recent years, qualitative studies on Asian nurses working in Western countries have flourished.[6,10–20] These studies not only "renewed" the previously little-heard voices of Asian nurses but also expanded the geographical boundary beyond the United States.

However, systematic searches revealed no scholarly efforts to synthesize the available research except one systematic review that evaluated studies on black (African and Caribbean) and minority ethnic (Asian) nurses in the United Kingdom.[21] Essentially, this review concludes that the experiences of black and minority ethnic nurses is "generally poorly researched"[21(p50)] and there is a "lack of comprehensive literature concerning experiences of overseas black and minority ethnic nurses in the UK."[21(p54)] In addition, it identifies "a notable lack of empirical studies with gaps in knowledge, theory, and methodology"[21(p54)] and suggests a need for "rigorous, high-quality research."[21(p53)] However, the limitations of this review in context of the purpose of this metasynthesis are apparent: (*a*) its focus on how to conduct a rigorous systematic review rather than the substantive issues encountered by black and minority ethnic nurses; (*b*) its exclusion of studies conducted outside the United Kingdom; and (*c*) its inclusion of nonresearch literature.

The absence of a metasynthesis of the experiences of Asian nurses working in Western countries indicates a cross-disciplinary knowledge gap. The purpose of this metasynthesis is to provide cumulative insight into the collectively lived experiences of these Asian nurses in order to advance nursing knowledge and to inform practice, policy, and future research. For the purpose of this study, *Asian nurses* are defined as nurses whose home countries are in Asia.

■ Methods

Metasynthesis is a method of synthesizing findings from qualitative studies. According to Sandelowski and colleagues, metasynthesis refers to "the theories, grand narratives, generalizations, or interpretative translations produced from the integration or comparison of findings from qualitative studies."[22(p366)] Specifically, metasynthesis refers to translating qualitative studies into each other so that a grand narrative or interpretation can emerge that is more than a sum of the parts.[22] Unlike meta-analysis where the purpose is to

reduce findings (ie, data), the purpose of metasynthesis is to allow for an enlarged interpretation.[22]

PROCEDURES

Systematic searches through the Cumulative Index to Nursing and Allied Health Literature (CINAHL), MEDLINE, PsychINFO, Sociological Abstracts, and ERIC were performed in consultation with an experienced health sciences librarian. To minimize bias against nonpublished research literature, a search through ProQuest Dissertations and Theses was also conducted. The following terms and their variations and combinations were used as search terms: "Asian nurses," "foreign nurses," "foreign-born nurses," "internationally educated nurses," "internationally recruited nurses," "international nurses," "immigrant nurses," and names of a half dozen Asian countries or regions such as Korea and Taiwan. These electronic searches did not set any specific cutoff dates; the last search was performed in July of 2006. In addition, ancestral searches (ie, tracing relevant studies through references in qualified studies) were conducted. Finally, targeted journals that had published studies on the topic were hand-searched. Two criteria were set for inclusion in this metasynthesis: (*a*) empirical studies published in English that had a qualitative research design or contained qualitative data and (*b*) studies that focused on the experiences of Asian nurses working as clinicians in Western countries.

Types of qualitative research designs had no effect on selection. For a qualified study using a mixed method design or an overall quantitative design with a qualitative component, only data from the qualitative portion of the study were included for synthesis. For studies that included both Asian nurses and nurses from other countries, only data specifically identified from Asian nurses were incorporated. When the nationalities of included nurses could not be determined, efforts were

inclusion.

made to contact the primary author of the original study for clarification to make an inclusion or exclusion decision. As a result, a few qualitative studies had to be excluded because of the inability to separate the qualitative data among groups of international nurses, even though the author(s) had a blanket statement indicating nurses from Asian countries made up part of the samples. For one study, the primary author refused to disclose the national origins of participating nurses because of concern with confidentiality since the sample was very small.

SAMPLE

Sampling in the real world is rarely simple and clear-cut. For this metasynthesis, studies based on the same sample but reporting different aspects of research findings were counted separately; however, they were grouped together in analyses to conserve space. This situation applied to several studies.[9] [11,20] When it was impossible to differentiate data from Asian nurses and data from nurses coming from other countries in the original report of 2 studies,[10,11] an inquiry was made. Based on an e-mail reply from the primary author (O. Alexis, [oalexis@brookes.ac.uk] e-mail, July 28, 2006) indicating the applicability of all the identified themes to Asian nurses, both studies were included in this metasynthesis. Despite repeated efforts, one master of science thesis study from the University of Birmingham in the United Kingdom could not be obtained to evaluate for inclusion. The final sample for this metasynthesis included 14 studies.

DATA ANALYSIS

The established 7-phase procedures proposed by Noblit and Hare[23(pp26–29)] were employed in this metasynthesis. In phase 1, this researcher determined the studies to include on the basis of the above 2 selection criteria. In phase 2, the researcher identified what was relevant to the purpose of this metasynthesis. In phase 3,

the researcher read and re-read all the selected studies to become engaged with the results and contexts. In phase 4, how the selected studies were related to one another was examined. Several procedures were undertaken in this phase: (*a*) making a list of key metaphors (ie, "themes," "concepts," or "phrases") from each study; (*b*) identifying relations among these metaphors (ie, "reciprocal," "refutational," or presenting a "line of argument"); and (*c*) making initial assumptions of the relationships among the selected studies. After comparing all the metaphors from the selected studies, it was determined that the relationships among these metaphors were reciprocal because they were about similar things in similar "directions." In phase 5, the selected studies were translated into each other by juxtaposing the key metaphors. "Translations are especially unique syntheses, because they protect the particular, respect holism, and enable comparison. An adequate translation maintains the central metaphors and/or concepts of each account *in their relation to other key metaphors or concepts* in that account" (original emphasis).[23(p28)] In phase 6, the translations were synthesized. This involved "putting together" a whole that was more than what the each individual study implied. In phase 7, this researcher expressed the synthesis through written word. During the working process of the 7 steps, the advice from Sandelowski and colleagues was kept in mind:

> Qualitative metasynthesis is not a trivial pursuit, but rather a complex exercise in interpretation: Carefully peeling away the surface layers of studies to find their hearts and souls in a way that does the least damage to them. Synthesists must analyze studies in sufficient detail to preserve the integrity of each study and yet not become so immersed in detail that no useable synthesis is produced.[22(p370)]

■ Results

Demographic and methodological characteristics of all the studies included in this metasynthesis are provided in Tables 1 and 2. Out of

Table 1. Demographic Characteristics of the Participants of Individual Studies in the Metasynthesis[a]

Study	Sample Size	Age	Marital Status	Gender	Time in Host Country	Religion	Type of Program Graduated From	Nationality of Asian Nurses
Alexis & Vydelingum (2004, 2005a)	12[b]	...	...	F = 7 M = 5	...	...	...	Philippines
Allen & Larsen (2003)[c]	67 (11 Asians)	25–61	...	F = 58 M = 9	Mean = 3.8 y	...	...	Philippines India Pakistan
Daniel et al. (2001)	24	...	...	F = 23 M = 1	Group 1 = 3 mo Group 2 = 2 wk	...	...	Philippines
Davison (1993)	10	42–59	...	F = 10	5–24 y	Mainly Catholic	BSN = 6 MSN = 2 PhD = 2	Philippines
Dicicco-Bloom (2004)	10	40–50	M = 10	F = 10	20–25 y	Christian	Diploma	India
Lopez (1990)	10	...	M = 7 S = 3	F = 9 M = 1	<2 y = 4 4–6 y = 3 >10 y = 3	Catholic	Mostly BSN	Philippines
Matti & Taylor (2005)	12[d]	...	...	7 M = 5	9 mo–2 y	...	...	India Philippines
McGonagle et al. (2004)	10	...	...	F & M	>3 mo	...	...	Philippines
Miraflor (1976)[e]	405	21 to >60	M = 205 S = 190 Sp = 3 W = 6	F = 384 M = 21	A few mo	Mainly Catholic	5-yr BSN = 112 4-yr BSN = 53 4-yr diploma = 238	Philippines

Study	N	Age	Marital Status	Gender	Experience	Religion	Education	Country
Spangler (1991)	26	25–51	...	F & M	<5 y = 14 5–10 y = 7 >10 y = 5	Mainly Catholic	BSN = 23 Diploma = 3	Philippines
Withers & Snowball (2003)[f]	45	25–39	...	F = 31 M = 12	3–18 mo	...	...	Philippines
Yi (1993) Yi & Jezewski (2000)	12	25–57	M = 8 D = 1 S = 3	F = 12	1–23 y	Christian = 10	MSN = 3 BSN = 5 Diploma = 4	Korea

[a]Under "Marital Status": M = married; S = single; Sp = separated; D = divorced; W = widowed. Under "Gender": F = female; M = male.
[b]This figure included an unspecific number of nurses from South Africa, the Caribbean, and Sub-Saharan Africa.
[c]The demographical profile reported here is for the total sample (N = 671) due to the unavailability of specific demographical data on the 11 Asian nurses.
[d]This figure included an unspecified number of non-Asian nurses.
[e]Sum of subcategory figures under "Marital Status" is not equal to 405 due to missing data in the original study.
[f]Sum of subcategory figures under "Gender" is not equal to 45 due to missing data in the original study.

Table 2. Methodological Characteristics of Included Studies in the Metasynthesis

Study	Discipline Published in	Country	Data Analysis Method	Research Design and Data-Collection Method
Alexis & Vydelingum (2004, 2005a)	Nursing	United Kingdom	Thematic analysis	Phenomenology (focus group)
Allen & Larsen (2003)	Nursing	United Kingdom	Thematic analysis	Phenomenology (focus group)
Daniel (2001)	Nursing	United Kingdom	Thematic analysis	Phenomenology (focus group)
Davison (1993)	Asian American studies	United States	Thematic analysis	Oral history (interview)
Dicicco-Bloom (2004)	Nursing	United States	Content analysis and critical case analysis	General descriptive design (interview)
Lopez (1990)	Education	United States	Thematic analysis	General descriptive design (interview)
Matti & Taylor (2005)	Nursing	United Kingdom	Thematic analysis	General descriptive design (semistructured interview)
McGonagle et al. (2004)	Allied health	Ireland	Thematic analysis	Phenomenology (focus group)
Miraflor (1976)[a]	Education	United States	Thematic analysis	Quantitative design with qualitative component (open-ended questions in questionnaire)
Spangler (1991)	Nursing	United States	Leininger's Ethnonursing Phases of Qualitative Data Analysis (Thematic analysis via induction)	Ethnonursing (ethnonursing interview, observation)
Withers & Snowball (2003)[b]	Nursing	United Kingdom	Thematic analysis	Mixed method design (semistructured interview)
Yi (1993) and Yi & Jezewski (2000)	Nursing	United States	Constant comparative method	Grounded theory

[a]Only qualitative data from this quantitative study were included for analysis.
[b]Only qualitative data from this mixed method study were included for analysis.

the 14 studies, 4 were doctoral dissertations, 1 was master's thesis, and the rest (9) were research reports. The disciplines or fields represented by the selected studies were nursing, education, Asian American studies, and allied health. These studies took place in 3 countries (United States, United Kingdom, and Ireland), involving nurses from 4 Asian countries (India, Korea, Pakistan, and the Philippines). The most frequently used research design was phenomenology ($n = 5$) and general descriptive design (ie, qualitative descriptive studies without identifying a specific research design) ($n = 3$), followed by grounded theory ($n = 2$), ethnonursing ($n = 1$), oral history ($n = 1$), mixed method design ($n = 1$), and quantitative design with a qualitative component ($n = 1$). In addition, a detailed table of metaphors, themes, and concepts from the 14 studies was constructed and translated into each other, using Noblit and Hare[23] as outlined above (Table 3). What follows is a descriptive and interpretive report of the lived experiences of Asian nurses under 4 overarching themes.

THEME 1: COMMUNICATION AS A DAUNTING CHALLENGE

Communication is critical in healthcare settings, especially for nurses who work with patients around the clock to conduct assessment, plan, coordinate, and deliver care, and evaluate interventions. By definition, communication is the creation of *shared* meaning and understanding. However, because of a variety of factors, Asian nurses encounter an array of difficulties that hinder their ability to communicate.

Unfamiliarity with Accents and Informal Language Usage. All of the included studies except one[16] documented language difficulties of Asian nurses, including agonizing experiences, especially during the initial period following their arrival in a new country. No matter how well Asian nurses thought they were prepared linguistically, they still found themselves not prepared enough to meet the

communication needs in a foreign country. For many Asian nurses, language was a major obstacle for survival, both at work and in other aspects of their lives, particularly during the initial time after arrival.

The communication difficulties came from unfamiliar accents; usage of slang, idioms, jargon, abbreviations; recorded shift reports; and idiosyncratic physicians' handwriting.[6–12,15,17,19,20] Difficulties also rose from differences between the "book English" they learned formally in their home countries and the "street English" used in the new country.[7] For instance, to newly arrived Filipino nurses, the euphemistic use of "potty"(for "bedpan") was new; the British use of "theater" for "operating room" was unheard of; and the idiomatic use of the words such as "hell" as in "You are a hell of a good worker" was seemingly paradoxical and puzzling to their linear interpretation. Another example was the response "Uh-huh" because different tones had different and even opposite meanings.

Frequently, communication difficulty was compounded by frustration, stress, and psychological breakdown, and prevented Asian nurses from performing at their best, especially with regard to patient care, leaving them with a deeply saddened feeling of inadequacy, shame, and self-pity. From time to time, they questioned their ability to "handle" the new job and wondered "Why am I here?" Somatic symptoms were also reported from the associated distress.[9] At its worst, communication deficiency led to downward psychological spiral such as depression and resulted in job termination.[7]

Communication deficiency not only affected the effectiveness and efficiency of care delivery to patients but also impacted patients' families and the healthcare team in a variety of ways. In extreme cases, patients refused care by Asian nurses merely because of their inability to create mutual understanding.[7] Such incidents were painful, humiliating, and devastating because such refusals were interpreted by the involved nurses as incompetence to fulfill the basic duties for which they were hired. Moreover, Asian nurses tended to take such events

Table 3. Individual Study Metaphors as Related to 4 Overarching Themes[a]

Study	Communication Challenges	Differences in Nursing Practice	Marginalization, Discrimination, and Exploitation	Cultural Differences
Alexis & Vydelingum (2004, 2005a)	Communication difficulties with patients and peers	Organization of care and its delivery; not prepared to provide ADLs for patients; focus on paperwork rather than delivery of care	Being seen as "other"; feeling unwelcome, not appreciated, and not belonging; no one would listen to complaints; lack of support from British peers & training opportunities; unfair treatment; lack of equal opportunity for promotion; had to prove self; being bullied & fear of being reported and reprisal	Lack of cultural preparation for United Kingdom and what to expect; feeling of being displaced and thrown into a different world
Allen & Larsen (2003)	Communication compromised by dialects, accents, colloquialism, intonation and style of talking; communication issue as stigma; being labeled "different" and "difficult" due to language deficiency	Nursing qualifications unrecognized; narrower scope of practice leading to feeling of being deskilled; humiliated to provide ADLs; different legal framework; focus on paperwork rather than care	Language barrier as vehicle for discrimination; felt exploited during induction and adaptation period; continuing exploitation after registration when negotiating employment status; being paid for one grade while being asked to take on responsibilitie of a higher grade; undesirable working hours; backstabbing and policed by carers; not being accepted by patients—lack of appreciation, respect & trust; feeling of discrimination; manipulated & bullied by care assists	Negative UK attitude and treatment of the elderly; unaware of existence of care homes; tiers of bureaucracy to get registered; high living cost and tax

Dicicco-Bloom (2004)			Discrimination for being immigrant nonwhite female nurses in a gendered profession; alienation at work; marginalization, exploitation, and racism at workplace	Culturally uprooted; valuing family less by Americans; struggle to retain women's traditional role in Asian family
Davison (1993)	Communication barriers; language as an area of tension		Marginalization/discrimination as "foreigners": substandard wage, undesirable shifts, passed over for promotion; not allowed to speak Tagalog during work break, treated with hostility and retaliation, demot on for speaking Tagalog; nursing as a gendered profession: Asian women as exotic and sexual objects; constant fight against stereotyping	Hard-to-understand "American way of life" and culture: elderly abandonment, loose moral, lack of discipline, and "crumbling" of families; culture as another area of tension
Daniel (2001)	Difficulty understanding jargons, medications, abbreviations, and accents of staff and patients	Different role of family; nursing physically demanding; common use of verbal orders; different names of medications; different procedures for dispensing medications; specialization in nursing; legal issues in nursing practice.		Low social status of the elderly

(continued)

Table 3. *(Continued)*

Study	Communication Challenges	Differences in Nursing Practice	Marginalization, Discrimination, and Exploitation	Cultural Differences
Lopez (1990)	Communication deficiency: slang, "street English" vs "book English," fear of phone conversation; difficulty expressing self	Differences in nurses' role: bedside care vs paperwork; doing vs talking; respect and gratitude vs disrespect and lack of respect from patients; rejection from patients; risk of being sued	No one at airport to meet newly arrived Filipino nurses; lack of trust; frustration with "testy" US nursing aides; suffering quietly; had to earn right to be heard; differential treatment; hostility toward foreign nurses; jealousy; favoritism; rejection by patients and physicians	Lack of understanding of US culture, social skills, and assertiveness; hard to admit "Don't know;" speaking up as challenge
Matti & Taylor (2005)	Language and communication deficiency as a 2-way issue: due to colloquialism and accents	Not used to providing basic care to patients; feeling devalued and deskilled: skills not being recognized or utilized	Feeling not being trusted for performing some clinical procedures	Cultural differences between UK and home country; induction not specific to foreign nurses' needs
McGonagle et al. (2004)[b]	Difficulties with language, documentation & terminology (ie, abbreviation and jargon)	Irish nurses less autonomous; less focused on patients' physical needs; confusion regarding intellectual disability and mental illness		Little family involvement in care of sick family members; perception of institutionalization of elderly as uncaring and unjust

Miraflor (1976)	Language and communication ranked as top issue: taking phone orders, intonation, accent, and physician's handwriting	Learning to use modern equipment, machines, and supplies	Being taken advantage of by nursing aides; not respected as team leaders by nursing aides	Buying on credit, fast pace of life; "Dutch treat"; concept of "first come, first served"; American concept of time; open expression of affection; pervasive exposure of sex in media; disrespect for the elderly; direct communication style
Spangler (1991)	Language difficulties: slang, accent; had to talk in native language	Heavy workload; inability to provide adequate care; reducing care to technical tasks and its contribution to non-caring behaviors; impact of bureaucracy, standards and policies of regulatory agencies.	Mistrust by US nurses; had to prove self; had to "put up with a lot"; had to settle for less desirable shifts; prohibited from speaking Tagalog in work area; abuse; manipulated by patients; made to float to other clinical areas more frequently; frustration with heavier work load	Conflicts resulting from cultural differences; differences in interaction and relational style; differences in lifestyle

(continued)

Table 3. *(Continued)*

Study	Communication Challenges	Differences in Nursing Practice	Marginalization, Discrimination, and Exploitation	Cultural Differences
Withers & Snowball (2003)	Communication issues: idioms, abbreviations, slang, unfamiliarity with British accent	Differences in nurse's role; not allowed to perform certain procedures	Unfair treatment from colleagues and patients; cultural imposition: not allowed to speak own language; exploitation and bullying; fear to report abuse	Unassertiveness
Yi (1993) and Yi & Jezewski (2000)	Language deficiency as most challenging for successful adaptation	Different role of nurse and family; focus of care: needs of patients (Korea) vs diseases (United States)	Difficult relations with patients, peers, nurse aides, and supervisors; not being respected and accepted as leader by nursing aides; nonassertiveness and kind nature being taken advantage of; emotions over unfair treatment affecting health; being reported to supervisor behind back	Difficulty dealing with interpersonal conflicts; different communication styles

[a]ADLs indicates activities of daily living; Tagalog, most frequently spoken native language of the Philippines.
[b]Study took place in a learning disability service clinical setting.

personally because of their cultural upbringing and socialization. What made this feeling of inadequacy even worse was the cognitive dissonance with their self-perceived image as caring, compassionate, and competent professionals.[7,9,24]

Telecommunication as Most Challenging.
Verbal communication over the telephone was reported as the most nerve-racking experiences for Asian nurses. Fear of making medical errors from communication mistakes and from other situational factors such as a medical emergency or talking to an awakening on-call physician at an early morning hour could magnify the experienced stress due to absence of nonverbal cues for validation as evidenced by the following reflexive reaction: "During the first few days on the job, I ran to the bathroom when the phone rang."[9(p93)]

Domino Effects of Communication Deficiency.
Language barrier virtually affected every other aspect of Asian nurses' experiences. First, it affected their confidence in themselves and stripped them of their dignity in extreme cases when they felt embarrassed because they could not express themselves adequately.[8–10,24] To save "face," Yi[9] documented that a Korean nurse was too frightened to ask questions, which could potentially cause harm to her patients. Second, it further reinforced the stereotype of Asian nurses that they were shy, unassertive, and not tough enough to be leaders. However, when a Filipino nurse did not fit into the stereotype, she was labeled as un-Filipino because she was "not quiet."[6(p31)] Third, language deficiency had a vicious cycle: the less Asian nurses spoke because of fear of making mistakes, the longer it took for them to develop a command of the language. Furthermore, language improvement was inherently associated with improvement in professional knowledge and interpersonal skills.[9] Unfortunately, some Asian nurses never overcame the language barrier and had to take a lower level position, quit nursing, or even return to their home countries.[7] These outcomes were regarded not only as catastrophic failures to the involved nurses but also as bringing shame to the nurses' families and even home countries.

Accent and Communication Deficiency as Grounds for Discrimination.
Language was a key factor for distress to Asian nurses because accent was unjustly used as a "social marker" for stigmatization.[12] The intense emotions were palpable in the following comment by a Filipino nurse working in a New Jersey hospital: "They [American nursing staff] hate our accent. That's why they don't want to work with us. Although they don't say that, you just sense it."[7(p84)] Although some Filipino nurses lived and worked in the host country for more than 10 years, they still encountered "accent discrimination." [6(p30)] Being labeled "different" or "difficult" because of an unfamiliar accent or language deficiency was frequently used as a vehicle for discrimination. In some cases, this also gave their Western peers a "legitimate" excuse for not trying to understand.

Clashes between Asian nurses and their Western peers regarding language were constant. In an extreme case, a Filipino nurse had to resort to litigation to regain her civil rights to speak her indigenous language in the staff lounge during breaks.[6] On the surface, communication medium appeared to be the concern; in fact, these conflicts revealed deeper issues—intolerance, imposition, and the seemingly paradoxical coexistence of superiority and insecurity on the part of American nurses.

Lack of communication proficiency also negatively affected Asian nurses' ability to fight for their own rights: "Some people tell us, 'Why don't you speak up?' Maybe because we have a hard time in speaking in English, that's why."[24(p185)] On the other hand, learning to "speak the same language" facilitated the acceptance of Asian nurses by their Western peers, and hence, their socialization and integration. It also served as an indicator of their acculturation level. For example, when a Filipino nurse expressed frustration with "Oh my god," her American peer was very excited to tell her that she "had become Americanized."[7(p90)]

THEME 2: DIFFERENCES IN NURSING PRACTICE

Role of the Nurse. One of the first differences Asian nurses discovered was the autonomy granted by laws and regulations as well as the accountability in Western nursing.[15] Initially, it was surprising for them to learn that nurses in Western countries functioned much more independently. However, they were also appalled that family members did not provide or assist with activities of daily living (ADLs) at all and depended completely on the nursing staff for meeting such needs.[9–12,15,19,20] Both professionally and culturally, they were not used to providing ADLs because those basic needs were taken care of by families in Asian countries. Asian family members regard providing such basic and intimate care for their loved one as their privilege. Consequently, many Asian nurses perceived providing ADLs as being deskilled, humiliating, demoralizing, and a waste of their education as evidenced by the following statements: "I feel degraded and frustrated having to wash patients"[10(p15)]; "I did not expect that life as a nurse would go around words like pee, loo, and poo."[19(p285)]

In addition, many Asian nurses were not prepared for the physical and psychological demand in taking care of heavy and dependent Western patients, referring to their weight and high acuity.[15] Furthermore, they were highly critical of the approach to nursing where the focus was perceived to be on the disease process rather than on the needs of patients and holistic care. They were frustrated to see nursing being reduced to technical tasks that contributed little to bedside care. To them, the most important role of the nurse was to provide bedside care that incorporated the hands, mind, heart, and soul.[9,24] Nursing was to give hands-on care with compassion, relieve suffering, and help with the healing process. It should never be merely a series of mechanical tasks. For instance, the sampled Filipino nurses in Spangler's study[24] felt an "obligation to care" and emphasized patients' physical comfort as their central concern. To them, caring was expressed by "doing," especially spending time with patients.

Meanwhile, Asian nurses were shocked by the amount of paperwork required institutionally and legally. Not surprisingly, such emphasis on documentation was perceived as "putting the cart before the horse" as criticized by a Filipino nurse: "Nursing is bedside care, not paper work. Here in the U.S. the prestige is when you are away from the bedside. Actual patient care is relegated to the nurses' aide."[24(p206)] Because of fast work pace, heavy paper work, and understaffing, many Asian nurses felt torn between providing quality patient care and getting everything done on time, which often lead to stress, job dissatisfaction, changing job, or even leaving the profession once for all.

Scope of Practice. Quickly, Asian nurses learned that some routinely performed procedures in their home countries such as cannulation, venipuncture, and collecting arterial blood might not fall within the legal practice in some Western countries such as the United Kingdom.[15] Consequently, they felt that patients under their care suffered needlessly because of procedure delays. Such restriction also affected their job satisfaction because of the perception of being treated less like professionals.

Technological and Legal Environment. Asian nurses had to get to know quickly the 3 Ps: protocols, procedures, and policies, as well as new healthcare technologies to adapt to a more automated healthcare environment.[8] While the use of advanced technology was largely true in America, it was disappointing to find that healthcare technologies in some Western countries such as the United Kingdom were not as advanced as expected.[12] On the other hand, the legal framework within which Western healthcare operated was dramatically different.[7,15] For example, the emphasis on documentation took on added legal importance because "If it is not charted, it didn't happen." Given the prevalence of litigation, many Asian nurses quickly learned to practice what this researcher called "defensive nursing" to minimize the margin of error and thus liability for both themselves and their employers. However, during the process, fear, stress, and distress could take their toll: "You have more at stake here. If you administer a medication a doctor ordered and it's wrong, you are liable since you are the one that gave it."[6(p33)] The Western notions of legality and accountability were unfamiliar and even foreign to them at the beginning of their first job.

THEME 3: MARGINALIZATION, DISCRIMINATION, AND EXPLOITATION NURSING AS A GENDERED PROFESSION

The vast majority of Asian nurses were females (Table 1). Because of the social perception of women as the weaker and less powerful gender, stereotypes of Asian women, and the simple fact of being in a foreign country, Asian nurses were exposed to a host of vulnerabilities and frequently became targets of marginalization, discrimination, and exploitation.[6–7,10–12,16–17,19] On a cultural level, Asian nurses collectively felt "otherness" or a lack of sense of belonging because of cultural differences or lack of sufficient cultural knowledge to fit in; hence, they felt disfranchised from their coworkers.[6,10,11,16] For instance, one Indian nurse related a disheartening experience: "Nobody learned my name for 4 months when I first came, and when they did it . . . they shortened it and pronounced it wrong. I finally stopped correcting them."[16(p26)]

To some degree, the unassertiveness of Asian nurses contributed to what this researcher termed "professional silence and invisibility"— the lack of professional representation and leadership positions in the healthcare hierarchy, and hence the lack of perceived political clout in the collective consciousness of the host country. Asian nurses (and Asians in general) as a group were taught in their home cultures not to challenge authorities or "rock the boat."[7,9,24] They also had high expectations of others and of themselves and expected that their preceptors and supervisors would take on a mater-

nal role, treating them like a *parang kapatid* (like a sister) or an "adopted mother." These "messages" internalized through primary socialization were incongruent with dominant Western values and norms. The following excerpt from a Filipino nurse demonstrated how long she had to suffer needlessly before feeling accepted enough to request what she needed to do her job adequately:

> I am only 4′11″ and the operating tables were almost at the level of my neck. Even with the use of a stool I could hardly see what was going on with the surgery. I could not anticipate very well the instruments that the surgeons needed. They were frustrated and so was I. After the surgery I would go to the bathroom and cry. It was after 3 years that I felt I really belonged to the OR and therefore I had the right to ask for a higher stool.[7(pp87–88)]

Unfair Treatment and Lack of Equal Opportunity. Asian nurses were frequently passed over for career opportunities and believed that race determines promotion.[6,16] In addition, in some situations Asian nurses were paid substandard wages,[6] or unfairly compensated for a lower position while being asked to take on responsibilities of a higher one.[12] Moreover, they felt that they were discriminated against because of their skin color and "foreignness": "We can change some of our outlook, our values, but we cannot change our looks, our accents. No matter how egalitarian Americans claim to be, we know that they are not color blind . . ."[24(p208)] Although many Asian nurses wanted to fight against injustice, they felt powerless and uncertain about the outcome. Some did fight, but at the expense of personal health.[9]

Bullying and Sexual Harassment. At times, Asian nurses were taken advantage of by their Western employers, coworkers, and even subordinates.[6–7,9–12,19] Receiving the "worst" patient assignment, being given the most undesirable work shift, and being assigned to work during holidays were not uncommon. In extreme cases, Asian nurses were targets of bullying by prejudicial patients, physicians, peers, supervisors, and even their subordinates. Furthermore, there was outright harassment as Asian nurses were perceived as exotic and sexual objects. One Filipino nurse encountered a white patient who asked whether he could bring her home as a maid with a sexual overtone and profound ignorance that the Philippines was so backward that the entire country was connected by dirt roads. This Filipino nurse fought back courageously by replying with a laugh: "You cannot afford to hire me."[6(p22)] At other times, Asian nurses told stories of being backstabbed such as being reported to management without their knowledge, being policed by their white peers, intentional withholding critical information by white peers, and a lack of appreciation and recognition for what they could contribute.[12] *We Need Respect,* the title of a recent report on the experiences of IRNs in the United Kingdom commissioned by the Royal College of Nursing, projected the voices of these nurses, including those from Asia—loud and clear.[12]

Having to Prove Self. Asian nurses believed they had to prove themselves to their patients, peers, and supervisors in order to win their trust and support.[10–12,17] Until then, there was frequent doubt about their worth and competence. Such apprehension and suspicion were particularly hurtful when patients under their care were dubious about the medications given to them and checked with their white peers behind their back.[12]

THEME 4: CULTURAL DIFFERENCES CULTURAL DISPLACEMENT

Asian nurses felt "uprooted" culturally and "being thrown into a different world," especially during their initial transition after arrival.[10–11,16] Meanwhile, they experienced mounting pressure to "re-root" in the new culture. The feeling of being torn between 2 cultures was best captured by the metaphor from an Indian nurse as "a foot here, a foot there, a foot nowhere"[16(p28)] and as a

"rupture"[16(p29)] with her homeland. The sense of cultural displacement was frequently made worse by the fact that a majority of Asian nurses left their close-knit families behind. Lopez reported that one Filipino nurse spent an average of $500 monthly on telephone fees to relieve her nostalgia.[7]

Asian nurses were challenged to understand the host culture and adjust to new ways of life.[6–9,24] During this adaptation process, their own values, beliefs, and cultural norms unavoidably clashed with those of Western societies as the 2 systems of thinking were likened to "oil and water."[14(p57)] These cultural differences ranged from different concepts of time (ie, "American time" equaling to "punctuality") to different communication styles, foods, and ways of life and customs such as "Dutch treat" and buying things on credit. In addition, they were not used to the "loose morality"(eg, being naked in the street, permeation of sex in the media), lack of discipline, and the "crumbling" of the family in Western societies.[8]

Negativity Toward the Elderly. Asian nurses were not prepared culturally for the perceived lack of respect for the elderly such as "Calling elders by their first name"[8(p75)] and for the perceived maltreatment of the elderly.[15] Moreover, they resented what they perceived as the "elder abandonment" when frail parents were institutionalized in nursing homes with few visitations from their families or without family members being at the bedside when they were hospitalized. This perceived lack of family obligation and compassion was regarded as the ultimate shame and social evil of Western societies.

Interpersonal Challenge. To a large extent, interpersonal challenge had its "roots" in the cultural upbringing of Asian nurses, who were taught to avoid conflicts at all cost in order to maintain harmony.[7] Culturally, Asian nurses came from collectivistic cultures where "we" and "us" came before "I" and "me." Therefore, to say "No" was socially unacceptable, especially to people with seniority and authority. To challenge physicians when necessary was expected in the Western nursing culture, but very hard to learn for Asian nurses, even though they realized that it was a legal and professional requirement.

In addition, Asian nurses quickly found out that their "all-yes" habitual mentality frequently brought them unnecessary work and even trouble in the real world because their kindness and tendency to accommodate were taken advantage of and even abused. Interestingly, the most intense conflicts were with nursing aides, especially those of African American background, rather than with their peers, supervisors, or physicians.[7,9] Asian nurses were particularly resentful if their subordinates refused to follow their directions because obedience to authority was expected according to the ways they were brought up.[6–9,24]

Inadequate training on leadership and management skills such as delegation and conflict resolution[8] was another barrier to building productive working relationships. In addition, many Asian nurses operated under their culture-based assumption that every employee was motivated, who was willing and ready to carry out duties as specified in one's own job description. Moreover, the cultural belief that it was an insult to someone if he or she had to be told to perform his or her regular duties also affected Asian nurses' management behaviors. However, frequently this culture-based expectation proved to be a un-starter at Western workplaces, particularly with many less motivated or unmotivated nursing aides.

■ Discussion

GENDER, RACE, CULTURE, AND INTERPERSONAL DYNAMICS

Gender, race, and culture are at the crux of one's identity and impact interpersonal interactions profoundly; therefore, they are salient categories of analysis. The lived experiences

of Asian nurses working in Western countries cannot be fully understood without looking through these 3 different lenses simultaneously. Essentially, their experiences were framed by these 3 dimensions of one's identity and humanity as well as their intricate interactions in the ever-changing physical, technological, legal, and interpersonal contexts in Western countries. It is from this framing that meanings of their experiences are defined and dynamics of relationships understood.

What Asian nurses went through was a *gendered* experience. Such experiences are crystallized in the metaphoric advertisement: "Your cap is your passport."[14(p61)] The socially constructed image of women in general and Asian women in particular affected not only the perceived status of Asian nurses but also treatment by their Western employers and the people they interacted with. This metasynthesis suggested that as women, Asian nurses were more vulnerable to social injustice and sexual harassment. Moreover, Asian nurses perceived that they had little power to change the status quo, particularly given the foreign contexts. The gendered experiences of Asian nurses in this metasynthesis validated similar experiences by minority foreign nurses documented in numerous Western countries.[11,14,25] Moreover, their gendered experiences were furthermore compounded by race and culture. As Thurston and Vissandjee pointed out: ". . . gender interacts with other Symbolic Institutions—in particular race, class, and sexuality—to form hierarchies of inclusion and exclusion, is never seen alone, and is essential to understanding the organization of society."[26(p232)]

What Asian nurses went through was also a *racial* experience. They reported sabotaging attempts aiming to set them up for failure; documented double standards, exploitation, and abuse; witnessed intolerance and unrelenting discrimination; and encountered the "glass ceiling," all because of their skin color. Perhaps, the worst example racial discrimination was against 2 Filipino nurses who were convicted of poisoning, murder, and conspiracy at the Veteran Affairs Hospital in Ann

Arbor, Mich, in 1976 and later were acquitted in a sensational national trial. Consequently as a group, Filipino nurses suffered from public suspicion about their professional intentions and even death threat.[14]

Furthermore, the glass ceiling effect was validated by longitudinal data in a study indicating that the vast majority of internationally educated nurses in the United States held staff nurse positions, which increased from 71.2% to 76.7% during 1977–2000, while their proportions in management positions declined from 6.2% to 2.7% during 1984–2000.[27] Hawthorn also found that immigrant nurses from non–English-speaking countries were not only much less likely to advance beyond the entry-level registered nurse position but also disproportionately concentrated in stigmatized geriatric units.[28] The documented experiences of Asian nurses in this metasynthesis revealed that racial equality in Western countries remain merely a myth. In light of the increasing reports of discrimination against nonwhite foreign nurses in Australia, Canada, the United Kingdom, and the United States,[3,12,14,16,25,29,30] one has to conclude that institutional racism still exists.

Lastly, what Asian nurses went through was also a *cultural* experience. The cultural heritage of Asian nurses was a mixed blessing, serving as both a barrier and a resource to their transition. Frequently, Asian nurses were puzzled and frustrated as to what part of "themselves" to give up and what part to retain during the adaptation process. This was an intense, and frequently agonizing, intrapersonal process involving soul searching, resolution of values conflicts, and even self-negation to seek and establish a new personal, professional, and cultural identity. Data indicated that Asian nurses had to change *who they were* in varying degrees in order to adapt successfully to the new culture and work environment. However, changing oneself was a challenge that was at least formidable to some but monumental to others.

Language is one of the most important carriers and exemplars of culture. Essentially, language functioned as both a symbol and a tool for Asian nurses. As a symbol, language and its associated properties such as accent gave away their "foreignness" and frequently served as a social marker, thus offering a handy vehicle for prejudice and discrimination.[28] As a tool, language served as a fundamental instrument for survival and adaptation both at work and in daily life in a new culture.

The meanings and dynamics of the precarious relationships between Asian nurses and African American nurse aides in the US healthcare environment cannot be fully understood unless the frequently cited conflicts are put into the sociopolitical, economic, and cultural contexts.[31] Control of the work environment is at the core of these conflicts. The underlying factors go far beyond the simple explanations of different accents, language use such as "Black English," and ways of relating to one another,[8] as well as cultural differences such as work ethics.[24] On the one hand, African Americans find themselves at the bottom of the American society. The position of African Americans nurse aides in the US healthcare system reflects their socioeconomic status in the American society at large. They often have the most physically challenging jobs but the lowest pay. Many of these African American nurse aides are single parents with limited education and work at multiple jobs to make ends meet. Their work and daily struggles are vividly portrayed in Diamond's classic ethnography of American nursing home care—*Making Gray Gold*.[32] Compounding the situation is the ingrained memory of slavery and the painful fight for civil rights in US history. The feeling that the system has failed them can be overwhelming, often accompanied with a sense of powerlessness and hopelessness. Frequently, a spark is all that is needed to trigger an explosion of their frustration and anger. A simple, delegated task from a newly arrived Asian nurse, who is a "foreigner" with less-than-fluent English and a hard-to-understand accent but a higher position and salary, could well be "the last straw on the camel's back."

On the other hand, several factors on the part of Asian nurses also contribute to the surfacing and development of these conflicts. First, brought up in hierarchical cultures, Asian nurses expect obedience from subordinates. Furthermore, culturally Asian nurses avoid interpersonal conflicts if at all possible. However, oftentimes such avoidance behaviors enable African American nurse aids to become more testy and demanding. Second, they are thrown into the preexisting, predominant black-white racial politics that play out in the workplace daily. However, unaware of the interpersonal dynamics that are affected by the racial politics beyond hospital walls and situational factors, Asian nurses are caught completely unprepared and clueless as to how to effectively handle disobedience and subsequent conflicts. Third, Asian nurses are perceived as having multiple vulnerabilities and weaknesses that have further contributed to their ineffectiveness as team leaders: language deficiency, status as "aliens," job insecurity as contracted foreign nurses, less seniority as new comers, soft voice, and the small physical stature.

IMPLICATIONS FOR KNOWLEDGE DEVELOPMENT, CLINICAL PRACTICE, AND POLICY MAKING

Implications for Nursing Knowledge Development. Asian nurses working in Western countries encounter a host of unique challenges that ultimately affect their adaptation as reported above. Consequently, the experiences and adaptation of Asian nurses in Western countries are likely to be different from those of non-Asian nurses, at least in some aspects. Consequently, this metasynthesis provides a starting point for the development of a midrange theory regarding Asian nurses' adaptation to the Western healthcare environment. This theory is expected to provide the foundation for theory-based interventions to improve the integration of Asian nurses into the Western healthcare environment. In addition, such theoretical advancement will contribute substantively to the knowledge base related to "transition" as

one major area of inquiry in nursing research.[33] Finally, the research on the lived experiences of immigrant Asian nurses has opened new areas of inquiry into the dynamics of interpersonal relationships: How does the "failure" of some Asian nurses affect other immigrant nurses? What are the relationships between native-born Asian nurses and immigrant Asian nurses? How do immigrant nurses from different countries interface with each other? Is there any "reverse discrimination" against white nurses, especially in healthcare settings where immigrant nurses concentrate?

Implications for Practice. In light of this metasynthesis, several issues need to be addressed regarding the current orientation and transitional programs for IRNs. First, apart from the general facility orientation, there should be a tailored transitional program for IRNs that specifically addresses their needs such as the differences in nursing practice, with detailed elaborations on legality, policies, and procedures and their implications. The importance of explaining these differences cannot be overestimated because they directly affect patient safety and quality of care. Second, Western healthcare employers need to develop and implement support mechanisms to facilitate the adaptation and integration of IRNs. Such measures should include mentoring programs such as the "buddy system," which proved effective in enhancing the adaptation of Asian nurses, and hence, their retention and success. Third, cultural competence training that facilitates mutual understanding of culture-based values, beliefs, expectations, and behavioral and communication patterns is also needed. For Asian nurses, such training needs to be included in their prearrival recruitment programs.

However, how to prepare Asian nurses to handle inevitable interpersonal conflicts remains a serious challenge, especially when such conflicts are rooted in history and framed by socioeconomic forces that are beyond institutional control. At the minimum, Asian nurses should be made aware of the potential conflicts arising from racial tension in the new country prior to their arrival. In addition, exercises such as role-play to practice how to handle these emotionally charged situations in a high-stress environment will be helpful. A working knowledge of the history, people, and sociopolitical system of the host country and building a repertoire of interpersonal skills will certainly help in dealing with the unavoidable conflicts.

Meanwhile, Western employers need to understand that language acquisition is a lengthy process that takes years of learning and practice. Asian nurses have varying levels of language skills that differ from individual to individual and from one source country to another. For nurses from the Philippines and India, the language issues might be less profound since English is one of the official languages and most nurses from these 2 countries were trained in English nursing programs. However, for nurses from non–English-speaking Asian countries such as Korea, language barriers could be more challenging. Similarly, acquisition of a working knowledge about a new culture also requires years of immersion and accumulation through persistent efforts.

Implications for Policy Making. The documented experiences of Asian nurses in this metasynthesis underscore the central issue of social injustice and the imperative to address it head-on. The included studies reported widespread discriminatory practices and behaviors in one form or another. Oftentimes, discrimination was covert and subtle; other times, it was explicit and outright. To a large extent, the prejudice and discrimination against Asian nurses reflect the deeply rooted intolerance for, and injustice against, racial and ethnic minorities in Western societies and nurses from these groups. Although the eradication of racism is a long-term goal in nursing, both Western governments and employers need to determine what more can be done at the societal and

institutional levels. Could Western governments make and implement policies on recruitment, credentialing, employment nondiscriminatory to immigrant nurses, including those from Asia? Although many of these policies are already in place, they exist merely on paper in many cases, with wide variations in their interpretation and execution. At the institutional level, can Western employers implement programs on cultural diversity and competence to cultivate a more tolerable, welcoming workplace environment and to facilitate the communication between Asian nurses and those they work with? More importantly, could specific measures be institutionalized to prevent or minimize discrimination in hiring, performance evaluation, compensation, and so forth so that antidiscrimination is not merely empty lip service or calculated political tactic?

■ Conclusions

Asian nurses constitute the largest group of immigrant nurses working in Western countries. For the foreseeable future, the number and share of Asian nurses in the global migration of nurses are likely to continue to increase. This metasynthesis of the lived experiences of Asian nurses working in Western countries encapsulates their challenges, agonies, and struggles for personal and professional identity and social justice. To a large extent, the story of Asian nurses is an integral part of the collective experiences of international nurses from other parts of the world and parallels those of immigrant women. The lived experiences of Asian nurses must be first documented and examined before any effective interventions can be designed and implemented to facilitate their adaptation and integration. However, when gender, race, and culture intersect, the dynamics of relationships of the involved groups will inevitably be complex, and defies simple, linear explanations and easy solutions.

Funding for this research was provided by the Small Faculty Fund, University of Connecticut. The author thanks Drs Barbara Jacobs, Carolyn Yucha, Cheryl Bowles, Michele Clark, and Nancy Menzel for critiquing an earlier version of this manuscript. Thanks also go to Drs Ola Fox, Paulette Williams, Barbara Schneider, and Tish Smyer for sharing their insight and to the 3 anonymous reviewers for their valuable comments.

Yu Xu, PhD, RN, CTN, University of Nevada at Las Vegas School of Nursing, 4505 Maryland Parkway, Las Vegas, NV 89154 (mailto:yu.xu@unlv.edu).

REFERENCES

1. Aiken LH, Buchan J, Sochalski J, Nichols B, Powell M. Trends in international nurse migration. *Health Aff.* 2004;23(3):69–77.
2. Buchan J, Calman L. *The Global Shortage of Registered Nurses: An Overview of Issues and Actions.* Geneva: International Council of Nurses; 2004.
3. Kingma M. *Nurses on the Move: Migration and the Global Health Care Economy.* Ithaca, NY: Cornell University Press; 2006.
4. Health Resources and Services Administration. Preliminary findings: 2004 national sample survey of registered nurses. http://bhpr.hrsa.gov/healthworkforce/reports/rnpopulation/preliminaryfindings.htm. Accessed July 6, 2006.
5. Buchan J. Filipino nurses in the UK: A case study in active international recruitment. *Harv Health Policy Rev.* 2006;7(1):113–120.
6. Davison MA. *Filipina Nurses: Voices of Struggle and Determination* [master's thesis]. Los Angeles, CA: University of California; 1993.
7. Lopez N. *The Acculturation of Selected Filipino Nurses to Nursing Practice in the United States* [dissertation]. Philadelphia, PA: University of Pennsylvania; 1990.
8. Miraflor CG. *The Philippine Nurses: Implications for Orientation and In-Service Education for Foreign Nurses in the United States* [dissertation]. Chicago, IL: Loyola University of Chicago; 1976.
9. Yi M. *Adjustment of Korean Nurses to United States Hospital Settings* [dissertation]. Buffalo, NY: State University of New York; 1993.
10. Alexis O, Vydelingum V. The lived experiences of overseas black and minority ethnic nurses in the NHS in the south of England. *Divers Health Soc Care.* 2004;1(1):13–20.
11. Alexis O, Vydelingum V. The experiences of overseas black and minority ethnic nurses in the NHS

in an English hospital: a phenomenological study. *J Res Nurs.* 2005a;10(4):459–472.
12. Allan H, Larsen JA. *"We Need Respect": Experiences of Internationally Recruited Nurses in the UK.* London: Royal College of Nursing; 2003.
13. Allan H, Larsen JA, Bryan K, Smith PA. The social reproduction of institutional racism: internationally recruited nurses' experiences of the British health services. *Divers Health Soc Care.* 2003;1:117–125.
14. Choy CC. *Empire of Care: Nursing and Migration in Filipino American History.* Durham, NC: Duke University Press; 2003.
15. Daniel P, Chamberlain A, Gordon F. Expectations and experiences of newly recruited Filipino nurses. *Br J Nurs.* 2001;10(4):254,256,258–265.
16. DiCicco-Bloom B. The racial and gendered experiences of immigrant nurses from Kerala, India. *J Transcult Nurs.* 2004;15(1):26–33.
17. Matiti MR, Taylor D. The cultural lived experience of internationally recruited nurses: a phenomenological study. *Divers Health Soc Care.* 2005;2 (1):7–15.
18. Mc Gonagle C, Halloran SO, O'Reilly O. The expectations and experiences of Filipino nurses working in an intellectual disability service in the Republic of Ireland. *J Learn Disabil.* 2004;8 (4):371–381.
19. Withers J, Snowball J. Adapting to a new culture: a study of the expectations and experiences of Filipino nurses in the Oxford Radcliffe Hospitals NHS Trust. *NT Res.* 2003;8(4):278–290.
20. Yi M, Jezewski MA. Korean nurses' adjustment to hospitals in the United States of America. *J Adv Nurs.* 2000;32(3):721–729.
21. Alexis O, Vydelingum V. Overseas black and minority ethnic nurses: a systematic review. *Nurse Res.* 2005b;12(4):42–56.
22. Sandelowski M, Docherty S, Emden C. Qualitative meta-synthesis: issues and techniques. *Res Nurs Health.* 1997;20:365–371.
23. Noblit GW, Hare RD. *Meta-ethnography: Synthesizing Qualitative Studies.* Newbury Park, CA: Sage;1988.
24. Spangler Z. *Nursing Care Values and Caregiving Practices of Anglo-American and Philippine-American Nurse Conceptualize within Leininger's Theory* [dissertation]. Detroit, Mich:Wayne State University; 1991.
25. Omeri A, Atkins K. Lived experiences of immigrant nurses in New South Wales, Australia: searching for meaning. *Int J Nur Stud.* 2002;39:495–505.
26. Thurston WE, Vissandjee B. An ecological model for understanding culture as a determinant of women's health. *Crit Public Health.* 2005;15(3):229–242.
27. Xu Y, Kwak C. Comparative trend analysis of characteristics of internationally educated nurses and U.S. educated nurses (1977–2000). *Int Nurs Rev.* 2007;54:78–84.

28. Hawthorn L. The globalization of the nursing workforce: barriers confronting overseas qualified nurses in Australia. *Nurs Inq.* 2001;8(4):213–229.

29. Hagey R, Choudhry U, Guruge S, Turrittin J, Collins E, Lee R. Immigrant nurses' experience of racism. *J Nurs Sch.* 2001;33(4):389–394.

30. Turrittin J, Hagey R, Guruge S, Collins E, Mitchell M. The experiences of professional nurses who have migrated to Canada: cosmopolitan citizen-ship or democratic racism? *Int J Nur Stud.* 2005; 39(6):655– 667.

31. McFerson HM. *Blacks and Asians: Crossings, Conflict and Commonality.* Durham, NC: Carolina Academic Press; 2006.

32. Diamond T. *Making Gray Gold.* Chicago, Ill: University of Chicago Press; 1992.

33. Schumacher K, Meleis A. Transitions: a central concept in nursing. *Image J Nurs Sch.* 1994;26(2): 119– 127.

Older Adults' Response to Health Care Practitioner Pain Communication

Grant Application to NINR, Summary Sheet, and Letter of Response to Reviewer Comments

Deborah Dillon McDonald

Form Approved Through 09/30/2007

OMB No. 0925-0001

Department of Health and Human Services Public Health Services ### Grant Application *Do not exceed character length restrictions indicated.*	**LEAVE BLANK—FOR PHS USE ONLY.**

Type	Activity	Number	
Review Group		Formerly	
Council/Board (Month, Year)		Date Received	

1. TITLE OF PROJECT *(Do not exceed 81 characters, including spaces and punctuation.)*

Older Adults' Response to Health Care Practitioner Pain Communication

2. RESPONSE TO SPECIFIC REQUEST FOR APPLICATIONS OR PROGRAM ANNOUNCEMENT OR SOLICITATION ☐ NO ☒ YES
(If "Yes," state number and title)

Number: PA-03-152   Title: Biobehavioral Pain Research

3. PRINCIPAL INVESTIGATOR/PROGRAM DIRECTOR   New Investigator ☐ No ☒ Yes

3a. NAME (Last, first, middle) McDonald, Deborah Dillon	3b. DEGREE(S) BS MS PhD	3h. eRA Commons User Name

3c. POSITION TITLE
Associate Professor

3d. MAILING ADDRESS *(Street, city, state, zip code)*
The University of Connecticut
School of Nursing
231 Glenbrook Road, Unit 2026
Storrs, CT 06269-2026

3e. DEPARTMENT, SERVICE, LABORATORY, OR EQUIVALENT
School of Nursing

3f. MAJOR SUBDIVISION
N/A

3g. TELEPHONE AND FAX *(Area code, number and extension)*
TEL: 860-486-3714   FAX: 860-486-0001

E-MAIL ADDRESS:
deborah.mcdonald@uconn.edu

4. HUMAN SUBJECTS RESEARCH ☐ No ☒ Yes	4b. Human Subjects Assurance No. FWA00007125	5. VERTEBRATE ANIMALS ☒ No ☐ Yes
	4c. Clinical Trial ☒ No ☐ Yes	4d. NIH-defined Phase III Clinical Trial ☒ No ☐ Yes	5a. If "Yes," IACUC approval Date	5b. Animal welfare assurance no. A3124-01

4a. Research Exempt ☒ No ☐ Yes   If "Yes," Exemption No.

6. DATES OF PROPOSED PERIOD OF SUPPORT *(month, day, year—MM/DD/YY)*		7. COSTS REQUESTED FOR INITIAL BUDGET PERIOD		8. COSTS REQUESTED FOR PROPOSED PERIOD OF SUPPORT	
From	Through	7a. Direct Costs ($)	7b. Total Costs ($)	8a. Direct Costs ($)	8b. Total Costs ($)
5/01/06	4/30/08	$100,000	$148,000	$175,000	$259,000

9. APPLICANT ORGANIZATION

Name   University of Connecticut

Address   Office for Sponsored Programs
438 Whitney Road Ext., Unit 1133
Storrs, CT 06269-1133
Telephone: 860-486-3622
Fax: 860-486-3726; Email: osp@uconn.edu

10. TYPE OF ORGANIZATION

Public: ❙ ☐ Federal ☒ State ☐ Local
Private: ❙ ☐ Private Nonprofit
For-profit: ❙ ☐ General ☐ Small Business
☐ Woman-owned ☐ Socially and Economically Disadvantaged

11. ENTITY IDENTIFICATION NUMBER
06-0772160

DUNS NO. 614209054   Cong. District Second

12. ADMINISTRATIVE OFFICIAL TO BE NOTIFIED IF AWARD IS MADE

Name   Carol Welt, PhD
Title   Executive Director & Assist. V. Prov. Research
Address   Office of Sponsored Programs
438 Whitney Road Ext., Unit 1133
Storrs, CT 06269-1133

Tel: 860-486-8704   FAX: 860-486-3726
E-Mail: carol.welt@uconn.edu

13. OFFICIAL SIGNING FOR APPLICANT ORGANIZATION

Name   Carol Welt, PhD
Title   Executive Director & Assist. V. Prov. Research
Address   Office of Sponsored Programs
438 Whitney Road Ext., Unit 1133
Storrs, CT 06269-1133

Tel: 860-486-8704   FAX: 860-486-3726
E-Mail: carol.welt@uconn.edu

14. PRINCIPAL INVESTIGATOR/PROGRAM DIRECTOR ASSURANCE: I certify that the statements herein are true, complete and accurate to the best of my knowledge. I am aware that any false, fictitious, or fraudulent statements or claims may subject me to criminal, civil, or administrative penalties. I agree to accept responsibility for the scientific conduct of the project and to provide the required progress reports if a grant is awarded as a result of this application.

SIGNATURE OF PI/PD NAMED IN 3a.
(In ink. "Per" signature not acceptable.)   DATE

15. APPLICANT ORGANIZATION CERTIFICATION AND ACCEPTANCE: I certify that the statements herein are true, complete and accurate to the best of my knowledge, and accept the obligation to comply with Public Health Services terms and conditions if a grant is awarded as a result of this application. I am aware that any false, fictitious, or fraudulent statements or claims may subject me to criminal, civil, or administrative penalties.

SIGNATURE OF OFFICIAL NAMED IN 13.
(In ink. "Per" signature not acceptable.)   DATE

PHS 398 (Rev. 09/04)   Face Page   **Form Page 1**

Principal Investigator/Program Director (Last, First, Middle):   McDonald, Deborah Dillon

DESCRIPTION: See instructions. State the application's broad, long-term objectives and specific aims, making reference to the health relatedness of the project (i.e., relevance to the **mission of the agency**). Describe concisely the research design and methods for achieving these goals. Describe the rationale and techniques you will use to pursue these goals.

In addition, in two or three sentences, describe in plain, lay language the relevance of this research to **public** health. If the application is funded, this description, as is, will become public information. Therefore, do not include proprietary/confidential information. **DO NOT EXCEED THE SPACE PROVIDED.**

How practitioners communicate with patients about their pain has been overlooked as a factor contributing to effective pain management. Eliciting important pain information from patients enables practitioners to prescribe more specific pain treatments, and significantly decrease pain. The aim of our study is to test the effect of practitioners asking patients an open-ended question about pain that does not encourage a socially desirable response. A posttest only double blind experiment will test how the phrasing of health care practitioners' pain questions, open-ended and without social desirability bias; closed-ended and without social desirability bias; or open-ended and with social desirability bias, affects the pain information provided by people with chronic pain. Three hundred community dwelling older adults with chronic osteoarthritis pain will be randomly assigned to one of the three practitioner pain communication conditions. Older adults will watch and verbally respond to a videotape clip of a practitioner asking the patient about their pain. The clips will be identical except for the pain question asked by the practitioner. After responding to the pain question, all of the older adults will respond to a second videotape clip of the practitioner asking if there is anything further they want to communicate. The older adults will then respond to a third videotape clip asking if there is anything further they want to communicate about their pain. Responses to the three videotape clips will be audiotaped. To control for pain differences between participants, the Brief Pain Inventory Short Form will be administered to measure present pain intensity and pain interference with functional activities. Participants' audiotaped responses will be transcribed and content analyzed using a priori criteria from national guidelines to identify communicated pain information and omitted pain information important for osteoarthritis pain management. The three groups will be compared for the communicated pain information and omitted pain information while controlling for present pain intensity and pain interference with activities. The goal is to identify practitioner pain communication strategies that allow patients to describe pain information important for guiding effective pain management, and to substantiate what pain information is missed when practitioners use less effective pain communication. The results will provide empirically tested communication strategies that can be used in practitioner and patient pain communication.

PERFORMANCE SITE(S) (organization, city, state)

University of Connecticut School of Nursing, Storrs, CT
P.C. Smith Towers, Hartford, CT
Betty Knox Apartments, Hartford, CT
Capitol Towers, Hartford, CT
Fireside Apartments, Bridgeport, CT
Harborview Towers, Bridgeport, CT
Park Ridge I and II, New Haven, CT
Tower One/Tower East, New Haven, CT

Principal Investigator/Program Director (Last, First, Middle):   McDonald, Deborah Dillon

KEY PERSONNEL. See instructions. *Use continuation pages as needed* to provide the required information in the format shown below.
Start with Principal Investigator. List all other key personnel in alphabetical order, last name first.

Name	eRA Commons User Name	Organization	Role on Project
McDonald Deborah Dillon		University of Connecticut	PI
Katz, Leonard		University of Connecticut	Statistical Consultant
Rosiene, Joel		Eastern CT State Univ.	Computer Consultant
Maura Shea		University of Connecticut	Graduate Assistant
Leonie Rose		University of Connecticut	Graduate Assistant

OTHER SIGNIFICANT CONTRIBUTORS

Name	Organization	Role on Project
N/A		

Human Embryonic Stem Cells   ☒ No   ☐ Yes
If the proposed project involves human embryonic stem cells, list below the registration number of the specific cell line(s) from the following list:
http://stemcells.nih.gov/registry/index.asp. *Use continuation pages as needed.*

If a specific line cannot be referenced at this time, include a statement that one from the Registry will be used.

Cell Line

Disclosure Permission Statement. Applicable to SBIR/STTR Only. See SBIR/STTR instructions.   ☐ Yes   ☐ No

PHS 398 (Rev. 09/04)   Page 3   **Form Page 2-continued**
Number the *following* pages consecutively throughout
the application. Do not use suffixes such as 4a, 4b.

The name of the principal investigator/program director must be provided at the top of each printed page and each continuation page.

RESEARCH GRANT
TABLE OF CONTENTS

Appendix *(Five collated sets. No page numbering necessary for Appendix.)*

Appendices NOT PERMITTED for Phase I SBIR/STTR unless specifically solicited. .... ☒

Check if Appendix is Included

Number of publications and manuscripts accepted for publication *(not to exceed 10)*   5

Other items (list):

Brief Pain Inventory Short Form

Demographic Form

Principal Investigator/Program Director (Last, First, Middle): McDonald, Deborah Dillon

BUDGET JUSTIFICATION PAGE
MODULAR RESEARCH GRANT APPLICATION

	Initial Period	2nd	3rd	4th	5th	Sum Total (For Entire Project Period)
DC less Consortium F&A	100,000 *(Item 7a, Face Page)*	75,000				175,000 *(Item 8a, Face Page)*
Consortium F&A						
Total Direct Costs	100,000	75,000				$ 175,000

Personnel

Deborah Dillon McDonald, RN, PhD, Principal Investigator (Y1-20% & 50% summer; Y2-20% & 50% summer) will be responsible for the overall administration and completion of the project. She will collaborate with the videotape production company to produce the health care practitioner videotape clips. She will consult with Dr. Rosiene to program the laptop computer with touch screen. She will train and supervise the GA. She will prepare the sites for data collection and maintain contact with sites throughout the study. She will conduct the content analysis with the GA, statistically analyze the data in consultation with Dr. Katz, write, and submit manuscripts reporting the findings.

Leonard Katz, PhD, Consultant (Y2-1% effort) will advise the PI regarding statistical analyses.

Joel Rosiene, PhD, Consultant (Y1-5% effort) will program the laptop computer with the SuperLab 3.0 software and insert the health care practitioner videotape clips as the experimental manipulation. He will test the program and resolve any programming issues. He will remain available for consultation in the event of future programming problems.

TBA, Graduate Assistant (Y1-8 mos., 20 hrs/wk; Y2-4 mos., 20 hrs/wk; Y2-4 mos., 10 hrs/wk) will recruit eligible older adults, provide informed consent, data collect, debrief, and compensate the older adults. The GA will also transcribe the audiotaped responses. The GA will content analyze the data with the PI, enter the data into a SPSS data base, and clean the data to remove input errors.

Explanation for Budget Deviation
The increased budget by $25,000 during year one is due to the cost of video development and the need for the 20 hour per week GA during eight months.

Consortium

N/A

Fee (SBIR/STTR Only)
N/A

Principal Investigator/Program Director (Last, First, Middle): McDonald, Deborah Dillon

BIOGRAPHICAL SKETCH

Provide the following information for the key personnel and other significant contributors in the order listed on Form Page 2.
Follow this format for each person. **DO NOT EXCEED FOUR PAGES.**

NAME Deborah Dillon McDonald	POSITION TITLE Associate Professor
eRA COMMONS USER NAME	

EDUCATION/TRAINING *(Begin with baccalaureate or other initial professional education, such as nursing, and include postdoctoral training.)*

INSTITUTION AND LOCATION	DEGREE *(if applicable)*	YEAR(s)	FIELD OF STUDY
Marycrest College, Davenport, IA	BSN	1975	Nursing
University of Connecticut, Storrs, CT	MS	1981	Nursing
Columbia University, New York, NY	PhD	1990	Social Psychology

A. Positions and Honors

1975-1978	Navy Regional Medical Center, Long Beach, CA; Lieutenant in Nurse Corps
1978-1979	Hartford Hospital, Hartford, CT; Staff
1981-1983	Elms College, Chicopee, MA; Assistant Professor of Nursing
1983-1986	University of Connecticut, Storrs, CT; Assistant Professor of Nursing
1988-1990	National Center for Nursing Research Pre-doctoral Fellowship at Columbia University, New York, NY; Pre-doctoral Fellow
1990-present	University of Connecticut, Storrs, CT; Associate Professor

B. Selected Peer-Reviewed Publications

McDonald, D. (1993). Postoperative narcotic analgesic administration: A pilot study. *Applied Nursing Research. 6*, 106-110.

McDonald, D. (1994). Gender and ethnic stereotyping and narcotic analgesic administration. *Research in Nursing & Health, 17*, 45-49.

McDonald, D. (1996). Nurses' memory of patient's pain. *International Journal of Nursing Studies. 23*, 487-494.

McDonald, D., & Sterling, R. (1998). Acute pain reduction strategies used by well older adults. *International Journal of Nursing Studies, 35*, 265-70.

Wessman, A., & McDonald, D. (1999). Nurses' personal pain experiences and their pain management knowledge. *Journal of Continuing Education in Nursing, 30*, 152-157.

McDonald, D. (1999). Postoperative pain after hospital discharge. *Clinical Nursing Research, 8*, 347-359.

McDonald, D., McNulty, J., Erickson, K., & Weiskopf, C. (2000). Communicating pain and pain management needs after surgery. *Applied Nursing Research, 13*, 70-75.

McDonald, D., Freeland, M., Thomas, G., & Moore, J. (2001). Testing a preoperative pain management intervention for elders. *Research in Nursing & Health, 24*, 402-409.

McDonald, D. & Weiskopf, C. (2001). Adult patients' postoperative pain descriptions and responses to the Short-Form McGill Pain Questionnaire. *Clinical Nursing Research, 10*, 442-452.

Tafas, C., Patiraki, E., McDonald, D. & Lemonidou, C. (2002). Testing an instrument measuring Greek nurses' knowledge and attitudes regarding pain. *Cancer Nursing, 25* (1), 1 – 7.

Principal Investigator/Program Director (Last, First, Middle): McDonald, Deborah Dillon

McDonald, D., Pourier, S., Gonzalez, T., Brace, J., Lakhani, K., Landry, S. & Wrigley, P. (2002). Pain problems in young adults and pain reduction strategies. *Pain Management Nursing, 3*(3), 81-86.

McDonald, D. & Molony, S. (2004). Postoperative pain communication skills for older adults. *Western Journal of Nursing Research, 26*, 836 – 852, 858 - 859.

Patiraki - Kourbani , E., Tafas , C., McDonald , D., Papathanassoglou , E., Katsaragakis , S. & Lemonidou , C. (2004). Greek nurses' personal and professional pain experiences. *International Journal of Nursing Studies, 41*, 345-54.

McDonald, D., Thomas, G., Livingston, K. & Severson, J. (2005). Assisting older adults to communicate their postoperative pain. *Clinical Nursing Research, 14*, 109-126.

McDonald, D., LaPorta, M., & Meadows-Oliver, M. (2006). Nurses' response to pain communication from patients: A post-test experimental Study. *International Journal of Nursing Studies*.

C. Research Support

National Institute of Nursing Research, 1R21NR009848-01, 3/16/06 – 3/15/08, McDonald PI
Older Adults' Response to Health Care Practitioner Pain Communication
The aim of our study is to test the effect of practitioners asking patients an open-ended question about pain that does not encourage a socially desirable response.

Donaghue Foundation, 10/1/01 – 10/1/02; McDonald PI
Assisting Elders to Communicate their Pain After Surgery
The goal of the study was to refine our videotape intervention teaching older adults about postoperative pain communication and pain management, and test the effects of the videotape intervention on the pain outcomes of older adults after major surgery.

National Institute of Nursing Research, 1 R15 NR04876-03, 5/1/99 – 10/1/01; McDonald PI
Postoperative Pain Communication Skills for Older Adults
The goal of the study was to develop a videotape intervention teaching older adults about postoperative pain communication and pain management, and test the effects of the videotape intervention on the pain outcomes of older adults after major surgery.

University of Athens, Athens, Greece, 11/98 – 1/03; McDonald Co-Investigator
Nurses' Knowledge Regarding Pain and Cancer Patients' Reports of Pain Control
The goal of the study was to test the construct validity, test-retest reliability, and internal consistency of the Greek version of the Nurses' Knowledge and Attitudes Survey Regarding Pain (NKASRP) with Greek nurses, as phase I in a series of studies examining how to improve pain outcomes for cancer patients in Greece.

Principal Investigator/Program Director (Last, First, Middle): McDonald, Deborah Dillon
Resources

Clinical: We will recruit and conduct the study at seven independent living elder housing sites throughout Connecticut. The urban sites in Bridgeport, New Haven and, Hartford, CT increase the opportunity to include Black or African Americans, Hispanic and Asian elders. The sites include P.C. Smith Towers, Capitol Towers, and the Betty Knox Apartments in Hartford, CT; Park Ridge I and II and Tower One/Tower East in New Haven, CT; and Fireside Apartments and Harborview Towers in Bridgeport, CT. The sites contain from 193 to 248 housing units each, insuring a large group of older adults for our study.

Computer: The PI has a Dell Pentium 4 computer 2.4 GHz with 256 MB RAM, loaded with SPSS-13.0 and Word 2000 professional operating system; and a Hewlett Packard LaserJet5 printer in her university office. Additional computer resources are available through the Center for Nursing Research (CNR) in the School of Nursing at the University of Connecticut. Fourteen new Dell computers each with Intel Pentium 4 processor 520's are available. There are two HP LaserJet IV printers, one HP LaserJet III printer, one HP LaserJet 1200, one HP LaserJet 5L printer, one Laser Jet 1100 printer, and an HP Office jet 5110 all-in-one copier, scanner, and printer. All computers have direct access to the university mainframe computer, the university library system, and the Internet. Software programs available on the PCs in the CNR relevant for our study include: Power and Precision, QRS N6 (NUD*IST), and SPSS 12.0.

Office: The PI has a private university office, telephone, and four locked filing cabinets. Various support personnel are available through the Center for Nursing Research at the School of Nursing. Work-study students, graduate assistants, and secretaries are available for assisting with all aspects of a research project. In addition, a program for doctoral study in the School of Nursing offers a pool of well-qualified graduate nursing students from which to select a research assistant for the study.

Other: The Seven Seas Film Company located in Madison, CT will produce the three videotape clips of the health care practitioner asking the older adults about their pain, the two follow up videotape clips, and the test videotape that will be used to adjust the audibility of the videotapes for each participant. Seven Seas produced our 15-minute documentary style pain communication videotape tested with older adults and reported in McDonald, et al., (2005). Seven Seas has produced films for the Public Broadcasting Service (PBS) and major universities.

MAJOR EQUIPMENT: List the most important equipment items already available for this project, noting the location and pertinent capabilities of each.
The University of Connecticut School of Nursing offers access to additional equipment. There are multiple copiers (i.e. Cannon IR3300, Savin 4060 SP, all with sorter and stapler, a color scanner (HP Office jet 9130), a color printer (Hewlett Packard color laser jet 5550hdn) and two independent fax lines. In addition to readily available equipment, there is ample conference meeting space and facilities for use in research projects.

Principal Investigator/Program Director (Last, First, Middle): McDonald, Deborah Dillon

A. Specific Aims

Management of patients' pain is one of the most enduring challenges facing all health care practitioners. Assessment of pain is now an assumed standard of practice required by the Joint Commission for Accreditation of Health Care Organizations. Pain communication between patients and practitioners provides a critical link for the assessment and management of pain.

Inadequate pain communication between patients and health care practitioners[1-3] can result in sustained or increased pain for patients.[4] Researchers have shown that pain remained undiagnosed for 53% of patients with moderate pain and 30% with severe pain during their primary care outpatient visit,[5] indicating that pain was not addressed despite a pressing need to talk about pain. Nearly half of the people reported moderate levels of acute[6] or chronic pain[7] in two recent surveys. Communicating about pain involves more than use of pain assessment measures. Hospitalized patients did not consider responding to a numerical pain intensity scale equivalent to communicating about pain.[2] Effective pain communication involves talking with patients in ways that permit patients to more fully discuss salient aspects of their pain experience. Research is needed to test communication strategies that enhance patient and practitioner communication about pain.

The aim of this study is to test how practitioners' pain communication affects the pain information provided by older adults. The study will specifically test the effect of asking an open-ended question about pain that does not direct a socially desirable response. We suspect that a question about pain presented in what might be perceived as a social exchange ("How are you feeling?") might not be sufficient to elicit clinically meaningful and important information if patients perceive a social, rather than a clinical, source of the question.

Hypothesis

Older adults asked about their pain with an open-ended question without social desirability bias will describe more important pain information and omit less information than older adults asked about their pain with a closed-ended question without social desirability or an open-ended question with social desirability bias.

To test the hypothesis, three videos will be developed that portray a health care practitioner asking participants about their pain in one of three different ways: open-ended without social desirability, closed-ended without social desirability, and open-ended with social desirability. Older adults with chronic osteoarthritis pain will be randomly assigned to watch and respond to one of the three videos. The second and third parts of the videos, after the first part of questioning, will be the same. All participants will next watch and respond to the second part of the video with the practitioner asking if there is anything further participants want to communicate in general, and then the third part with the practitioner asking if there is anything further they want to communicate about their pain. Participants' audio taped responses will be content analyzed for important included and omitted pain information.

Older adults with chronic pain due to osteoarthritis will be randomly assigned to one of the three practitioner pain communication conditions. Present pain will be measured with the counterbalanced Brief Pain Inventory Short Form (BPI-SF) to statistically control for pain differences between participants evident after random assignment while controlling for the timing of the BPI-SF. Participants' audio taped responses will be content analyzed using a priori criteria from the American Pain Society[8] guidelines for the management of pain in osteoarthritis to identify pain communication content important for osteoarthritis pain management, and important omitted pain information. The three groups will be compared for the included and omitted pain information while controlling for pre-existing, current pain intensity and pain interference with activities. The immediate goal is to identify practitioner pain communication strategies that allow patients to describe important pain information that can more effectively guide pain management, and significantly reduce or eliminate pain. The long-term goal is to incorporate empirically tested, theory driven pain communication strategies into health practitioner curricula and patient education.

PHS 398/2590 (Rev. 09/04)   Page 14
—

Principal Investigator/Program Director (Last, First, Middle): McDonald, Deborah Dillon
B. Background and Significance

Communication About Pain Management

Effective pain communication involves more than practitioners encouraging patients to identify when patients have pain. An intervention that encouraged terminally ill patients to talk with their physicians about their pain showed that 43.4% of patients continued to have a pain problem at hospital discharge, and less than half received a pain intervention.[9] Interventions that only encourage patients to talk about their pain might be inadequate for promoting pain communication. Increased communication between patients and practitioners was not associated with increased pain relief, perhaps because communication was restricted to discussing pain treatments, and asking the patient to alert practitioners when pain occurred.[10] Clinical contexts where routine pain communication should be part of standard practice continue to demonstrate deficiencies in pain communication. Physicians discussed pain during only 72% of the outpatient palliative care visits, and initiated the pain topic only half of the time.[11] Cancer patients and family caregivers have clearly identified the need for improved communication with their health care practitioners.[12] Patients and practitioners need research-based support to help them communicate about pain in ways that lead to greater pain relief for patients.

Reasons for the inadequate pain communication might be directly attributable to the way that practitioners speak with patients. Constructing pain assessment questions in the form of social conversation (i.e. "How are you today?") encourages patients to respond in a socially desirable manner by suppressing their pain concerns.[3,13] These types of approaches might be seen as directing social exchange rather than soliciting important clinical assessment data. Giving little attention to patients' reports of pain, and controlling pain communication by interrupting patients, minimizing or dismissing the reports of pain, and curtailing patient responses to yes/no responses were techniques observed to be used by physicians in a descriptive study of oncology patients consulting with their physicians.[13] Again, these methods to ask for pain information are more directing in soliciting a response than merely asking a patient, "tell me about your pain." Physicians challenged and attempted to disconfirm biological explanations for the pain, insisting on psychological explanations when talking with chronic pain patients who had no apparent medical reason for their pain.[14] When subjected to practitioner statements suggesting where the pain might be felt, patients reported significantly more referred pain, and more intense pain.[15] The preceding communication techniques thwart complete and accurate pain discussions between patients and practitioners. Randomized controlled clinical trials are needed to link specific pain communication strategies to patient outcomes.

Patient factors impact pain communication. Patient factors include low expectations for pain relief,[16-17] reluctance to bother busy staff,[3,12,18] concern about repercussions from staff if patients complain about pain,[4] fear of addiction to opioids,[17,19-20] fear of unpleasant opioid side effects,[3,19-21] belief that health care providers innately know best how to manage their pain;[17] and general lack of information about pain management, and difficulty articulating pain management needs.[4] Hospitalized patients reporting more intense pain communicated about their pain more often, but were less satisfied with the information communicated by the nurse. Older adults communicated less about their pain, but voiced greater satisfaction with the information provided by nurses.[2] When given the opportunity, many patients clearly describe their pain (e.g. "my leg is going to burst," "someone turning a knife under my skin."[22] Patients have the ability to clearly communicate their pain, but multiple barriers continue to restrain patients from communicating about pain with practitioners.

Principal Investigator/Program Director (Last, First, Middle): McDonald, Deborah Dillon

Pain Communication Interventions

Promising interventions to assist patients to describe their pain have been tested, such as individual coaching prior to an office visit,[23] and combinations of written scripts and individual coaching.[24] Both interventions resulted in a significant decrease in pain. These findings suggest that patients can be assisted to effectively communicate their pain and receive interventions that significantly reduce their pain. The cost of the individual coaching interventions might limit the widespread use of coaching interventions. Both studies involved patients with cancer pain. Individual coaching interventions for patients with different pain etiologies might not be as effective in eliciting more responsive pain management from practitioners.

Practitioner Influence in Health Care Communication

Health care communication research, conducted mainly in psychology and medicine, provides insight about pain management communication. The Bayer Institute for Health Care Communication literature review on health care practitioner and patient communication identified only six medical studies that examined eliciting patients' agenda.[25] All six were limited to descriptive medical studies. Primary care physicians interrupted opening statements by their patients during 77% of the visits, and patients completed only 1 out of 52 interrupted statements.[26] Physician communication remained virtually unchanged 12 years later when physicians again interrupted 72% of the opening statements.[27] Physicians using problem defining communication skills, which included starting off with an open-ended question to delineate the patient's problem, identified significantly more patients with emotional distress than physicians not taught problem defining skills. Six months later patient distress remained significantly reduced for patients of physicians using problem defining communication skills.[28] Female physicians use more positive statements, more psychosocial information giving, more active partnership behaviors, but also more closed-ended questions during office visits.[29] The ability to gather or omit potentially important information from patients is influenced by how health care practitioners communicate with patients.

Patient Influence in Health Care Communication

Descriptive and intervention studies have examined patients' contribution to their health care interaction. During a family practice office visit, younger, more educated, and more anxious patients who asked more questions received more diagnostic health information. Patients who asked more questions and expressed more concern received more treatment information from their physicians.[30] Similarly, parents of pediatric patients received more information when they asked more questions and expressed more affect.[31] Patients communicated more and provided more biomedical and psychosocial information, promoted more partnership building, and talked more positively with female physicians.[32] Patients trained via a booklet and coaching to talk with their family practice physicians asked more questions about medically related topics, elicited more information from the physician, and provided more information about their medical problems than untrained patients.[33] Women either prompted to think about their questions prior to seeing their women's health physician or informed that the physician was open to questions were significantly more likely to ask all of the questions that they wanted compared to women in a control group.[34] Participants who watched a video with a patient either asking questions or making disclosures communicated more than participants who watched a video without patient interaction.[35] Patients who prior to their office visit were instructed to think about the instructions the physician gave them during the visit, imagine carrying out the instructions, and to ask the physician questions about problems that they anticipated, communicated significantly more than patients not given any additional instructions, or patients instructed that the physician was open to answering questions.[36] Preliminary evaluation of a community based intervention teaching people how to communicate with their physician by teaching them communication skills and helping them practice the skills was associated with a moderate increase in

Principal Investigator/Program Director (Last, First, Middle): McDonald, Deborah Dillon

patient confidence for communicating with the physician.[37] The variety of successful communication interventions indicates that people can successfully communicate with their health care practitioners when supported to do so.

Linking increased practitioner and patient communication with improved health outcomes substantiates the impact of communication during health care interactions. Patients with diabetes, hypertension, ulcer disease, and breast cancer were tested during three randomized controlled trials and a nonequivalent control trial respectively for the effect of an intervention to improve communication by patients during health care visits.[38] The intervention for each study consisted of providing each patient with individualized information about their medical care, and coaching about actively communicating during the visit. The communication techniques included more effective ways to ask questions, keeping focused on the medical care, and negotiating skills. Improved hemoglobin A1c and lowered diastolic blood pressure resulted from more patient control, less physician control, more negative affect expressed by both, more information seeking by patients, and more patient communication. How patients with chronic health problems communicate with practitioners during their health care visits can directly impact their health outcomes. The success of the individualized coaching intervention demonstrates that patients with different chronic health problems can be assisted to communicate more effectively and impact their health outcomes. The resource intensity of the intervention remains a drawback.

Pain Communication and Health Practitioner Curricula

Practitioner pain management education has been the major means for improving pain outcomes, but medical and nursing curricula have generally not included education about pain communication beyond pain assessment (e.g. Giamberardino[39]), even though experts have identified pain communication skills as an essential component of training in medical education.[40] The benefit of increased education in pain communication was provided by a recent study with pediatric residents.[41] An 18-hour educational intervention teaching physicians a more patient centered approach when communicating about pain problems with patients with fibromyalgia found that patients felt that they were allowed to fully discuss their pain,[42] perhaps because of a Hawthorne effect for the physicians, or low expectations by patients. This resource intensive intervention supported increased pain communication between patients and practitioners, but the specific communication strategies that promoted the full discussion remain unclear, and the effect on patient pain outcomes was not measured. Further research is needed to test specific pain communication strategies essential for practitioner pain management education.

Communication Theory Attuning Strategies

Communication Accommodation Theory (CAT) has been used to guide causal research about communication behaviors with older adults.[43] CAT describes the motivations and behaviors of people as they adjust their communication in response to their own needs and the perceived behavior of the other person.[44-45] Paying attention to the other person when communicating provides useful information that can enhance communication. This attention has been termed attuning strategies.[46] Attuning strategies include discourse management and interpersonal control strategies. Discourse management strategies involve evaluating the social aspects of the communication interaction, such as selecting and sharing a topic. Interpersonal control strategies pertain to identifying the relationship between the communicators.

Within the context of pain management communication CAT provides strategies that practitioners can use to enhance communication with patients. For example, practitioners could use a topic sharing discourse management strategy by using an open-ended question to inquire about pain to allow patients more freedom to respond in the way they feel most helpful in communicating their pain. An interpersonal control strategy by practitioners would be to avoid phrasing questions about pain in a socially desirable way, clarifying that the pain communication is taking place within a health care rather than a social context. Testing how different strategies affect pain communication between practitioners and patients can lead to more effective use of the communication strategies to decrease pain.

Summary the Literature Review

Pain communication has emerged as an important, but poorly understood aspect of pain management. Descriptive studies document problems with pain communication and patient related barriers to pain communication. Clinical trials have demonstrated the benefits of resource intensive coaching interventions for patients prior to office visits. An extensive pain communication education intervention with physicians did not clarify if pain was adequately discussed, or how individual communication strategies affected pain communication. Our study addresses gaps in pain communication research by using theory based pain communication strategies in a rigorously designed study to test how older adults' respond to different types of health care practitioner pain communication.

C. Preliminary Studies

In nine studies, the PI has investigated different aspects of practitioner and patient communication that might affect pain management. A summary of the findings from the nine studies includes:

∞ nurses' administration of opioids after surgery is related to the patients' race and gender;[47]
∞ some nurses may not attend to their patients' specific pain information, and consequently either omit this pain information or recall it incorrectly;[48]
∞ many older adults do not plan to talk in the hospital with their practitioners about their pain;[49]
∞ adults have difficulty communicating their pain to their health care providers after
∞ surgery;[3]
∞ postoperative pain after discharge continues to plague many adults and might be decreased if adults understood more about pain management and possessed more effective pain communication skills;[50]
∞ a majority of postoperative patients used exact Short-Form McGill Pain questionnaire sensory or affective words or synonyms to describe their postoperative pain;[51]
∞ a slide show teaching older adults about postoperative pain communication and pain management helped decrease postoperative pain;[52]
∞ a video teaching pain communication and pain management assisted older adults to experience less sensory pain during the early postoperative period;[53]
∞ a refined video teaching pain management and pain communication skills assisted older adults to experience less pain interference with sleep during the first postoperative day.[54]

The nine studies represent a wide range of methods, including post-test only experiments, patient surveys using audio taped interviews, and content analysis. Five manuscripts,[3,49-50,53-54] contained in Appendix A, provide more detailed accounts of our research.

Summary

The processes used in conducting these studies have provided excellent preparation for the implementation of the proposed research. We have recruited and retained over 320 participants during our previous pain management studies. We have worked exclusively with older adults during four of our recent studies, three of which were randomized controlled trials that provided us with the expertise needed to conduct our proposed experiment. Our experience with refining our video intervention teaching older adults how to communicate with practitioners about pain has prepared us to develop the videos in our proposed study as a way to standardize our experimental manipulations. Our experience in conducting content analyses with participants' responses provides us with the skill required for content analysis of participants' responses in our proposed study. We are well prepared to conduct our proposed study, if the science is deemed sound.

We have established pain communication between the practitioner and patient as an integral part of achieving pain relief. The results from our three pain communication intervention studies indicate that closer scrutiny of pain communication is needed to identify communication strategies that exert the greatest effect on patients and practitioners. We need to directly test specific communication strategies in order to clarify which communication strategies encourage older adults to describe important information, and what important information is missed when health care practitioners use ineffective communication strategies. Research based communication skills provide a more powerful way to help practitioners and older adults communicate about pain problems.

D. Research Design and Methods

Our study takes the novel approach of testing patients' responses to being asked about their pain to determine what important information people communicate. Our innovative use of national osteoarthritis pain management guidelines to analyze the clinical importance of the information communicated by the older adults further strengthens our proposed study. In particular we are interested in knowing whether important pain information is omitted when practitioners use closed ended questions and/or socially phrased questions that might direct responding. Practitioners need to be aware if pain information is gained or lost when different communication strategies are used to talk about pain. The attuning strategies from CAT provides the theoretical framework for our study, allowing us to test two aspects of how well CAT describes the dynamic process of participating in a health care conversation about pain.

Design

A posttest only double blind experiment will test how the phrasing of health care practitioners' pain question, open-ended without social desirability, closed-ended without social desirability, or open-ended with social desirability bias, affects the pain information provided by older adults with chronic osteoarthritis pain. To control for the measurement effect, half of each of the three groups will respond to the Brief Pain Inventory Short Form (BPI-SF) before watching the videos, and the remaining half after responding to the final video. Table 1 depicts the research design.

Sample

Older adults may be even more vulnerable to pain communication difficulties with health care practitioners.[2,49] Inclusion criteria for the sample size of 300 consists of community dwelling adults, age 60 and older who speak, read, and understand English and who have self identified osteoarthritis pain. Exclusion criteria consists of the presence of self identified malignant pain. Older adults with malignant pain might communicate differently due to the life-threatening context of pain associated with a cancer diagnosis. A small effect size is indicated when no previous effect size is available to base the sample size estimate upon.[55] A total sample size of 300 is needed for a multivariate analysis of covariance (MANCOVA) with three groups (open-ended without social desirability, closed-ended without social desirability, or open-ended with social desirability bias), two dependent variables (pain information included and pain information omitted), .05 level of significance, .80 power, and small estimated effect size.[56] Over 20 million Americans have osteoarthritis.[57] More than 80% of older adults over 75 have osteoarthritis.[58] The feasibility is high for recruiting the required sample size.

Table 1
Research Design

Group		Measurements						
R open-ended and without social desirability bias (a) BPI	Xa	O1	X2	O2	X3	O3	
R open-ended and without social desirability bias (a)	Xa	O1	X2	O2	X3	O3	BPI
R closed-ended and without social desirability bias (b) BPI	Xb	O1	X2	O2	X3	O3	
R closed-ended and without social desirability bias (b)	Xb	O1	X2	O2	X3	O3	BPI
R open-ended and with social desirability bias (c) BPI	Xc	O1	X2	O2	X3	O3	
R open-ended and with social desirability bias (c)	Xc	O1	X2	O2	X3	O3	BPI

R   = Random assignment
BPI = Brief Pain Inventory measure for covariates, pain intensity and interference with activities
Xa = Video with open-ended without social desirability bias
Xb = Video with closed-ended without social desirability bias
Xc = Video with open-ended with social desirability bias
O1 = Verbal response to the video clip practitioner pain question
O2 = Verbal response to the video clips about additional information in general
O3 = Verbal response to the video clips about additional information specific to pain
X2 = General additional information question
X3 = Pain specific additional information question

Procedure

We will first describe the overall procedure to provide context for our video experimental manipulation. We will then describe our measures, followed by our plans for content analyses and statistical analyses.

Recruitment.

Eligible older adults will be recruited from independent housing sites in Hartford, Bridgeport, New Haven, and suburban areas of Connecticut. The registered nurse doctoral student graduate assistant (GA) will screen for eligibility, give the older adult an enlarged print copy of the informed consent, and secure informed consent. Screening will include asking participants to self identify if they experience pain from osteoarthritis. To avoid priming participants about how to describe their pain, a yes/no question will be used to screen for osteoarthritis pain, "Do you have pain from osteoarthritis?" Participants will also be asked if they have any cancer pain, "If you have been diagnosed with cancer, do you have any pain from cancer?" Participants with malignant pain will be excluded from the study. Participants will be asked their age. Consenting, eligible participants will be automatically randomized to one of the three conditions by the SuperLab 3.0 computer software program, keeping the GA blind to the condition.

A cover story will be given to each older adult to increase experimental realism and to decrease the introduction of response bias. Participants will be told that the study is testing the feasibility of helping people prepare for their health care office visit while waiting in the office for their appointment. The GA will make the following statement. "We are testing whether asking patients to respond to a video of a health care practitioner asking questions about your health prior to an office visit helps you communicate better during the office visit."

Our cover story provides experimental realism by providing a credible reason for asking older adults to watch and respond to a computer video clip of a health care practitioner. Closely approximating a real life clinical situation increases the likelihood that responses from participants will be similar to their responses to health care practitioners during actual pain communication in the clinical setting. Successful patient coaching interventions prior to office visits have been reported,[24] making the cover story more credible.

Experimental Manipulation and Measurement.

The use of a video clip to provide the experimental manipulation strengthens the study by controlling for differences that occur across repeated live presentations of the same condition, strengthening fidelity[59] to the treatment. The use of video clips controls for any experimenter demand effects by standardizing the way participants are asked about pain in each condition. The use of the health care practitioner title increases the applicability of the findings to both nurse practitioners and physicians. Each of the three video clips will be subjected to a review panel of primary care nurse practitioners and physicians to determine the face validity of the practitioner posed question, and the similarity of other aspects of the clips. The use of the video clip reduces the cost of an additional GA to personally administer the experimental manipulation.

Our method avoids the problem of using patient analogues,[60] people who are asked to imagine themselves as having chronic pain. Responses from patient analogues might not be generalized to people with chronic pain, because patient analogues might not accurately grasp the experience of chronic pain.

The GA will test the audio tape recorder to insure that participants' voices are clearly and completely recorded. The GA will explain that the participant is going to watch three video clips of a health care practitioner on the computer screen and verbally respond to the practitioner's question in each clip before proceeding to the next clip. The participant's response will be audio taped. Participant will be instructed to touch any area of the screen to proceed to the next question, after they have responded to each question. We chose a touch screen for the increased ease of use especially for older adults with osteoarthritis in their hands. The final screen will instruct participants to press the buzzer placed on the table beside the computer to signal the GA to return to the room. After providing the instructions, the GA will use a test video to adjust the sound to a comfortable, audible level for each participant. The GA will start the audio tape recorder, press the computer to start the video clip and then leave the room. There will be a 15 second delay before the video clip begins. During that time, the participant will be randomly assigned to one of the three conditions through use of the SuperLab 3.0 software. The computer software can be programmed to randomly assign treatments to participants, and provide an experimental treatment (the video tape clips). The ability to use video clips as stimuli and randomly assign older adults to condition make the software a valuable resource for our study.

The randomized video clip will begin and the condition will be audio-recorded allowing the PI to later determine the participant's condition. The participant will respond to the practitioner's question about their pain, and the verbal response will be audio taped. The question will consist of one of the following, corresponding to the three experimental conditions.
- ∞ Tell me about your pain, aches, soreness, or discomfort. (open-ended and without social desirability)
- ∞ What would you rate your pain, aches, soreness, or discomfort on a 0 to 10 scale with 0, no pain, and 10 the worst pain possible? (closed-ended and without social desirability bias)
- ∞ How are you feeling? (open-ended and with social desirability bias)

The second part of each practitioner video will consist of the practitioner asking all participants, "What else can you tell me?" The third and final part of the practitioner video will consist of the practitioner asking, "What else can you tell me about your pain, aches, soreness or discomfort?" Responses to all three questions will be audio-recorded. Participants will be instructed by the GA to press the screen

PHS 398/2590 (Rev. 09/04)   Page 21

to proceed to the next question, after fully responding to each question. The final screen will instruct participants to press the buzzer placed beside the computer after responding to the third and final question. The buzzer will signal the GA to return to the room. A separate audiotape will be labeled for each participant.

Brief Pain Inventory Short Form (BPI-SF) Pain Measure.
The GA will orally administer the BPI-SF to measure participants' pain at the present time. Measuring participants' present pain with the BPI-SF allows us to control for pain differences across participants. Participants might learn how to better describe their pain by responding to the BPI-SF, but might also respond differently to the BPI-SF after viewing and responding to the videos. We will randomly counterbalance the BPI-SF measure to control for these potential learning effects. Fifty participants from each of the three experimental groups will respond to the BPI-SF after responding to the final video. The remaining 50 participants from each group will respond to the BPI-SF prior to watching the first video (experimental manipulation). The PI will randomize timing of the BPI-SF with a computer program for random assignment and compile a list that indicates, by order of entry into the study, whether the BPI-SF will be administered prior to watching the videos or after responding to the third and final video.

Demographic information will be measured last. The GA will orally ask the demographic questions and record responses on a demographic form. The BPI-SF, and demographic form will be coded with the same number used to identify the participant's audiotape.

Upon completion of all of the measures, the following protocol will be followed by the GA for participants who report present pain intensity on the BPI-SF at a level of four or greater. The GA will encourage the older adults to talk with their health care practitioner about their pain problem. If participants state that they do not have a health care practitioner, the name, location and telephone number of nearby accredited ambulatory care clinics will be given in writing to participants, with encouragement to make an appointment. If participants state that they have no health care insurance to pay for an office visit, the name, location and telephone number of a nearby sliding scale community health clinic will be given to them in written form.

Debriefing.
After completing the demographic information, the GA will debrief each participant. Participants will be thanked for their help. The debriefing will first include checking for hypothesis guessing by asking participants what they thought the study was about. Data from any participants guessing what the study was about will be marked and will not be used in the analysis. The study will be completely explained to participants, along with the reason for the deception. Participants will be checked for any concern or distress about the deception used in the study, and reminded that they are free to withdraw from the study. Participants will be asked not to discuss the study with people living in the housing development, because they might participate in the study. Participants will be asked if they have any questions or comments to make about the study. Participants will be thanked for their participation in the study, given a personal copy of the Arthritis Foundation publication, *Managing Your Pain*,[61] compensated for their time with a $20 money order, and informed that their participation has been completed.

Video Clip Experimental Manipulation
A video clip presented on a touch screen equipped laptop computer monitor will be used for the experimental manipulation. Prior to leaving the room, the GA will adjust the sound, using a video clip not associated with the experimental manipulation with the same sound volume of the three

PHS 398/2590 (Rev. 09/04)   Page 22

experimental video clips. The GA will adjust the sound volume to a level that allows each participant to clearly hear the video.

A brief health care office visit scene will be depicted. The same practitioner will be videoed for each of the three conditions. The conditions will be identical except for how the practitioner asks patients about their pain. Each condition will start out with the practitioner entering the examination room and sitting down in a chair to face the camera (participant). The practitioner will say, "Hello, I am going to ask you some questions about your health." After a slight pause, the practitioner will ask about the participant's pain (the experimental manipulation). The practitioner will use the same volume, voice inflection and nonverbal communication when asking each of the three questions. The three video clips will be reviewed by a group of five primary care nurse practitioners and primary care physicians for face validity and for equality of practitioner nonverbal behavior and verbal behavior such as tone, and voice inflection.

The practitioner will ask only one question in each condition. The three questions representing each of the three conditions are as follows:
- ∞ Tell me about your pain, aches, soreness, or discomfort. (open-ended and without social desirability)
- ∞ What would you rate your pain, aches, soreness, or discomfort on a 0 to 10 scale with 0, no pain, and 10 the worst pain possible? (closed-ended and without social desirability bias)
- ∞ How are you feeling? (open-ended and with social desirability bias)

An alternative approach would be to embed the pain questions within a more prolonged discussion by the practitioner. Further discussion would burden participants with a longer time to complete the study. Additional general health care discussion would also require participants to reveal personal health information unnecessary for the purposes of the study. To increase privacy of health information and decrease burden for participants, we chose to place the pain question at the beginning of the discussion. It would be reasonable for a practitioner to ask older adults with osteoarthritis pain about their pain at the beginning of the visit.

We also chose to leave the health care practitioner credentials ambiguous, rather than specifying the practitioner as a physician or a nurse practitioner. The ambiguity allows us to extend the applicability of the findings to both physicians and nurse practitioners.

Measures

Content Analysis of Included Pain Information.
Participants' verbal response to the practitioner's pain question will be audio taped and transcribed for content analysis. Content analysis for included pain information is described in the section on content analysis.

Content Analysis of Omitted Information.
Two questions will be used to measure additional information that participants communicate, when given the opportunity. After responding to the practitioners' pain question, all of the older adults will watch and listen to a second video clip of the practitioner asking, "What else can you tell me?" Next all participants will respond to a third video clip of the practitioner asking the participant, "What else can you tell me about your pain, aches, soreness or discomfort?" Responses to both questions will be audio taped and transcribed for content analysis. Participant responses to additional information might be increased if measured in a face-to-face interview. Use of the same practitioner

PHS 398/2590 (Rev. 09/04)   Page 23

video clip format decreases the confounding influence of different measurement methods. Content analysis for omitted pain information is described in the content analysis section.

Brief Pain Inventory Short Form (BPI-SF).

The GA will use the BPI-SF to measure participants' present pain intensity and present pain interference with activities. The BPI-SF was developed to examine the prevalence and severity of pain in the general population.[62] The BPI-SF consists of 15 questions that measure pain location, intensity, pain treatment, and the effect of pain on mood and every day activities. The first question asks if the person has had any pain today. An anterior and posterior body diagram allows the respondent to shade areas where they feel pain and mark with an "X" the area that hurts the most. Respondents rate their worst, least, and average pain in the past 24 hours using a 0 – 10 numeric rating scale with 0, no pain, and 10, pain as bad as you can imagine. They also rate their pain right now. An open-ended question asks what treatments or medications they are receiving for their pain. Respondents then rate the percent of relief they received from the treatments in the past 24 hours. The seven remaining questions evaluate how pain has interfered with activities including general activity, mood, walking, work, relations with others, sleep and enjoyment of life. Anchors for the 0 – 10 scale consist of 0, does not interfere and 10, completely interferes. Zalon[63] compared the BPI-SF with the Short Form McGill Pain Questionnaire (SF-MPQ) with a group of surgical patients. The correlation between the BPI-SF and the SF-MPQ for pain over the previous 24 hours was .61, $p < .001$, supporting concurrent validity. Cronbach's alpha for the overall BPI-SF has been reported as .77 to .87.[54,63] The BPI-SF is in Appendix B.

Demographic Form.

Older adults' demographic information will be measured last. The GA will ask participants to provide the following information: age, gender, race, ethnic group, marital status, highest completed education, if they are currently followed by a health care practitioner for their osteoarthritis and osteoarthritis related pain. The Demographic Form is in Appendix C.

Content Analysis

Krippendorff's[64] components for content analysis will be used to conduct the content analysis of older adults' responses to the practitioner's question about pain and the two follow up questions. The content analysis components include unitizing, sampling, coding, and inferring. The way in which each of the components will be used in the analysis is described below.

Unitizing.

The unit of analysis for the content analysis will be any word or phrase that describes one of the a priori criteria. One point will be given for each word or phrase describing a criterion. Repeated use of the same word or phrase will be counted only the initial time to avoid inflating the communication score. Each distinctly different word or phrase about the same criterion will be credited with one point. The statement, "I start each day off by taking two Tylenol and placing a hot pack on my knee while I eat my breakfast." would be coded for current pain treatments with one point for the Tylenol and one point for the hot pack. One additional point would be coded for the word knee, which addressed the pain location criterion.

Sampling.

All transcripts of older adults' response to the way that the nurse practitioner asked them about their pain will constitute the sample for content analysis of included pain information. The initial practitioner question will be skipped over on the audiotape and omitted from the transcript. The persons conducting the content analysis will remain blind to participants' condition until the content

Principal Investigator/Program Director (Last, First, Middle): McDonald, Deborah Dillon

analysis is complete, at which time the experimental condition will be identified directly from the audiotape. Text will be read at the level of words and phrases to identify important content for management of osteoarthritis pain. The same process will be used for responses to the practitioner question asking if there is anything further they want to say (omitted pain information). The same process will be used a third time for responses to the final practitioner question about if there is anything further about their pain that they would like to say (omitted pain information).

Coding.
The American Pain Society (2002) *Guidelines for the Management of Pain in Osteoarthritis, Rheumatoid Arthritis, and Juvenile Chronic Arthritis*[8] will be used to identify important osteoarthritis pain management content included or omitted from older adults' transcribed responses to the practitioner's pain communication question. The Guidelines are the culmination of expert review of the Cochrane Collaboration Reviews, additional published systematic reviews, American Pain Society (APS) commissioned reviews, and reviews conducted by the expert 10 member interdisciplinary panel and APS staff. The a priori osteoarthritis pain management criteria include:

1. Type of pain (nociceptive/neuropathic);
2. Quality of pain;
3. Pain source;
4. Pain location;
5. Pain intensity;
6. Duration/time course;
7. Pain affect;
8. Effect on personal lifestyle;
9. Functional status;
10. Current pain treatments;
11. Use of recommended glucosamine sulfate;
12. Effectiveness of prescribed treatments;
13. Prescription analgesic side effects;
14. Weight management to ideal body weight;
15. Exercise regimen, or physical therapy and/or occupational therapy;
16. Indications for surgery.

QRS N6 (NUD*IST) will be used to manage the content analysis and organize the coded data. The node system will be composed of the a priori codes listed above. Included pain communication content (responses to the first practitioner question) will be coded by highlighting the content and marking the content with a number representing the criterion. The criterion number will be placed at the end of the word or phrase (e.g. pain in my right knee 4; I take Tylenol extra strength10; The Tylenol dulls the pain a little bit 12). A subscript will indicate if the item is the first, second, and so on item for the criterion described by that participant. After coding each participant's responses, the coder will check all coded content on the same criterion to identify repeated instances of coding identical content. Identical content will be coded only one time for each participant. The same procedure will be used to code omitted pain communication content (responses to the second and third practitioner questions). Content will be coded separately for the second question and for the third practitioner question.

Reducing.
Coded data will be entered into an SPSS database. The number of distinct content for each criterion will be entered into the database. Separate sets of variables will be entered for content analyzed from responses to the practitioner pain question, responses to the practitioner's general

follow up question, and responses to the practitioner's pain specific follow up question. Frequencies will be used to further reduce the data. The included pain communication score will be calculated by summing all of the important pain content described by participants in response to the practitioner pain question (first question). The omitted important pain information will be calculated by summing all important pain content described by participants in response to the practitioner's two follow up questions.

Inferring.

The American Pain Society (2002) *Guidelines for the Management of Pain in Osteoarthritis, Rheumatoid Arthritis, and Juvenile Chronic Arthritis*[8] provides the research-based criteria for coding the data. The PI will train the GA to conduct the content analysis. The PI and the GA will independently code all of the responses, remaining blind to participants' conditions. The PI and GA will compare the codes. The PI will document each instance of coding disagreement. Disagreements will be resolved through discussion. Inter-rater reliability will be calculated, as described in the analysis section.

Summary of the Methods

Older adults with chronic osteoarthritis pain will be randomly assigned to one of three practitioner pain communication conditions. Participants will watch and verbally respond to a video clip of a practitioner asking them about their pain with either an open-ended question without social desirability bias; closed-ended question without social desirability bias; or open-ended question with social desirability bias. All participants will respond next to a video clip of the practitioner asking them if there is anything further they want to say, and finally to a video clip of the practitioner asking them if there is anything more about their pain that they want to say. The GA will administer the BPI-SF to half of each of the three groups prior to watching the videos, and to the remaining half of each group after responding to the final video, to measure and control for present pain differences in participants across groups, and to counterbalance the effect of the BPI-SF measure. Verbal responses to all three video clips will be audio taped and transcribed. Important included pain information (responses to the first video) and omitted pain information (responses to the second and third videos) will be content analyzed by two trained independent raters, blind to participants' conditions. A priori criteria derived from national osteoarthritis pain management guidelines will be used to code the responses. Our methods provide a context with strong experimental realism to test theory driven pain communication skills for the effect on information included and omitted by older adults important in managing osteoarthritis pain.

Analysis

The characteristics of the sample will be summarized and described with frequencies, (and means and standard deviations for interval level measures) for the descriptive data. These data includes age, gender, race, highest education completed, and if participants are currently followed by a health care practitioner for their osteoarthritis and osteoarthritis related pain.

Inter-rater reliability will be calculated using Krippendorff's alpha to compare the equivalence of coding between the independent raters, the PI and GA. Krippendorff's alpha is calculated by the following formula, $\alpha = 1 - (D_o/D_e)$ where D_o is the measure of observed disagreement and D_e is the measure of the disagreement expected by chance. Krippendorff's alpha corrects for chance, and can be used with large sample sizes.[64]

A check for randomization to condition will be conducted prior to the main analyses to test for significant pre-existing differences between older adult participants in the three conditions:

1. health care practitioner open-ended without social desirability bias pain question;
2. health care practitioner closed-ended without social desirability bias pain question;
3. health care practitioner open-ended with social desirability bias pain question.

Analyses of variance (ANOVA) will test for age differences between the three groups. Cross tabulation using the chi-square statistic will be used to test for differences between the groups for gender, race, ethnicity, highest education achieved, followed/not followed for osteoarthritis by a health care practitioner, and followed/not followed for osteoarthritis pain by a health care practitioner.

The timing effect of the BPI-SF will be tested by ANOVAs on the variables of pain intensity, interference with activities, and responses to practitioner questions about pain (included and omitted information). Each ANOVA will have two factors (groups and timing) and their interaction. Thus, a single ANOVA will test for group differences on a specific dependent variable, timing differences, and the possibility of an interaction, i.e., that one of the groups showed a stronger timing effect than the other. However, a strong interaction is not expected.

Hypothesis

Hypothesis: Older adults asked about their pain with an open-ended question without social desirability bias will describe more important pain information and omit less information than older adults asked about their pain with a closed-ended question without social desirability or an open-ended question with social desirability bias.

The hypothesis will be tested with a multivariate analysis of covariance (MANCOVA). The grouping variable consists of three groups: 1. health care practitioner open-ended without social desirability bias pain question; 2. health care practitioner closed-ended without social desirability bias pain question; 3. health care practitioner open-ended with social desirability bias pain question. The two participant response measures will comprise the input for the multivariate vectors for comparison. The two response measures include: 1. the content analysis summed scores of important osteoarthritis pain information described by the participant in response to the practitioner's pain question; and 2. important omitted pain information measured by responses to the second and third questions about any further information. Present pain intensity and pain interference with activity will be used as covariates to control for pain differences between participants. If timing of the BPI-SF is significant, timing of the BPI-SF will be entered as a covariate. If important pre-existing group differences occur during the preliminary analyses, the variable will also be used as an additional covariate to adjust for the differences. Descriptive discriminant function analysis (DFA) following significant results from the MANCOVA will provide a multivariate way to interpret group differences that result from MANCOVA,[65] maintaining a more rigorous analysis than possible with post hoc univariate analyses. Post hoc DFA involves examination of the correlation between the discriminant function and the pain communication variables, examination of the canonical discriminant function coefficients for lack of redundancy, interpretation of the group centroids, and group membership classification.

Summary of the Analyses

A summary of the data analysis includes: 1) describing and summarizing the participating older adults with descriptive statistics and frequencies; 2) computing the inter-rater reliability for coding participant responses; 3) checking that randomization to condition resulted in no significant differences between the groups; 4) checking that the timing of administering the BPI-SF had no significant effect; 5) testing the hypothesis related to important pain information provided and omitted by participants with a MANCOVA, using present pain intensity and pain interference with activities as covariates, and using DFA as a multivariate technique to interpret the differences if the MANCOVA is significant.

Study Summary

Our study provides an innovative controlled test of how older adults respond to pain communication strategies used by health care practitioners. Following informed consent, older adults with osteoarthritis pain will be randomly assigned to one of three groups. Participants will watch and verbally respond to: (1) one of three video clips of a practitioner asking them about their pain (a. open-ended and without social desirability bias, b. closed-ended and without social desirability bias, or c. open-ended and with social desirability bias); (2) a video clip asking, "What else can you tell me?" (3) a video clip asking, "What else can you tell me about your pain, aches, soreness or discomfort?" All responses to the videos will be audio taped. The GA will counterbalance the BPI-SF measure by orally administering the BPI-SF to a randomly selected half of each of the three groups prior to the videos, or after responding to the final video. The GA will administer the demographic measure as the final measure. The GA will debrief each participant, thank them for their contribution to the study, and compensate each person for their time with a $20 money order and a copy of the Arthritis Foundation *Managing Your Pain* publication. Content analysis will be conducted on the transcribed audiotapes to identify important pain information included in the response to the initial pain question (included information), and important information included in the response to the two follow up questions (omitted information). The summed scores for included and omitted information will be entered into the MANCOVA comparing the three groups for differences in older adult pain communication responses, using current pain intensity and pain interference with activities as covariates. The goal is to identify practitioner pain communication strategies that allow patients to describe pain information important for guiding effective pain management, and to substantiate what pain information is missed when practitioners use less effective pain communication. The results will provide empirically tested theory based communication strategies that can be used in pain communication education for patients. Our study has the potential to inform curriculum across a number of health care practitioner groups, including nursing and medicine. Effective communication between older adults and health care practitioners provides the link for significantly reducing or eliminating pain. Table 2 presents the timeline for completing our study.

Table 2
Study Timeline

Activity	Time						
	5/1/06	8/1/06	9/1/06	8/31/07	12/1/07	3/1/08	4/30/08
1. Video clips developed, reviewed for face validity, & edited	X_1						
2. SuperLab software loaded & tested		X_2					
3. GA trained, data collected & transcribed			X_3				
4. Content analysis				X_4			
5. Statistical analyses					X_5		
6. Manuscript preparation						X_6	
7. R21 final report							X_7

Note. The time for a listed activity extends from the start date of that activity to the start date of the following activity.

Continuation Format Page
—

Principal Investigator/Program Director (Last, First, Middle): McDonald, Deborah Dillon
E. Human Subjects Research

Overview

The study involves the participation of community dwelling older adult with osteoarthritis pain but no cancer pain (malignant pain). The risks, adequacy of protection, and potential benefits will be presented, followed by the importance of the knowledge that might be gained. The GA will recruit older adults from elder independent housing sites in Hartford, New Haven, Bridgeport, and suburban areas in Connecticut.

1. Risk to the Subjects

Human Subjects Involvement and Characteristics.

The GA will recruit community dwelling adults, age 60 and older who have osteoarthritis pain but no malignant pain who speak, read, and understand English. Recruitment will be through housing newsletter announcements, posted materials, and direct contact in the public areas of the housing sites. We selected Hartford, Bridgeport, and New Haven as sites for our study to increase representation of Black or African American, Hispanic, and Asian Americans. Older adults interested in participating in the study will be screened for eligibility, receive informed consent, and make an appointment for the GA to conduct the study in the older adults' home. Older adults will be recruited until a total of 300 eligible participants have completed the 15-minute study. The age range is anticipated to be from 60 to 90.

Before beginning the study, the GA will again provide oral informed consent and include written consent with an enlarged print consent form. The GA will instruct the participant to listen and respond in turn to each of three separate video tape clips and press the buzzer after responding to the third and final video clip. Participants will be randomly assigned to one of the three treatment conditions by the SuperLab 3.0 software. All responses will be audio taped. When the participant is ready, and after the video sound level has been adjusted, the GA will start the video clip and leave the room. The first video will begin 15 seconds later. A video clip of a health care practitioner will ask participants about their pain in one of three ways. After responding to the practitioner, participants will touch the screen and view and listen to the practitioner ask them, "What else can you tell me?" After responding to the practitioner, participants will touch the screen again and view and listen to the third and final clip of the practitioner asking them, "What else can you tell me about your pain, aches, soreness or discomfort?" After completing their response, participants will ring the buzzer and the GA will return to the room and turn off the audio tape recorder. The GA will orally administer the BPI-SF to measure present pain, if the BPI-SF was not administered prior to the videotapes, and administer the Demographic Form as the final measure. The GA will then debrief the participant, checking for hypothesis guessing, more fully explaining the study, assessing for any discomfort, and requesting that they do not talk about the study in case others wish to participate. Participation in the study will be complete after the debriefing. Participants will be thanked and given the Arthritis Foundation publication, *Managing Your Pain*,[61] and a $20 money order for participating in the study. Older adults are exclusively studied because they have been identified as having more difficulty in communicating about their pain.[49] The 80% incidence of osteoarthritis in people over 75[58] makes older adults highly vulnerable to pain problems, and a high priority for pain communication studies. Osteoarthritis occurs much less frequently in younger and middle aged adults, and is unlikely to occur in children.

Source of Materials.

Three instruments will be used to gather individually identifiable data for the purpose of the study. The GA will audiotape participants' verbal responses to the three videos which will be content

PHS 398/2590 (Rev. 09/04)   Page 29

analyzed to extract the two dependent variables, included and omitted important pain information. The GA will orally administer the BPI-SF to measure the two covariates, present pain intensity, and pain interference with activities. The GA will orally administer the Demographic Form to record demographic variables including age, gender, race, ethnic group, marital status, highest completed education, if they are currently followed by a health care practitioner for their osteoarthritis and osteoarthritis related pain. Names will not be linked to the data. A number code will be used to link the audio taped responses and the responses to the BPI-SF and the Demographic Form for each participant. The GA will be absent from the room when participants are audio taped. Only the PI and GA will have access to the data. The audiotapes and the written data will be kept locked in the PI's office at the University of Connecticut. The data will be analyzed on the PI's university office computer, which is secured with password protection. The data will be collected specifically for the proposed study.

Potential Risks.

The intervention involves minimal risk. The practitioner questions comprising the experimental manipulation are commonly used questions about pain that participants have likely responded to before during health care visits. The BPI-SF questions about pain include common areas of pain assessment such as pain intensity, and how the pain interferes with daily activities. The entire study takes approximately 15 minutes to complete. The study will take place in the older adults' homes at a time convenient for them. All participants will be debriefed to check for any psychological discomfort with the study, and to allow participants to withdraw if they so wish. If at any time older adults do feel burdened, they are free to withdraw from the study.

2. Adequacy of Protection Against Risks

Recruitment and Informed Consent.

The GA will recruit participants through housing newsletter announcements, posted materials and direct contact in the public areas of the independent elder housing sites. Older adults interested in participating in the study will be screened for eligibility, receive informed consent, and make an appointment for the GA to conduct the study in their home.

The GA will use the cover story that we are testing the feasibility of helping people prepare for their health care office visit while waiting in the office for their appointment. The GA will make the following statement. "We are testing whether asking patients to respond to a videotaped health care practitioner asking questions about your health just prior to an office visit helps you communicate better during the office visit." The mild deception is warranted to increase the experimental realism and decrease response bias. The GA will explain that the study involves privately watching three brief video clips of a practitioner asking them health questions on a laptop computer screen. Participants will verbally respond after each clip and responses will be audio taped. When they have finished responding to the third clip, the GA will return to the room and ask them questions about pain problems, and general information such as their age and marital status. Their participation will then be complete and no other contact will be requested. The entire study takes about 15 minutes. No names will be linked with any information provided by participants. All information will remain confidential. The information will be kept secure in the University of Connecticut office of Deborah Dillon McDonald. Older adults will be reminded that participation is voluntary. They do not have to be in the study if they do not wish to be. They can withdraw from the study at any time without risk. They will be given an enlarged type copy of the written consent form to keep. The consent form will contain the name and contact office telephone number of the PI and the University of Connecticut IRB, if participants have questions. Older adults willing to participate will be asked to sign the consent form after reviewing the form and receiving informed consent from the GA.

Protection Against Risk.

Several safeguards have been designed into the study to protect participants from risk. The GA will not be present in the room while participants respond to the video clips. After completing the demographic information, each participant will be debriefed by the GA. The study will be completely explained to participants, along with the reason for the mild deception. Participants will be checked for concern or distress about the mild deception, and reminded that they are free to withdraw. No names will be written on any of the collected data. Identification numbers will be assigned by the GA and used to link the three sources of data from each individual. All collected data will be kept confidential and will be locked in the PI's university office.

A referral protocol will be followed in cases where participants describe moderate or greater present pain problems (pain levels of 4 or greater on the 0 to 10 BPI-SF). The protocol will include the registered nurse GA encouraging: (1) the person to contact their primary care provider to assess and treat the problem; (2) if the person has no primary care provider, a list of names and telephone numbers of local accredited ambulatory care clinics will be given if the person; (3) if the person has no insurance, the name and telephone number for a local community health clinic providing sliding scale health care will be given to the person.

3. Potential Benefits of the Proposed Research to the Subjects and Others

Testing how older adults respond to the way health care practitioners ask them about their pain, and whether important information is included or omitted provides a critical starting point for educating patients and practitioners about more effective ways to communicate about pain. Patients who are able to communicate important information about their pain are more likely to be prescribed more effective pain treatments and achieve greater pain relief. Consumer pain management resources such as the Mayday Foundation web site and existing coaching interventions could easily incorporate the communication strategies. The effective pain communication strategies could be incorporated into nursing, medical, pharmacy, and allied health curricula.

Older adults participating in the study might become more aware of the importance of communicating important aspects of their pain to their health care practitioner. The experience of responding to the practitioner might provide a helpful rehearsal for talking with their health care practitioner. The BPI-SF indicates several important components for pain assessment that participants could include when discussing their pain problems. All participants will be given a copy of the Arthritis Foundation *Managing Your Pain* 2003 publication. The publication provides helpful information for decreasing osteoarthritis pain, and has been approved by the American College of Rheumatology. A registered nurse GA will collect the data. The GA will use the referral protocol to encourage participants to get effective treatment for their pain, if participants describe moderate or greater pain intensity.

The risks are minimal for older adult participants. The study takes place in participants' homes at a time convenient to them. We use a mild deception to maintain experimental realism and to avoid response bias. Participants are debriefed and given the opportunity to withdraw from the study at any time, including after the debriefing. The burden for participants is low. The time requirement is 15 minutes, and only verbal responses are required.

4. Importance of Knowledge Gained

Pain communication has been identified as important for effective pain management, but specific communication factors contributing to effective pain management have not been tested. Our study takes the novel approach of testing specific pain communication skills derived from Communication Accommodation theory attuning strategies, for the effect on important included and omitted pain information described by older adults with osteoarthritis pain. Previous pain communication research has generally taken a macro approach, testing general pain communication content and/or increasing patients' confidence in communicating with their health care practitioner. We take a micro approach and link the effect of two specific pain communication strategies, discourse management (open ended/closed ended) and interpersonal control (with social desirability/without social desirability bias), to pain information identified by the American Pain Society[8] as important information in the management of osteoarthritis pain. Our study provides the opportunity to advance our understanding of pain communication by testing Communication Accommodation theory, and improve pain management by incorporating into health care practice the simple strategies tested in our study. The strategies can be taught to health care practitioners and older adults with chronic pain. The results might have implications for acute pain and malignant pain communication.

The risk for older adult participants is minimal. Participation requires only 15 minutes. Older adults are asked to respond to questions similar to those encountered during their usual health care.

Inclusion of Women and Minorities

Selection criteria for our study include women and minorities. Our selection criteria include any community dwelling adult age 60 or older and who have pain from osteoarthritis who can speak, read, and understand English. Osteoarthritis commonly occurs with adults, age 60 and older.[8] People with cancer pain are excluded from the study. Older adults are more vulnerable to problems communicating about their pain. Osteoarthritis is a pain producing condition that crosses gender, racial, and ethnic groups, with high incidence in the older adult population. Women and men will both be recruited for the study. The selection criteria include Hispanics, and also include African or Black Americans, Asian Americans, and members of other minority groups.

In an effort to include more participants from minority groups, independent living housing sites will be included from Bridgeport and New Haven, Connecticut. According to the most recent census data, Bridgeport consists of 30.8% Black or African Americans, and 31.9% Hispanic, and New Haven consists of 37.4% Black or African Americans, and 21.4% Hispanic or Latinos.[66-67] We expect that recruitment in these two cities will increase the ethnic and racial representation of our sample.

Principal Investigator/Program Director (Last, First, Middle):   McDonald, Deborah Dillon

Targeted/Planned Enrollment Table

This report format should NOT be used for data collection from study participants.

Study Title: Older Adults' Response to Health Care Practitioner Pain Communication

Total Planned Enrollment: 300

TARGETED/PLANNED ENROLLMENT: Number of Subjects			
Ethnic Category	**Sex/Gender**		
	Females	**Males**	**Total**
Hispanic or Latino	25	12	37
Not Hispanic or Latino	184	79	263
Ethnic Category: Total of All Subjects *	209	91	300
Racial Categories			
American Indian/Alaska Native	4	2	6
Asian	8	4	12
Native Hawaiian or Other Pacific Islander	4	2	6
Black or African American	35	14	49
White	156	71	227
Racial Categories: Total of All Subjects *	207	93	300

* The "Ethnic Category: Total of All Subjects" must be equal to the "Racial Categories: Total of All Subjects."

Principal Investigator/Program Director (Last, First, Middle): McDonald, Deborah Dillon

Inclusion of Children

Exclusion of children from our study is justified because the research aim is to test how older adults with osteoarthritis pain respond to pain communication strategies used by health care practitioners. Older adults have been identified as more vulnerable to pain communication problems, and have a high incidence of osteoarthritis, a painful condition associated with aging. Children are much less likely to suffer from osteoarthritis pain, and would not allow generalization of data.

F. Vertebrate Animals

N/A

G. Literature Cited

1. Davis G, Hiemenz M, White T. Barriers to managing chronic pain of older adults with arthritis. *J Nurs Scholarsh.* 2002;*34*:121-6.
2. de Rond M, Wit R, Van Dam F, Muller M. A pain monitoring program for nurses: effects on communication, assessment and documentation of patients' pain. *J Pain Symptom Manage.* 2000;20:424-439.
3. McDonald D, McNulty J, Erickson K, Weiskopf C. Communicating pain and pain management needs after surgery. *Appl Nurs Res.* 2000;13:70-75.
4. Sherwood G, Adams-McNeill J, Starck P, Nieto B, Thompson C. Qualitative assessment of hospitalized patients' satisfaction with pain management. *Res Nurs Health.* 2000;23:486-495.
5. Bertakis K, Azari R, Callahan E. Patient pain in primary care: Factors that influence physician diagnosis. *Ann Fam Med.* 2004;2:224-230.
6. Apfelbaum J, Chen C, Mehta S, Gan, Tong J. Postoperative pain experience: Results From a national survey suggest postoperative pain continues to be undermanaged. *Anesth Analg.* 2003;97:534-540.
7. Leveille S, Ling S, Hochberg M, Resnick H, Bandeen-Roche K, Won A, Guralnik J. Widespread musculoskeletal pain and the progression of disability in older disabled women. *Ann Intern Med.* 2001;135:1038-46.
8. American Pain Society. Guidelines for the Management of Pain in Osteoarthritis, Rheumatoid *Arthritis, and Juvenile Chronic Arthritis.* Glenview, IL: American Pain Society; 2002.
9. Desbiens N, Wu A, Yasui, Y, Lynn J, Alzola C, Wenger N, Connors A, Phillips R, Fulkerson W. Patient empowerment and feedback did not decrease pain in seriously ill hospitalized adults. *Pain.* 1998;75:237-246.
10. Carlson J, Youngblood R, Dalton J, Blau W, Lindley C. Is patient satisfaction a legitimate outcome of pain management? *J Pain Symptom Manage.* 2003; 25(3):264-275.
11. Detmar S, Muller M, Wever L, Schornagel J, Aaronson N. Patient-physician communication during outpatient palliative treatment visits. *JAMA.* 2001;*285*: 1351-1357.
12. Kimberlin C, Brushwood D, Allen W, Radson E, Wilson D. Cancer patient and caregiver experiences: communication and pain management issues. *J Pain Symptom Manage.* 2004;28:566-578.
13. Rogers M, Todd C. The 'right kind' of pain: talking about symptoms in outpatient oncology consultations. *Palliat Med.* 2000;14:299-307.
14. Kenny D. Constructions of chronic pain in doctor-patient relationships: bridging the communication chasm. *Patient Educ Couns.* 2004;52:297-305.
15. Branch M, Carlson C, Okeson J. Influence of biased clinician statements on patient report of referred pain. *J Orofac Pain.* 2000;15:120-127.
16. Jairath N, Kowal N. Patient expectations and anticipated responses to postsurgical

PHS 398/2590 (Rev. 09/04)   Page 34

Principal Investigator/Program Director (Last, First, Middle): McDonald, Deborah Dillon

pain. *J Holist Nurs.* 1999;17(2);184-196.

17. Zalon M. Pain in frail, elderly women after surgery. *Image J Nurs Sch.*1997; 29, 21-26.
18. Manias E, Botti M, Bucknall T. Observation of pain assessment and management – the complexities of clinical practice. *J Clin Nurs.* 2002;11:724-733.
19. Schumacher K, West C, Dodd M, Paul S, Tripathy D, Koo P, Miaskowski C. Pain management autobiographies and reluctance to use opioids for cancer pain management. *Cancer Nurs.* 2002;25(2):125-133.
20. Ward S, Goldberg N, Miller-McCauley V, Mueller C, Nolan A, Pawlik-Plank D, Robbins A, Stormoen D, Weissman D. Patient-related barriers to management of cancer pain. *Pain.* 52: 319-324.
21. Kemper J. Pain management of older adults after discharge from outpatient surgery. *Pain Manage Nurs.* 2002;3(4):141-153.
22. Closs S, Briggs M. Patients' verbal descriptions of pain and discomfort following orthopaedic surgery. Int *J Nurs Stud.* 2002;39:563-72.
23. Oliver J, Kravitz R, Kaplan S, Meyers F. Individualized patient education and coaching to improve pain control among cancer outpatients. *J Clin Oncol.* 2001;19:2206-2212.
24. Miaskowski C, Dodd M, West C, Schumacher K, Paul S, Tripathy D, Koo P. Randomized clinical trial of the effectiveness of a self-care intervention to improve cancer pain management. *J Clin Oncol.* 2004;22:1713-1720.
25. White M, Bonvicini K. Bayer Institute for Health Care Communication *annotated bibliography for clinician patient communication to enhance health outcomes,* accessed 1/26/05, http://www.bayerinstitute.org/pdfs/biblio/CPC%20Bibliography-2-10-2005.doc; 2003.
26. Beckman H, Frankel R. The effect of physician behavior on the collection of data. *Ann Intern Med.* 1984;101:692-696.
27. Marvel M, Epstein R, Flowers K, Beckman H. Soliciting the patient's agenda have we improved? *JAMA.* 1999;281:283-287.
28. Roter D, Hall J, Kern D, Barker L, Cole K, Roca R. Improving physicians' interviewing skills and reducing patients' emotional distress. *Arch Intern Med.* 1995;155:1877-1884.
29. Roter D, Hall J, Aoki Y. Physician gender effects in medical communication a meta-analytic review. *JAMA.* 2002;288:756-764.
30. Street R. Information-giving in medical consultations: the influence of patients' communicative styles and personal characteristics. *Soc Sci Med.* 1991;32:541-548.
31. Street R. Communicative styles and adaptations in physician-parent consultations. *Soc Sci Med.* 1992;34:1155-1163.
32. Hall, J, Roter D. Do patients talk differently to male and female physicians? A meta-analytic review. *Patient Educ Couns.* 2002;48:217-224.
33. Cegala D, Post D, McClure L. The effects of patient communication skills training on the discourse of older patients during a primary care interview. *JAGS.* 2001;49:1505-1511.
34. Thompson S, Nanni C, Schwankovsky L. Patient-oriented interventions to improve communication in a medical office visit. *Health Psychol.* 1990;9:390-404.
35. Anderson L, DeVellis B, DeVellis R. Effects of modeling on patient communication satisfaction and knowledge. *Med Care.* 1987;25:1044-1056.
36. Robinson E, Whitefield M. Improving the efficiency of patients' comprehension monitoring: a way of increasing patients' participation in general practice consultations. *Soc Sci Med.* 1985;21:915-919.
37. Tran A, Haidet P, Street R, O'Malley K, Martin F, Ashton C. Empowering communication: a community-based intervention for patients. *Patient Educ Couns.* 2004;52:113-121.
38. Kaplan S, Greenfield S, Ware J. Assessing the effects of physician-patient interactions on the outcomes of chronic disease. *Med Care.* 1989;27:S110 – S127.

Principal Investigator/Program Director (Last, First, Middle): McDonald, Deborah Dillon

39. Giamberardino M. (Ed.). *Pain 2002 – an updated review refresher course syllabus 10th world congress on pain*. Seattle, WA: International Association for the Study of Pain; 2002.

40. Turner G, Weiner D. Essential components of a medical student curriculum on chronic pain management in older adults: Results of a modified Delphi process. *Pain Med*. 2002;3:240-252.

41. Roter D, Larson S, Shnitzky H, Chernoff R, Serwint J, Adamo G, Wissow L. Use of an innovative video feedback technique to enhance communication skills training. *Med Educ*. 2004;38: 145-157.

42. Moral R, Alamo M, Jurado M, Torres L. Effectiveness of a learner-centered training programme for primary care physicians in using a patient-centered consultation style. *Fam Pract*. 2001;18:60-63.

43. Ryan E, Hamilton J, See S. Patronizing the old: How do younger and older adults respond to baby talk in the nursing home? *Int J Aging Hum Dev*. 1994;39:21-32.

44. Fox S, Giles H. Accommodating intergenerational contact: A critique and theoretical model. *J Aging Stud*. 1993:7:423-451.

45. Giles H. Accent mobility. A model and some data. *Anthro Ling*. 1973;15:87-105.

46. Coupland N, Coupland J, Giles H, Henwood K. Accommodating the elderly: Invoking and extending a theory. *Lang Soc*. 1988;17:1-41.
Lawrence Erlbaum Associates Inc; 1988.

47. McDonald D. Gender and ethnic stereotyping and narcotic analgesic administration. *Res Nurs Health*. 1994;17:45-49.

48. McDonald D. Nurses' memory of patient's pain. Int *J Nurs Stud*. 1996;23:487-494.

49. McDonald D, Sterling R. Acute pain reduction strategies used by well older adults. Int *J Nurs Stud*.1998;35:265-70.

50. McDonald D. Postoperative pain after hospital discharge. *Clin Nurs Res*. 1999;8: 347-359.

51. McDonald D Weiskopf C. Adult patients' postoperative pain descriptions and responses to the Short-Form McGill Pain Questionnaire. *Clin Nurs Res*. 2001;10:442-452.

52. McDonald D, Freeland M, Thomas G, Moore J. Testing a preoperative pain management intervention for older adults. *Res Nurs Health*. 2001;24:402-409.

53. McDonald D, Molony S. Postoperative pain communication skills for older adults. *Wes J Nurs Res*. 2004;26:836-852.

54. McDonald D, Thomas G, Livingston K, Severson J. Assisting older adults to communicate their pain after surgery. *Clin Nurs Res*. 2005;14:109-126.

55. Cohen J. Statistical Power analysis for the Behavioral Sciences, 2nd ed., Hillsdale, NJ: Lawrence Erlbaum Associates, Inc; 1988.

56. Stevens J. *Applied Multivariate Statistics for the Social Sciences*. Mahwah, New Jersey: Lawrence Erlbaum Associates, Inc; 1996.

57. National Institutes of Health. National Institute of Arthritis and Musculoskeletal and Skin Diseases. *Handout on health: Osteoarthritis*. 2005. Accessed, 4/21/05, http://www.niams.nih.gov/hi/topics/arthritis/oahandout.htm.

58. Sharma L. Epidemiology of osteoarthritis. In Moskowitz R, Howell O, Altman R, Buckwalter J, V Goldberg eds. *Osteoarthritis: Diagnosis and Medical-surgical Management* (3rd ed., pp. 3 – 17). Philadelphia: Saunders; 2001.

59. Resnick B, Inguito P, Yahiro J, Hawkes W, Werner M, Zimmerman S, Magaziner J. Treatment fidelity in behavior change research: A case example. *Nurs Res*. 2005;54:139-143.

60. Roter D. Observations on methodological and measurement challenges in the assessment of communication during medical exchanges. *Patient Educ Couns*. 2003;50:17-21.

61. Arthritis Foundation. *Managing your Pain*. Atlanta, GA: Arthritis Foundation, Inc; 2003.

62. Daut R, Cleeland C, Flanery R. Development of the Wisconsin Brief Pain Questionnaire to assess pain in cancer and other diseases. *Pain*. 1983;17:197-210.

63. Zalon M. Comparison of pain measures in surgical patients. *J Nurs Meas*. 1999;7:135-152.

Principal Investigator/Program Director (Last, First, Middle): McDonald, Deborah Dillon

64. Krippendorff K. *Content Analysis an Introduction to Its Methodology.* 2nd ed. Thousand Oaks, CA: Sage Publications; 2004.
65. Huberty, C. *Applied discriminant analysis.* New York: Wiley; 1994.
66. U.S. Census Bureau. Profile of general demographic characteristics: 2000 data set: Census 2000 summary file1 (SF 1) 100-percent data geographic area: Bridgeport city, Connecticut, accessed 4/5/05, http://factfinder.census.gov/servlet/SAFFFacts?_event=ChangeGeoContext&geo_id=16000US0908000&_geoContext=&_street=&_county=Bridgeport&_cityTown=Bridgeport&_state=04000US09&_zip=&_lang=en&_sse=on&ActiveGeoDiv=&_useEV=&pctxt=fph&pgsl=010.
67. U.S. Census Bureau. Profile of general demographic characteristics: 2000 data set: Census 2000 summary file1 (SF 1) 100-percent data geographic area: New Haven city, Connecticut, accessed 4/5/05, http://factfinder.census.gov/servlet/SAFFFacts?_event=ChangeGeoContext&geo_id=16000US0952000&_geoContext=&_street=&_county=New+Haven&_cityTown=New+Haven&_state=04000US09&_zip=&_lang=en&_sse=on&ActiveGeoDiv=&_useEV=&pctxt=fph&pgsl=010

H. Consortium/Contractual Arrangements

N/A

I. Resource Sharing

N/A

J. Consultants

Leonard Katz, PhD, Consultant (Y2-1%) will advise the PI regarding statistical analyses.

Joel Rosiene, PhD, Consultant (Y1-5%) will program the SuperLab software and the videos onto the study laptop computer. He will test the software to randomize participants to condition, and present the videos.

Letters Confirming Role in the Project
Leonard Katz
Joel Rosiene

Letters of Commitment from Sites
P.C. Smith Towers and Betty Knox Apartments
Capitol Towers
Harborview Towers
Park Ridge I & II
Fireside Apartments
Tower One/Tower East

SUMMARY STATEMENT
(Privileged Communication)   *Release Date:* 11/03/2005

ALEXIS BAKOS
301.594.2542
bakosa@mail.nih.gov

Application Number: 1 R21 NR009848-01

MCDONALD, DEBORAH D PHD
UNIVERSITY OF CONNECTICUT
SCHOOL OF NURSING
231 GLENBROOK ROAD, UNIT 2026
STORRS, CT 06269-2026

Review Group: NSAA
Nursing Science: Adults and Older Adults Study Section

Meeting Date: 10/13/2005   *RFA/PA:* PA03-152
Council: JAN 2006   *PCC:* GXXAB
Requested Start: 05/01/2006
                                Dual IC(s): AG

Project Title: Older Adults' Response to Health Care Practitioner Pain Communication

SRG Action: Priority Score: 167
Human Subjects: 44-Human subjects involved - SRG concerns
Animal Subjects: 10-No live vertebrate animals involved for competing appl.
Gender: 1A-Both genders, scientifically acceptable
Minority: 1A-Minorities and non-minorities, scientifically acceptable
Children: 3A-No children included, scientifically acceptable
Clinical Research - not NIH-defined Phase III Trial

Project Year	Direct Costs Requested	Estimated Total Cost
1	100,000	148,000
2	75,000	111,000
TOTAL	175,000	259,000

ADMINISTRATIVE BUDGET NOTE: The budget shown is the requested budget and has not been adjusted to reflect any recommendations made by reviewers. If an award is planned, the costs will be calculated by Institute grants management staff based on the recommendations outlined below in the COMMITTEE BUDGET RECOMMENDATIONS section.

1R21NR009848-01 MCDONALD, DEBORAH

PROTECTION OF HUMAN SUBJECTS UNACCEPTABLE

RESUME AND SUMMARY OF DISCUSSION: The goal of this application is to identify practitioner pain communication strategies that allow patients to describe pain information important for guiding effective pain management and to substantiate what pain information is missed when practitioners use less effective pain communication. This is a very interesting new application form an experienced young investigator using a posttest-only double blind experiment to test type of provider communication on audio taped patient responses. The methods are highly innovative and the application is significant. The design and methods are creative and innovative and the analyses are appropriate to the aims of the project. There may be some introduced bias from the pre-intervention use of the BPI. And, the study protocol could be better presented. The previous work and commitment of this investigator to studying communication about pain and the well-prepared research team and strong environment bode well for the application.

DESCRIPTION (provided by applicant): How practitioners communicate with patients about their pain has been overlooked as a factor contributing to effective pain management. Eliciting important pain information from patients enables practitioners to prescribe more specific pain treatments, and significantly decrease pain. The aim of our study is to test the effect of practitioners asking patients an open-ended question about pain that does not encourage a socially desirable response. A posttest only double blind experiment will test how the phrasing of health care practitioners' pain questions, open-ended and without social desirability bias; closed-ended and without social desirability bias; or open-ended and with social desirability bias, affects the pain information provided by people with chronic pain. Three hundred community dwelling older adults with chronic osteoarthritis pain will be randomly assigned to one of the three practitioner pain communication conditions. Older adults will watch and verbally respond to a videotape clip of a practitioner asking the patient about their pain. The clips will be identical except for the pain question asked by the practitioner. After responding to the pain question, all of the older adults will respond to a second videotape clip of the practitioner asking if there is anything further they want to communicate. The older adults will then respond to a third videotape clip asking if there is anything further they want to communicate about their pain. Responses to the three videotape clips will be audiotaped. To control for pain differences between participants, the Brief Pain Inventory Short Form will be administered to measure present pain intensity and pain interference with functional activities. Participants' audiotaped responses will be transcribed and content analyzed using a priori criteria from national guidelines to identify communicated pain information and omitted pain information important for osteoarthritis pain management. The three groups will be compared for the communicated pain information and omitted pain information while controlling for present pain intensity and pain interference with activities. The goal is to identify practitioner pain communication strategies that allow patients to describe pain information important for guiding effective pain management, and to substantiate what pain information is missed when practitioners use less effective pain communication. The results will provide empirically tested communication strategies that can be used in practitioner and patient pain communication education.

CRITIQUE 1:

Significance: Pain communication between patient and practitioner are crucial if the patient's pain is to be adequately treated. This is particularly the case with conditions characterized by chronic pain such as osteoarthritis. Prior research has indicated that pain control is a problem for patients receiving acute care and for patients with chronic conditions characterized by pain who dwell in the community. This research will test communication strategies that can enhance patient and practitioner communication about pain, which could result in better pain control.

Approach: The aim of the study is straightforward, clear and testable. The importance of clear communication to pain control was highlighted in the background and significance section and prior research evidence supports this view. The principal investigator referenced nine studies focused on communication about pain between providers and patients in the preliminary studies section. A post-test only double blind experiment will be used for this study to test how the phrasing of health care practitionersí pain question (open-ended without social desirability, closed-ended without social desirability, or open-ended with social desirability bias) affects the pain information provided by older adults with chronic osteoarthritis pain. Power analysis supports the projected sample size of 300. The random assignment of subjects to the three conditions that will be assessed is a strength of the study as well as keeping the persons who will do the content analysis of data blind to the condition to which each subject will be responding. Use of video taped provider communication scenarios has the advantage of standardizing provider communication to which the subjects would respond. Audio taping of the participantís responses also will ensure that responses are more accurately captured for later analysis. The second part of each practitioner video as described will ask two open-ended questions ñ one more general and one focused on encouraging discussion about pain. This will allow all subjects to ultimately respond to open-ended without social desirability questions. However, this aspect of the intervention is not fully acknowledged in the discussion of the design and the data analysis. Randomization of the administration of the Brief Pain Inventory Short Form for administration prior to or after the presentation of the videos should control for learning effects. Reliability and validity information for the Brief Pain Inventory Short Form was given. The debriefing session should adequately allow for handling of hypothesis guessing and any distress about deception regarding the focus of the study because of the use of a cover story. The content analysis procedure described follows accepted standards. Use of the American Pain Society's "Guidelines for the Management of Pain in Osteoarthritis, Rheumatoid Arthritis, and Juvenile Chronic Arthritis" for coding data will also help to yield a more reliable content analysis process. The approaches to data analysis are detailed and appropriate the address the research hypothesis. Redundancy and some disorganization of content in the design section was sometimes confusing.

Innovation: Patient and provider communication about pain has been a research concern in health care for many years. The uniqueness of this study lies in its focus on assessing specific communication approaches with older persons suffering with chronic pain in the community. The use of videotaped scenarios to which subjects will respond about their pain is a rather unique methodological approach for collecting this type of data.

Investigators: The principal investigator has a track record of publications focused on pain assessment and communicating pain. She has prior NIH funding for a project focused on post-operative pain. She will collaborate with a psychologist who will assist with statistical analysis and with a computer consultant. The research team has the experience to successfully complete the proposed project.

Environment: The University of Connecticut has the research resources to support this project. Participants will be recruited from seven independent living elder housing sites throughout Connecticut. Letters of support are included from the seven sites. The Seven Seas Film Company will produce the three videotapes required for the study.

Overall Evaluation: The proposed study addresses an important area in health care – control of chronic pain in older adults with chronic conditions. The focus on communication about pain could be a cost-effective approach for helping to address this problem if specific communication strategies are found to aid pain control. The proposed study has many strengths including a straightforward and clearly explicated aim, a background section and preliminary studies supportive of the proposed study, a well designed experimental approach, a well operationalized independent variable, a carefully planned data collection protocol, appropriate content analysis procedures, and detailed plans for statistical analysis which should address the study hypothesis. The description of the study protocol was sometimes confusing due to repetitive content that could have been better organized. This is a relative minor limitation given the many strengths of the proposal.

Protection of Human Subjects from Research Risks: This study will require the participation of 300 community dwelling older adults with osteoarthritis pain who are age 60 and older. Recruitment strategies are described. Procedures for obtaining informed consent and protection against risks are generally adequate. However, participant responses will be audio taped for later analysis. No mention was made if or how these audio tapes would be destroyed after they are analyzed. If they are to be retained for any purpose, permission must be obtained from participants. Potential benefits to subjects and others and the knowledge to be gained also are adequate.

Inclusion of Women Plan: Both women and men will be included in the sample. It is expected that 207 (69%) of the 300 subjects will be women.

Inclusion of Minorities Plan: It is anticipated that 12% of the sample will be Hispanic, 16% African American, and 8% from other minority groups.

Inclusion of Children Plan: Participants will be 60 years of age or older. Older adults have been targeted for the study because they typically have more difficulty communicating their pain than younger persons.

Budget: The budget is justified and appropriate.

CRITIQUE 2:

Significance: This R21 application addresses the problem of inadequate pain communication between patients and health care practitioners that could result in undiagnosed pain due to omission of important information for treatment of pain. If the aims of the application are achieved, practitioners can be taught to use open-ended pain assessment questions such as "tell me about your pain" and not ask: "How are you feeling?" which has social desirability implications. The aims are to determine which communication strategies encourage older adults to describe important information and what information is missed with ineffective communication strategies.

Approach: The review of literature is integrated and organized and the argument for the study is well developed and logical. The Communication Theory Attuning Strategies is described, but more clarity is needed so that concepts of the research are linked to or explained by concepts of the theory. The posttest-only double blind experiment is strong with some ingenious video and software methods planned for randomization to groups and for providing the experimental videotape clips. Blindness of the graduate assistant to computerized random assignment and the method of starting the video after leaving the room are strengths of the innovative methodology.

The previous experience of the PI is varied but fairly strong with 9 studies of practitioner and patient communication that the PI claims prepared the team to conduct randomized controlled trials with older adults, develop standardized intervention videos, and to learn content analysis of participants' responses. Although the findings of the 9 studies are listed, they have not been tied together into a narrative that shows substantive support for conducting this study.

The posttest-only double blind design is strong but a flaw seems to be that half the sample will be randomly assigned to answer the Brief Pain Inventory (BPI) before the experimental test. In doing this they will answer 16 pain assessment questions that could strongly bias the amount of information given in response to the video. Even with randomization of the BPI sequence, it seems that the purpose of the study would be compromised. The investigators do not expect a timing effect (interaction) but responding to the BPI before the test would raise participant awareness of the DV, "important information" when subsequently answering the video questions. Since it seems less likely that they would respond differently to the BPI after the videos and since the BPI is not the major DV, why not simply administer the BPI after the video test for all participants to eliminate the threat introduced by counterbalancing? In addition there is inconsistency in the several reasons given for counterbalancing the assessment of pain intensity and interference with the BPI. These include: to control for present pain differences, for timing of the BPI, for timing differences, for the measurement effect, for the learning effect. On the other hand, counterbalancing would give some exploratory information. The threats to internal validity need to be carefully and consistently identified and minimized

The a prior osteoarthritis pain management criteria from the American Pain Society guidelines need further specification for use in this study. For example, the nociceptive/neuropathic type of pain needs to be operationally defined in terms of what kinds of participant responses will be categorized as each type. Direct questioning by a knowledgeable nurse might more accurately assess that differentiation. In addition, it is not clear what is included in the criterion, current pain treatments.

In general, the analysis procedures seem to answer the research question. However, the multivariate factor is not clear. It seems to be composed of the sum of "important information included" and the sum of "important information excluded," which intuitively may be two sides of the same coin.

Innovation: The study is innovative because it tests patients' responses to different ways of that health care personnel might ask about their pain. There are several very innovative features surrounding the video taped treatment, and the technological methods to randomly assign and maintain blindness.

Investigators: Dr. McDonald is an Associate Professor at the University of Connecticut and holds bachelors and masters degrees in Nursing. Her PhD is in Social Psychology from Columbia University in 1990. She received a pre-doctoral fellowship from the National Center for Nursing Research from 1988 –1990, but does not list the topic, so it is not clear whether the results were published. She also received an R15 award from NINR, 1999 – 2001, and has published the results. She has received two other grants, one from the Donaghu Foundation and one from the University of Athens in Greece with publications. She lists 14 publications that appear to be data based. Dr. Katz is a Professor at the University of Connecticut and has his PhD in Psychology from University of Massachusetts/Amherst. He is a consulting statistician at Mount Sinai Medical School in New York and will consult in Year 2 of this project regarding statistical analyses. Joel Rosiene is an Associate Professor of Computer Science at Eastern Connecticut State University. He will program the laptop computer with the software and insert the healthcare practitioner videotape clips as the experimental manipulation. The research team is well qualified to conduct this study.

Environment: The environment includes seven independent living elder housing sites in Connecticut that will ensure an adequate sample. The study will be conducted in the living quarters of the residents. There is support from University of Connecticut in terms of computer resources, personnel and offices in the school of nursing. As in a previous study, the Pi will work with the Seven Seas Film Company to produce videotapes needed for the study. Support is good for the accomplishment of the aims.

Overall Evaluation: This is a very interesting new application form an experienced young investigator using a posttest-only double blind experiment to test type of provider communication on audio taped patient responses. The methods are highly innovative and the study is very significant. The design and methods are creative and innovative and the analyses are generally appropriate to the aims of the project. The major strengths of the application are the innovative methods for blindness, randomization, and reliability of the intervention; the previous work and commitment of this investigator to studying communication about pain, the well-prepared research team and strong environment. Potential bias from the pre-intervention use of the BPI, lack of operational definitions of the coding criteria, and some inconsistencies are noted. There are some human subjects issues but inclusion of participants is adequate with respect to gender, minority group status and children.

Protection of Human Subjects from Research Risks: The application adequately addresses risks, protection against risks, benefits and importance of the knowledge to be gained. Debriefing the participants is thoughtfully planned, but it seems inappropriate to remind them at the end of the study that if they have distress or concern about the study, they are free to withdraw. Another comment is that the method of contacting the participants is not clear. This is a clinical trial but a data safety monitoring plan is not adequately presented.

Inclusion of Women Plan: The research involves 31% men and 69% women, although rationale was not given.

Inclusion of Minorities Plan: The research involves minorities and non-minorities: 76% white, 16% black, 12% Hispanic, 4% Asian, 2% Native Hawaiian or Other Pacific Islander, and 2% American Indian/Alaskan Native. Recruitment from nearby cities that contain 20% to 30% people of color will increase the ethnic and racial representation of the sample.

Inclusion of Children Plan: The research involves only/adults because osteoarthritis is a painful condition associated with aging and older adults are more vulnerable to problems communicating about their pain. The age range of the sample is 60 and older.

Budget: The requested budget is appropriate for the work.

CRITIQUE 3:

This is a proposal by a new investigator that proposes a novel approach to improving communication between older adults and their health care providers about pain. The design is a post-test only double-blind experiment to test how phrasing of health care practitioners' pain questions affect pain information provided by older adults with chronic osteoarthritis pain. The investigator makes the case for better communication skills on the part of providers. Recent renewed interest by the scientific community and foundations in the effectiveness of provider communication skills, including listening and questioning, in improving health care delivery provides support for a study of this nature. The failure of health care providers to adequately listen to patient's complaints of pain, coupled with known reluctance to adequately treat pain, high light the significance of this study topic. Study outcomes would have immediate application in provider and patient pain communication education. The investigator has experience [including an R15] in studying various aspects of pain and pain communication in a variety of populations. Further, she has amassed a group of collaborators that complement her own skills, including ideography, computerized randomization and experimental manipulation of video clip testing. Adequate resources are described, including agreement from a sufficient number of senior housing units to assure adequate sample size. On page 24 the investigator introduces for the first time the notion of (apriori criteria) for coding the qualitative data and these need more description and clarification; presumably they relate to the American Pain Society Guidelines which appear later. The study design is well developed and described with appropriate rationale for decisions. The need for use of mild deception is adequately addressed in the human subjects section and subjects will be debriefed. There are minimal risks.

THE FOLLOWING RESUME SECTIONS WERE PREPARED BY THE SCIENTIFIC REVIEW ADMINISTRATOR TO SUMMARIZE THE OUTCOME OF DISCUSSIONS OF THE REVIEW COMMITTEE ON THE FOLLOWING ISSUES:

PROTECTION OF HUMAN SUBJECTS (Resume): UNACCEPTABLE. The reviewers noted human subjects concerns because information provided on the Data and Safety Monitoring Plan is insufficient.

INCLUSION OF WOMEN PLAN (Resume): ACCEPTABLE. The reviewers concluded that the degree of inclusion of women is appropriate.

INCLUSION OF MINORITIES PLAN (Resume): ACCEPTABLE. The reviewers concluded that the inclusion of minorities is appropriate.

NSAA 7 1 R21 NR009848-01
MCDONALD, D

INCLUSION OF CHILDREN PLAN (Resume): ACCEPTABLE. The reviewers concluded that the exclusion of children is appropriate.

COMMITTEE BUDGET RECOMMENDATIONS: The reviewers recommended no changes in the budget.

NOTICE: The NIH has modified its policy regarding the receipt of amended applications. Detailed information can be found by accessing the following URL address: http://grants.nih.gov/grants/policy/amendedapps.htm

NIH announced implementation of Modular Research Grants in the December 18, 1998 issue of the NIH Guide to Grants and Contracts. The main feature of this concept is that grant applications (R01, R03, R21, R15) will request direct costs in $25,000 modules, without budget detail for individual categories. Further information can be obtained from the Modular Grants Web site at http://grants.nih.gov/grants/funding/modular/modular.htm

Deborah Dillon McDonald
Associate Professor
(O) 860-486-3714
(Email) Deborah.mcdonald@uconn.edu
12/16/2005

Alexis D. Bakos, PhD, MPH, RN,C
Program Director
Office of Extramural Programs
National Institute of Nursing Research
National Institutes of Health
Bethesda, MD 20892-4870

Dear Dr. Bakos,

Thank you for the opportunity to respond to reviewer comments regarding human subjects protection for our grant application 1R21NR008948-01, *Older Adults' Response to Health Care Practitioner Pain Communication.* The PI will keep the data for five years after completion of data analysis, at which time the PI will destroy the audiotapes and shred hard copies of the raw data. Older adults' permission to maintain the secured raw data will be requested in the consent form, and as part of the consent process. Participants will be fully informed about the study during the debriefing. We will remind participants of their option to withdraw from the study, giving them the opportunity to deny inclusion of their data once they are fully informed. We have included our Data and Safety Monitoring Plan below. Thank you for your valuable support and feedback.

Data and Safety Monitoring Plan

Data and safety monitoring will be described for the older adults and the data, which include the audiotape response, the transcripts; and written response to the BPI-SF and demographic form. The PI will be responsible for monitoring data and safety. The data will be kept secure in a locked file cabinet in the PI's private university office. Data entered into the computer for data analysis will be kept on the PI's private office computer with password protection. The professional transcriptionist will transcribe the anonymous audiotapes, and maintain confidentiality of the information. The PI and GA will maintain confidentiality of the audiotape and written data.

Adverse events are unlikely. The GA will be trained to detect adverse events such as distress about pain by gently probing for concerns and distress during the debriefing. The previously identified protocol for referring to a health care practitioner will be used if the GA identifies any older adult with a pain referral need. The GA will enter into an adverse events reporting log the participant identification number, a description of the adverse event, and the action taken to resolve the adverse event. The PI will immediately report adverse events to the University of Connecticut IRB.

The PI will keep the data for five years after completion of data analysis, at which time the PI will destroy the audiotapes and shred hard copies of the raw data. Older adults' permission to maintain the secured raw data will be requested in the consent form, and as part of the consent process. An annual report of the study will be made to the National Institute of Nursing Research and University of Connecticut IRB including a report of the data and safety monitoring.

Sincerely,

Deborah Dillon McDonald, RN, PhD
Principal Investigator

Carol Welt, Ph.D.
Executive Director & Assistant Vice Provost for Research

APPENDIX N

ANSWERS TO SELECTED RESOURCE MANUAL EXERCISES

■ Chapter 1

EXERCISE C.1: QUESTIONS OF FACT (APPENDIX A)

a. Yes, this was a study that systematically tested the efficacy of an intervention designed to reduce risk-taking behaviors and increase safety behaviors in school-aged children.
b. It was a quantitative study. The researchers systematically measured several outcomes (e.g., risk-taking, safety behavior, health behavior) using scales that yielded quantitative information.
c. The underlying paradigm was positivism/post-positivism.
d. Yes, the study involved the collection of information through the senses (i.e., through scrutiny of study participants' responses to series of questions).
e. The purposes of the study could best be described as prediction and control—the investigators examined possible methods of controlling (improving) children's risk-related behaviors.
f. This study was applied research—there was a practical problem that the researchers wanted to solve (i.e., a problem relating to avoidable risks and unsafe behaviors in schoolchildren).
g. Yes, this study directly addressed a question relevant to the preventive treatments for children. The results of this study, together with those from other similar studies, could provide guidance about

evidence-based programs to improve children's health and safety.

EXERCISE C.2: QUESTIONS OF FACT (APPENDIX B)

a. Yes, this was a systematic study of the breastfeeding promotion in a neonatal intensive care unit (NICU).
b. It was a qualitative study. The researcher used loosely structured methods to capture in an in-depth fashion the experiences of nurses and mothers with high-risk infants in the NICU, relative to the promotion of breastfeeding.
c. The underlying paradigm is constructivism (naturalism).
d. Yes, the study involved the collection of information through the senses (e.g., through conversations with nurses, through direct observation of practices in the NICU, and through scrutiny of documents in the NICU).
e. The purpose of the study can be described as exploration into the everyday world of NICU processes and transactions, with emphasis on actions and interactions relating to breastfeeding.
f. This study is best described as basic—to gain a better understanding of the structure and processes of the culture in a particular NICU. Interventions could, however, be designed that take the study findings into account.
g. This study addresses the EBP question described in the textbook as "Meaning

and Processes," that is, developing an in-depth understanding of the NICU environment and processes.

■ Chapter 2

EXERCISE C.1: QUESTIONS OF FACT (APPENDIX C)

a. The purpose of the evidence-based project was to develop, implement, and evaluate the effectiveness of a standardized nursing procedure to increase the identification of depression in family members of active-duty soldiers.

b. The setting for the project was a military family practice clinic located on a U. S. Army infantry post in Hawaii.

c. The project was guided by the Iowa Model of Evidence-Based Practice to Promote Quality Care.

d. The authors described the project as having *both* a problem-focused trigger and a knowledge-focused trigger. With regard to the former, the introduction indicated that "The absence in this clinic of a systematic method to screen family members of deployed soldiers for depression and the inability to estimate rates of depression in this clinical population were the problem-focused triggers for this project." They cited national standards and guidelines calling for the screening of all adults for depression in primary care settings as the knowledge-focused triggers.

e. There were three authors of this report, and presumably they were major team members on this project. Two authors were masters-prepared officers in the U. S. Army Nurse Corps, and the third was an instructor at the University of Hawaii. The article also indicates that a "multidisciplinary panel of stakeholders," which included advance practice registered nurses (APRNs), physicians, certified nurse assistants, RNs, a psychologist, and clinic administrators, formed the EBP team. It is not unusual for EBP project teams to comprise research and clinical staff, and to be multidisciplinary.

f. The report did not discuss implementation at length, but it did state that the project team was lead by a change champion (an APRN) and an opinion leader (a physician), who were persuasive and influential in the clinic. The article stated that "The EBP project received enthusiastic support throughout the organization and at the highest levels of nursing leadership."

g. Yes, the report described the study that was undertaken as a pilot study.

h. Yes, one of the purposes of this pilot study was to evaluate the effectiveness of the newly developed practice guideline for screening for depression.

EXERCISE C.2: QUESTIONS OF FACT (APPENDIX K)

a. Yes, the article by Han and colleagues described a systematic review undertaken to summarize evidence on interventions to promote mammography among ethnic minority women. Systematic reviews are an especially important type of preappraised evidence. The particular type of systematic review in this example was a meta-analysis.

b. The meta-analysis in this study integrated information from several studies, including RCTs, so evidence from this study would be at the top rung of the evidence hierarchy portrayed in Figure 2.1.

c. The researchers stated that "The aim of this study was to determine the effectiveness of the interventions for improving mammography screening among asymptomatic ethnic minority women" (Abstract). At the end of the introduction, they also noted that an aim was to update an earlier meta-analysis using studies published after 2000, and to specifically focus on minority women.

■ Chapter 3

EXERCISE B.2

a. Independent variable (IV) = participation versus nonparticipation in assertiveness training; dependent variable (DV) = psychiatric nurses' effectiveness
b. IV = patients' postural positioning; DV = respiratory function
c. IV = amount of touch by nursing staff; DV = patients' anxiety
d. IV = frequency of turning patients; DV = incidence of decubitus ulcers
e. IV = history of parents' abuse during their childhood; DV = parental abuse of their own children
f. IV = patients' age and gender; DV = tolerance for pain
g. IV = pregnant women's number of prenatal visits; DV = labor and delivery outcomes
h. IV = children's status of having or not having a chronic illness; DV = levels of depression
i. IV = gender; DV = compliance with a medical regimen
j. IV = participation vs. nonparticipation in a support group among family caregivers of AIDS patients; DV = coping
k. IV = time of day; DV = hearing acuity among the elderly
l. IV = location of giving birth—home versus hospital; DV = parents' satisfaction with the childbirth experience
m. IV = type of diet in the outpatient setting among patients undergoing chemotherapy; DV = incidence of positive blood cultures

EXERCISE B.5

a. Experimental studies would not be conducted in an ethnographic tradition.
b. In the study described, receipt of relaxation therapy would be the *in*dependent variable and pain would be the dependent variable.

c. In grounded theory studies, researchers do not study "lived experiences"—that would involve a phenomenological inquiry.
d. In phenomenological studies, there would not be an intervention.
e. In an experimental study, the data collection plan would be developed well in advance of introducing an intervention.

EXERCISE C.1: QUESTIONS OF FACT (APPENDIX D)

a. The lead researcher on this study was Robin Whittemore, a nurse researcher and associate professor at Yale University. Other team members included other nurse researchers and a biostatistician from Yale and an assistant professor from the Division of Behavioral Sciences and Community Health at the University of Connecticut. All team members of this interdisciplinary team have a doctoral degree.
b. At the end of the article, there is an acknowledgment section that lists members of the project team, in addition to the lead researchers (the authors). The list includes 18 people with a wide range of skills and backgrounds who had various roles on this complex project.
c. At the end of the article, there is a statement indicating that the study was supported by a grant from the National Institutes of Health—specifically from the institute called the National Institute of Diabetes and Digestive and Kidney Diseases.
d. The study participants were 58 adults at risk of diabetes, recruited from four nurse practitioner primary care practices.
e. The independent variable in this study was the alternative treatment conditions— the enhanced standard care program or a lifestyle program. The researchers *created* this independent variable. It is not, however, inherently an independent variable. For example, if both programs were available to

people in the community, one could ask questions about factors influencing people's choice of one program or the other. In such a situation, program type would be the dependent variable.

f. There were various dependent variables in this study. The researchers were interested in the effect of participating in one or the other program on clinical outcomes (weight change, waist circumference, insulin resistance, and lipid profiles), behavioral outcomes (nutrition and exercise), a psychosocial outcome (depression), and patient satisfaction. None of these is *inherently* a dependent variable. For example, exercise and nutrition could be studied as the *cause of* health problems, longevity, quality of life, and so on.

g. No, the report did not specifically use the terms independent or dependent variable, as is typical. The term "outcomes" was used in lieu of dependent variables.

h. The data in this study were primarily quantitative. Whittemore and colleagues *measured* their outcome variables in a form that yielded numeric information. However, some qualitative data were also collected to better understand the processes of implementing the intervention.

i. The researchers were interested in a possible cause-and-effect relationship: the relationship between participation in the intervention on the one hand and improved outcomes on the other.

j. This study was experimental. The researchers controlled the independent variable, and gave only some people the opportunity to participate in the lifestyle program.

k. Yes, this study involved an intervention.

l. Yes, Whittemore and colleagues analyzed most of their data statistically. However, there was also qualitative analysis of some data, notably interviews with the nurse practitioners who implemented the program.

m. Yes, an IMRAD-type format was followed. There was an introduction that provided an overview of the literature, described the

study purpose, and discussed the projects' significance. Both the Methods and Results sections had several subsections. Finally, there was a Discussion section with s subsection labeled "Conclusions."

EXERCISE C.2: QUESTIONS OF FACT (APPENDIX E)

a. The author of this article is Cheryl Tatano Beck, one of the co-authors of the textbook. She is a professor of nursing at the University of Connecticut and has a doctoral degree (DNSc).

b. No, Beck did not receive funding for this study. There were no endnotes or footnotes that acknowledged funding, as would typically be the case if the study had received financial support.

c. The study participants were 23 mothers of children with obstetric brachial plexus injuries (OBPI). Eleven mothers participated in the study over the Internet, and 12 were interviewed in person.

d. The key concept in this study was the mothers' experiences caring for a child with OBPI.

e. The data in this study were qualitative.

f. No specific relationships were under investigation in this study. The researcher focused on elucidating the mothers' experiences, not on relationships between the experience and other aspects of the women's lives.

g. Beck's study was a phenomenological study.

h. This study was nonexperimental.

i. There was no intervention in this study.

j. Qualitative researchers do not call their concepts variables, nor are their concepts "measured." Data relating to the key concept in this study were gathered via Internet and in-person interviews with women who had given birth to a child with OBPI.

k. The study involved primarily a qualitative (nonstatistical) analysis of the interview data, although the report did include a few simple descriptive statistics (averages

and percentages) that portrayed participants' characteristics, such as their age
and marital status.

l. Yes, the report followed the IMRAD
format. There was an introduction, a methods section, results section, and a discussion.

▪ Chapter 4

EXERCISE B.4

2a. IV = type of stimulation (tactile vs.
verbal); DV = physiological arousal
2b. IV = infant birth weight; DV = risk of
hypoglycemia
2c. IV = use vs. nonuse of isotonic sodium
chloride solution; DV = oxygen saturation
2d. IV = fluid balance; DV = success in weaning patients from mechanical ventilation
2e. IV = patients' gender; DV = amount of
narcotic analgesics administered
3a. IV = prior blood donation vs. no prior
donation; DV = amount of stress
3b. IV = amount of conversation initiated by
nurses; DV = patients' ratings of nursing
effectiveness
3c. IV = ratings of nurses' informativeness;
DV = amount of preoperative stress
3d. IV = drained vs. not drained with a
Jackson-Pratt drain; DV = incidence of
peritoneal infection
3e. IV = type of delivery (vaginal vs. cesarean);
DV = incidence of postpartum depression

EXERCISE C.1: QUESTIONS OF FACT (APPENDIX F)

a. The first two paragraphs of this report
stated the essence of the problem—
namely, that hospital readmissions for
patients with heart failure (HF) are potentially preventable, and that patients delay
responding the their HF.
b. The authors stated their purpose (their
specific objectives) at the end of the introduction, in a subsection labeled

"Conceptual Framework." Several purposes were stated, two of which were
descriptive and specifically used the verb
"describe": To *describe* the experience of
and the cognitive and emotional response
to the symptoms of decompensated HF
and to *describe* self-care behaviors prior
to seeking care for decompensated HF.
These descriptive questions do not, in
themselves, provide insight into whether a
qualitative or quantitative approach
would be used, and in fact, these researchers
gathered both qualitative and quantitative
data. The third aim was: To *determine* the
influence of sociodemographic, clinical,
cognitive, emotional, and social contextual factors on symptom duration. This
aim is consistent with a quantitative study
that examined relationships among variables, as was the case.
c. The report did not explicitly state research
questions, although they could be inferred
from the purpose statement. For example,
the question corresponding to the first
descriptive purpose might be: What are
the experience of and the cognitive and
emotional response to the symptoms of
decompensated HF?
d. No hypotheses were formally stated.
e. The aim concerning factors affecting
symptom duration could be the basis for
several predictions. For example, one of
the factors being examined in relation to
symptom duration was an emotional factor, anxiety. One hypothesis would be:
Patients with HF who are less anxious will
have longer duration of symptoms before
seeking help than patients who are more
anxious.
f. Yes, the researchers used hypothesis-
testing statistical tests.

EXERCISE C.2: QUESTIONS OF FACT (APPENDIX B)

a. The first paragraph indicated that the
research focused on the problem of breastfeeding promotion in neonatal intensive

care units (NICUs). The next two paragraphs elaborated on the problem, noting that maternity practices in the U.S. often impede breastfeeding and the uptake of evidence-based practice guidelines.

b. Cricco-Lizza stated the purpose in the abstract: Purpose: This study explored the structure and process of breastfeeding promotion in the NICU. This statement was reiterated in the very first sentence of the report, and again in the last sentence of the introduction.

c. Specific research questions were not articulated.

d. No hypotheses were stated—nor would they have been appropriate in this qualitative study.

e. No, no hypotheses were tested. Qualitative studies do not use statistical methods to test hypotheses.

■ Chapter 5

EXERCISE C.1: QUESTIONS OF FACT (APPENDIX K)

a. This review was a systematic review—a meta-analysis.

b. Yes, the introduction described a research problem that the researchers addressed. The problem might be stated as followed: Minority women face an unequal burden of breast cancer in the United States. In part, this may be attributable to lower use of mammography screening among minority women. Although many interventions promoting mammography screening among ethnic minority women have been tested, the evidence regarding the effectiveness of these interventions has not been systematically integrated.

c. Yes, there was a statement of purpose in the last sentence of the introduction: "The objective of the meta-analysis was to describe mammography intervention approaches used for ethnic minority

(Asian American, African American, and Hispanic) women in the United States." This is somewhat different from the objective stated in the abstract: "The aim of this study was to determine the effectiveness of the interventions for improving mammography screening among asymptomatic ethnic minority women."

d. The researchers used 4 different electronic databases in their literature search: Medline, CINAHL, PsychInfo, and Web of Science. Two members of the team independently searched these databases. The article also said that there were some manual "hand searches from reference collections" (although there is no indication of what those reference collections were).

e. The key words used in the search included *Asian, African American, Hispanic* or *Latino, breast cancer screening, mammography, experimental studies, interventions,* and *intervention studies*. These key words cover independent variables (intervention), dependent variables (breast cancer screening), and the population of interest.

f. Yes, the researchers restricted their search to English-language articles.

g. The researchers limited their search to articles published from 2000 onwards. The researchers did not explain this decision.

h. The researchers originally identified 749 citations that they assessed in greater depth for possible inclusion in their review.

i. The researchers established a series of explicit criteria about studies that could be included in the review. For example, the study had to involve efforts to increase mammography use among asymptomatic women, had to have been done in the United States, and had to have 40% or more of the participants be of an ethnic minority.

j. Ultimately, 23 studies were included in the meta-analysis.

k. All studies included in the review were quantitative—which is always the case in a meta-analysis.

EXERCISE C.2: QUESTIONS OF FACT (APPENDIX L)

a. Xu undertook a systematic review of studies relating to the experience of being an Asian nurse working in a western country. His review was a metasynthesis.

b. Xu began with a problem statement that noted that the nursing shortage throughout the world has resulted in the international recruitment of Asian nurses, but that little is known about the actual experiences of Asian nurses who work in western countries.

c. According to the report, Xu searched five mainstream electronic databases, including CINAHL, Medline, PsychINFO, Sociological Abstract, and ERIC (a database for education literature). He also searched Proquest Dissertations and Theses for nonpublished work. His efforts were not restricted to electronic database searches. Xu also used traditional "ancestry" type searches (i.e., retrieving studies cited in other relevant studies) and hand-searched journals that had a history of publishing research on the topic of interest. Xu also made efforts to interact with original researchers.

d. The key words used in the search included *Asian nurses, foreign nurses, foreign-born nurses, internally educated nurse, internationally recruited nurses, immigrant nurses,* and the names of specific Asian countries, such as Korea and Taiwan.

e. The report indicated that the search was restricted to English-language reports.

f. The report did not indicate how many references were initially retrieved using the stated search strategies, nor how many were discarded because they did not meet inclusion criteria. A total of 14 studies were actually included in the review.

g. The studies included in the review were either purely qualitative or there was a qualitative component within a study that included both qualitative and quantitative data.

h. The 14 studies in the review included a grounded theory study, an ethnography,

phenomenological studies, qualitative descriptive studies, and some studies that had both qualitative and quantitative components (mixed methods studies).

■ Chapter 6

EXERCISE C.1: QUESTIONS OF FACT (APPENDIX F)

a. Jurgens and colleagues used as a conceptual framework the Self-Regulation Model of Illness. This model was developed by health psychologists, primarily Howard Leventhal. An overview of this model can be found in a chapter on the Internet: http://media.wiley.com/product_data/excerpt/70/04700240/0470024070.pdf

b. The Self-Regulation model was not described in the textbook, but it is a model that has been used by other nurse researchers.

c. Yes, a schematic model of the Self-Regulation Model of Illness was included as Figure 1.

d. The key concepts in the model are: (1) physical stimuli (e.g., symptoms), (2) cognitive representation of illness (e.g., perceived causes), (3) emotional representation of illness (e.g., anxiety), (4) coping, (5) appraisal of the situation, and (6) response to the physical stimuli (symptoms)—seeking care.

e. According to the model, the decision to seek care is *directly* affected by a person's *appraisal* of the health threat and efficacy of coping, which are developed along both a cognitive and an emotional pathway.

f. The decision to seek care is *indirectly* affected by all of the factors that lead to an appraisal of the health threat, including the physical symptoms themselves, the person's level of anxiety, perceptions of causes and consequences of the threat, and the person's coping skills.

g. The report did not articulate formal conceptual definitions of each construct in the model. For example, there is no conceptual definition of "coping" or "anxiety." Nevertheless, the overall model was very well explained in a section of the article labeled "Conceptual Framework."

h. No, the article did not present formal hypotheses deduced from the conceptual model. The researchers stated that "We propose that delay in seeking care is due to the difficulty that HF patients experience in discerning the quality and meaning of their symptoms." A formal hypothesis might be: "HF patients who are less well able to detect and interpret their symptoms are more likely to delay seeking care." The researchers also said that a goal was to "determine the influence of sociodemographic, clinical, cognitive, emotional, and social contextual factors on symptom duration during this time." They did not state a hypothesis predicting *which factors* might affect symptom duration, such as: "Symptom duration will be greater among those who are older and have higher levels of anxiety." Symptom duration, a major dependent variable in this study, is not the endpoint in the conceptual model.

EXERCISE C.2: QUESTIONS OF FACT (APPENDIX E)

a. Beck's study has as its broad framework the tradition of phenomenology. As noted in the textbook, phenomenologists try to suspend preconceived views of the phenomenon when they begin their research. Yet, they are guided by a philosophical framework that purports that human experience is a property of the experience itself, not constructed by outside observers. Beck based her inquiry on a particular school of phenomenological thinking—that of Colaizzi. Aspects of Colaizzi's approach were summarized in Beck's article.

b. No, this study was not based on a model of nursing such as those described in the textbook.

c. Yes, Figure 2 of Beck's article included a schematic model that integrated the six themes she identified in analyzing her rich verbatim data. The figure was a good way to illustrate how the themes were integrated. The schematic model helped to summarize the major findings for readers. This model emerged from the data—it was not a model that was formulated prior to data collection.

d. The concepts in Beck's model were the six themes that emerged about the mothers' experience of caring for children with obstetric brachial plexus injuries.

e. This was a phenomenological study, no hypotheses were tested.

▪ Chapter 7

EXERCISE C.1: QUESTIONS OF FACT (APPENDIX A)

a. Yes, in the "Procedures" subsection, the researchers indicated that human subject approval was received from the Committee on Human Research of the University of California, San Francisco.

b. Yes, the study participants were minors and would be considered "vulnerable." All children in the study were 8 or 9 years old.

c. There is no reason to suspect that participants were subjected to any physical harm or discomfort or psychological distress. The goal was to increase the children's safety behaviors and decrease risk-taking. The content of the intervention, and the small-group format, does not appear stressful. The fact that participants did not drop out of the study over the course of the research suggests that participants and their parents were comfortable with the research.

d. It does not appear that participants were deceived in any way. Children and their parents were recruited through community outreach efforts and were told about the purpose of the study. Although parents were not participating directly in the program, they were kept fully informed through weekly information packets.

e. There is no reason to suspect any coercion was used to force unwilling people to participate in the study. The article noted that several people declined to participate because of the time commitment.

f. The report indicated that written consent was obtained from all parents, and verbal assent was obtained from all children. Presumably, given review by a human subjects committee, the consent form stated that participation was purely voluntary. It is not possible to determine the extent to which disclosure was "full," but there does not appear to be any reason to conceal information in this study

g. The article indicated that issues of confidentiality and "group rules" were discussed with the children. Presumably, statements regarding privacy and confidentiality were also made in the informed consent form.

EXERCISE C.2: QUESTIONS OF FACT (APPENDIX B)

a. Yes, the report indicates that approval for the study was granted by the "Human Subjects' Committees," presumably the committee in the children's hospital where the study took place and perhaps also (because *Committees* is plural) the committee of Cricoo-Lizza's institutional affiliation at the time of the research.

b. The focus of the study was nurses in the NICU, not the mothers or their infants. The nurses would not be considered vulnerable.

c. Participants were not subjected to any physical harm or discomfort. Nurses were observed performing their normal duties. It is possible that there was a certain degree of self-consciousness when the study started, but it is likely that the nurses became accustomed to the presence of the researcher, who was probably considered a colleague.

d. Participants were probably not deceived. The article states that "information was

provided to the nurses through the intranet, staff meetings, and individual encounters in the NICU." It might be noted, though, that observations were made "unobtrusively," meaning that nurses were not always aware that their interactions with families were under direct scrutiny—and presumably families were not aware either. Notification about the observations undoubtedly would have affected the very interactions of interest, and behaviors would likely have been atypical, undermining the study purpose. The nurses under observation knew that Cricco-Lizza was a nurse researcher who was interested in learning about their perspectives on infant feeding.

e. It does not appear that any coercion was involved.

f. The report stated that the researcher obtained written informed consent from the 18 key informants who were formally interviewed. Informed consent was not obtained from the 114 nurses who were considered "general informants," nor from any family members.

g. Cricco-Lizza stated that the interviews with key informants took place in a private room near the NICU. She did not explicitly discuss who had access to the audiotaped interviews or the transcripts, but it seems safe to presume that they were safeguarded. No names were used in the report. When verbatim quotes were presented in the report, she said things such as: "One nurse said" or "one key informant stated."

▪ Chapter 8

EXERCISE C.1: QUESTIONS OF FACT (APPENDIX D)

a. Yes, the study involved a test of a diabetes prevention program implemented in primary care settings by nurse practitioners (NPs).

b. Yes, the investigators compared two groups of people, all of whom were adults at risk of diabetes. One group received standard care plus an NP and nutrition session. The second group received the special intervention, a lifestyle program involving enhanced standard care and six NP sessions.

c. The design was a mixed design. The two treatment groups were compared in terms of key outcomes at the end of the study, but outcomes were also compared within each group before and after the 6-month intervention.

d. This study was longitudinal. Data were collected from study participants three times: before the intervention and then 3 months and 6 months after the intervention. (Lab values were only collected at baseline and 6 months.)

e. The study was undertaken in four NP primary care practice sites in New England. Two sites had the enhanced standard care and the other two had the lifestyle change program.

f. The primary methods of data collection were self-reports (e.g., health-promoting behaviors, depressive symptoms) and bio-physiologic methods (weight, lipids).

g. Yes, this was described as a pilot study, whose purpose was "to test the translation of the DPP [diabetes prevention program] modified specifically for NPs to deliver in the context of primary care." The specific aims included modifying the DPP collaboratively with NPs; evaluating the program's reach, implementation, and preliminary efficacy according to a framework called RE-AIM—which we discuss in Chapter 10; and to explore the relationship between weight loss and behavioral, psychosocial, and clinical outcomes.

EXERCISE C.2: QUESTIONS OF FACT (APPENDIX I)

a. No, this study did not involve an intervention.

b. Yes, this study compared the perceptions relating to the diagnosis and treatment of obstructive sleep apnea (OSA) among patients who were adherent versus nonadherent to continuous positive airway pressure (CPAP) therapy. The researchers also conducted a supplementary analysis in which married and unmarried patients were compared.

c. The study was longitudinal. Data were collected shortly after patients were diagnosed with OSA. They were interviewed again shortly after initiating CPAP treatment.

d. The sleep study was done in a Veterans Affairs medical center sleep clinic, and the interview data were mostly collected in the clinic as well.

e. Self-reports were the primary method of data collection in this study. However, the researchers also collected data from the CPAP machines regarding the number of hours per night participants adhered to the CPAP therapy.

f. No, this was not a pilot study.

■ Chapter 9

EXERCISE C.1: QUESTIONS OF FACT (APPENDIX A)

a. Yes, the purpose of the study was to evaluate the effects of an intervention (a 4-week behaviorally based program) for reducing risk-taking behavior and increasing safety behavior in school-aged children.

b. The design for this study was experimental.

c. Yes, an intent of the study was to examine whether participation in the special program *caused* improvements in children's outcomes, especially behavioral outcomes relating to health and safety.

d. The experimentally manipulated independent variable was participation versus nonparticipation in the special program. The dependent variables included several measures of children's health behaviors and other psychosocial constructs such as self-perceptions, health perceptions, coping, motivation, risk-taking behaviors, and safety practices.

e. Yes, randomization was used, although the report did not provide much information about the actual randomization procedure, except to say that a random numbers table was used. It appears that a basic randomization process was used (i.e., not a Zelen approach, PRPP, and so on).

f. The control group strategy was to use a wait-listed control group. Thus, the counterfactual in this study was the absence of the special intervention at the time the follow-up data were collected.

g. In this study, data were collected from experimental and control group members four times—at baseline and at 1, 3, and 6 months after the intervention. Thus, the specific design was a before–after (repeated measures) experimental design.

h. The design is a mixed design, with a focus on the between-subjects aspect because the primary goal was to compare outcomes for the experimental and control group members, who were not the same people. However, the researchers also showed changes within the group over time (Table 2).

i. It does not appear that any blinding was used in this study. Blinding to group status was not feasible in this study. In terms of blinding of data collectors, most data were collected by means of self-administered forms, not by an interviewer who could have affected responses.

j. Yes, the data were gathered four times over a 6-month period and so this study was longitudinal. It is also prospective: The independent variable was experimentally manipulated and *then* outcome data were gathered.

k. It is possible that there was a pilot study for this project. Pilot work was not specifically noted, however.

EXERCISE C.2: QUESTIONS OF FACT (APPENDIX F)

a. No, there was no intervention in this study.

b. The study design was nonexperimental. It had both descriptive components (e.g., What symptoms were frequently reported?) and correlational components (e.g., What factors were predictive of dyspnea duration before seeking care?).

c. The article did not articulate a cause-probing intent. The abstract, for example, says that the study purpose was *to describe* contextual factors related to elders' symptom recognition and response.

d. In the analyses focused on the prediction of dyspnea duration, dyspnea duration before seeking care was the dependent variable. There were several independent variables, including the person's age, gender, symptom distress, perceived seriousness of the symptom, and anxiety.

e. None of the variables in the study could be experimentally manipulated.

f. No, randomization was not used.

g. This is a descriptive correlational study. It could also be described as retrospective: Loeb was interested in retrospectively identifying the factors that might predict length of time before seeking care in a dyspnea experience.

h. No, blinding was not used in this study.

i. No, this study was cross-sectional, and it was not prospective.

▪ Chapter 10

EXERCISE C.1: QUESTIONS OF FACT (APPENDIX A)

a. Kennedy and Chen relied on randomization to treatment groups to control confounding variables. It is likely that statistical control was also used, but there were few details about the statistical analysis. To a lesser extent, it could also be said that confounders were controlled through homogeneity: All of the children were between the ages of 8 and 9, were White or Latino, and were in good health.

b. No, this study could not have used a crossover design. Once children learned the "lessons" from the intervention program, there would be no way for them to "unlearn" them.

c. Through randomization, virtually *all* of the children's characteristics (e.g., their socioeconomic status, number of siblings, educational achievement, height and weight, and so on) would have been controlled. Through homogeneity, age, health, and ethnicity were controlled (i.e., held constant).

d. According to the report, there was no attrition in this study—which is very unusual given the length of the intervention.

e. Yes, although the report did not state this explicitly, the analysis would have been done on an intention-to-treat basis because there was no attrition. In other words, in the analysis, all of the children in the analysis were maintained in the groups to which they were randomly assigned. When there is attrition, missing data are usually estimated (using sophisticated methods) so that the intention-to-treat analysis can proceed.

f. In this study, the researchers took some steps to enhance constancy of conditions. For example, the intervention was delivered in small groups of four to six children, the groups followed standardized protocols, and the interventionists were trained and retrained to enhance consistency across the four staff.

g. The intervention group got a distinct 4-week treatment, and the wait-list control group presumably was unexposed to the content of the intervention program. It is difficult to know, though, if the two conditions were as distinct as possible, and whether the intervention was as powerful as possible. The researchers found that the intervention and control groups were not different on a lot of outcomes at the end of the study. This could mean that four weekly 2-hour sessions was insufficiently powerful to affect the children's behavior, given the many other forces that affect the behaviors of interest (family, peers, teachers, media). Other threats to statistical conclusion validity are also possible.

h. Randomization typically reduces the threat of selection—the children in the two groups were presumably equivalent with regard to many characteristics. The report specifically states that the groups were similar in terms of the distribution of boys and girls, and of Whites and Latinos. Ideally, the report would have stated the equivalence of the two groups with regard to all of the outcomes as measured at baseline. Table 2 shows that the two groups had different mean scores at T1 on all of the variables of interest, but it does not indicate whether group differences were sufficiently large to be statistically significant.

EXERCISE C.2: QUESTIONS OF FACT (APPENDIX D)

a. The authors called their design a cluster-randomized design, which is a type of true experimental design. The design involved randomization of four nurse practitioner (NP) primary care practice sites to either an enhanced standard care program (two sites) or to a lifestyle program (two sites). However, with only four sites, the design has flaws that a traditional RCT does not. Randomization only "works" in terms of equalizing groups if the numbers are sufficiently large, and with only four sites, it would be imprudent to assume that the people in the two groups being compared were equivalent in every respect.

b. The independent variable for this study was participation in one type of program (lifestyle) versus the other (enhanced standard). The primary dependent variable was weight loss. Other outcomes included waist circumference, insulin resistance, lipid profiles, health-promoting behaviors (diet and exercise), depressive symptoms, and satisfaction with the program.

c. Yes, randomization was used to allocate the sites to either the standard or lifestyle program. The researchers presumably did not randomly assign individual patients to treatment conditions because of the risk of contamination between treatments. That is, if some people within a site were randomized to one treatment, they could have learned about the other treatment from friends, neighbors, or family members who were in the other group. Contamination could also occur through co-mingling of or communication between staff. And, from a practical point of view, it would have been extremely complicated to have randomization of patients within a given site.

d. The researchers relied primarily on randomization to control confounding characteristics, but they also relied on statistical control methods. The data analysis section specifically stated that "the two groups were compared on major variables to make certain that the cluster random assignment equally distributed the sample. Variables unequally distributed were controlled for in subsequent analysis."

e. Randomization of sites probably controlled many characteristics. We can see in Table 2 that the two groups were similar at baseline with regard to age, gender, clinical variables, behavioral variables, and depression. Yet the two groups were quite different with respect to race (the enhanced standard or control group was disproportionately Hispanic) and income (the control group was poorer). Presumably, these characteristics were statistically controlled in the analyses.

f. Yes, in the flow chart in Figure 1, we see that 58 people were randomly assigned to one of the two groups: 27 in the control condition and 31 in the lifestyle (treatment) condition. At the point of 6-month data collection, all of the control group members remained in the study, but

seven people had dropped out of the treatment group. Overall, then, attrition was 12% of those randomized and 22.5% of those in the treatment group.

g. Yes, the article specifically stated, in the data analysis section, that an intent-to-treat analysis was used, even though not everyone provided follow-up data. The researchers used a sophisticated analytic approach (mixed modeling), which can account for the missing values in the analysis.

h. The researchers did a commendable job in their efforts to address external validity in this study. Importantly, they used the RE-AIM framework to examine the "Reach" of the intervention. For example, they documented a fairly high response rate to in-person recruitment, and they noted the diversity of participants in terms of age, income, and ethnicity. Their main focus in this study was on "Efficacy," but they also examined the "Implementation" aspect of the intervention, and concluded that the intervention was amenable to implementation in real-world practice settings.

▪ Chapter 11

EXERCISE C.1

a. Clinical trial:
   • The Kennedy and Chen study in Appendix A could be described as a clinical trial— a randomized design was used to test an innovative intervention.
   • The Whittemore and colleague's study in Appendix D might be considered a Phase II clinical trial because it was a pilot test of an intervention, and information was sought about its feasibility, acceptability, and its potential for effectiveness in improving health outcomes for those at risk of type 2 diabetes.
   • The McGillion and colleague's study (Appendix H) could be described as a clinical trial—it involved a randomized

design to test the efficacy of an intervention for people with chronic cardiac pain.
b. Outcomes research:
- None of the studies in the appendices would be considered outcomes research.
c. Survey research:
- The Jurgens and colleague's study (Appendix F) could be considered as involving a survey.
d. Needs assessment:
- None of the studies in the appendices would be considered a needs assessment, although the Jurgens and colleague's study (Appendix E) could shed light on the needs of elders with heart failure symptoms.
e. Replication research:
- None of the studies in the appendices would be considered a replication, although the study by Whittemore and colleagues (Appendix D) was designed to test whether previously tested interventions could be translated to primary care settings.
f. Secondary analysis:
- None of the studies in the appendices would be considered secondary analyses.

EXERCISE C.2: QUESTIONS OF FACT (APPENDIX J)

a. No, the study by Kalisch and colleagues is not a clinical trial.
b. This study *evaluated* the Nursing Teamwork Survey with regard to its adequacy as a useful instrument, but this would not be considered evaluation research as the term is usually used.
c. This study is not an example of outcomes research. (The Nursing Teamwork Survey could, however, be used to measure aspects of *process* in an outcomes study.)
d. This study is not specifically a survey, but it is certainly true that a survey component was used to gather data for the psychometric analysis.

e. Yes, this study is a good example of methodologic research. The purpose of the study was not to gather evidence relating to a substantive problem (nursing teamwork), but rather to design and test an instrument that could be used in substantive research.
f. The study was nonexperimental. The researchers did not introduce an intervention or manipulate an independent variable.

■ Chapter 12

EXERCISE B.4

a. Multistage cluster sampling
b. Convenience sampling
c. Systematic sampling
d. Quota sampling
e. Simple random sampling
f. Purposive sampling

EXERCISE C.1

a. None of the studies used probability sampling.
b. Except for the study in Appendix C, all of the studies used convenience sampling. In Yackel and colleagues' EBP study, the sample would best be described as a consecutive sample: "All patients meeting the inclusion criteria were screened for depression . . ."
c. None of the studies used quota sampling.

EXERCISE C.2: QUESTIONS OF FACT (APPENDIX F)

a. The target population in Jurgen and colleague's study might be described as community-dwelling men and women aged 65 and older in the United States (or in northeastern United States) with heart failure (HF). The accessible population was patients aged 65 or older in tertiary care hospitals in Philadelphia and New York diagnosed with decompensated HF.

b. The eligibility criteria for the study included (a) hospitalized in an emergency department or as an inpatient, (b) having a diagnosis or decompensated HF, (c) age of 65 or older, (d) cognitively intact, (e) medically stable, (f) able to read and understand English, (g) willing to provide informed consent, and (h) living independently in the community and able to manage their illness by self-care.

c. The sampling method was nonprobability, specifically, sampling by convenience.

d. Specific recruitment strategies were not discussed in the paper (e.g., who did the recruiting, what prospective participants were told, how they were screened for eligibility, what percentage of those approached actually participated).

e. The researchers did not appear to do anything specific to increase the likelihood that their sample would be diverse or representative.

f. The total sample size was 77 participants.

g. The report indicated that the researchers performed a power analysis to estimate sample size needs, but the specifics of the power analysis were not provided. The article also stated that another criterion was used to estimate sample size needs—a criterion involving the number of cases needed for each independent variable (predictor) in the type of analysis that was performed. The paragraph on sample size concluded with the following, somewhat ambiguous statement: "The exploratory nature of the study, together with the ability to meet the aims, was factored into the determination of the sample of 77 participants."

■ Chapters 13

EXERCISE B.2

Score of Y = 11; score of Z = 26

EXERCISE B.3

A = acquiescence; B = none; C = extreme response set; D = naysayers' bias

EXERCISE C.2: QUESTIONS OF FACT (APPENDIX D)

a. Yes, there were self-report measures in the assessment of efficacy in this study. Variables measured through self-reports included participants' health-promoting behavior and their depressive symptoms. (Demographic information was also collected "using a standard form," and would also have involved self-reports.)

b. Specific questions from the self-report instruments were not described in the article.

c. The researchers' instruments appear to have included only closed-ended questions.

d. Yes, the researchers used two composite scales as measures of efficacy. The first was the Health-Promoting Lifestyle Profile (HPLP) II, specifically two subscales measuring exercise and nutrition behavior. The two subscales included 17 items "constructed on a 4-point Likert scale." Depressive symptoms were measured on the 20-item Center for Epidemiological Studies-Depression (CES-D) Scale. Each item is rated on a scale from 0 to 3 in terms of frequency in the previous week. Finally, the instrument included an item regarding number of minutes of exercise per week. (The researchers also collected self-report data on participant satisfaction using a 7-item summated rating scale.)

e. Specific information about the mode of data collection was not presented in the article, which simply stated that "All data were collected by trained research assistants." Presumably, the self-report data were gathered by self-administered questionnaires rather than by interviews.

f. It appears that all of the instruments used in this study were previously developed for use in other studies.

g. The researchers did not offer specific rationales for selecting the HPLP or CES-D, but they did provide information about the strong quality of these instruments. (Relevant measurement concepts for understanding instrument quality are discussed in the next chapter.)

h. No, the report did not mention the readability level of self-report instruments.

i. No, time required to complete the self-report instruments was not mentioned.

j. No, observational data (e.g., actual exercise behavior) were not gathered.

k. Several outcome variables were biophysiologic measures, including weight, waist circumference, insulin resistance (IR), glucose tolerance, cholesterol levels, and triglycerides.

l. Yes, the report provided an adequate amount of information regarding how the biophysiologic measurements were made and standardized. For example, the article noted that "After an 8-hour fast, participants had fasting insulin and glucose levels drawn, ingested a standard glucose load (75 g), and had insulin and glucose drawn at 120 minutes." The method of assessment was also described, together with a rationale.

m. The article stated that trained research assistants collected the data, except for the clinical outcomes that were collected by "experienced laboratory personnel." The specific qualifications and the training of the research assistants were not described, but page constraints undoubtedly affected the level of detail that was possible.

■ Chapter 14

EXERCISE C: QUESTIONS OF FACT (APPENDIX A)

a. Psychometric information about all of the instruments used to measure characteristics of both children and their parents who participated in the study was conveniently summarized in Table 1 of the article.

b. Internal consistency reliability, as assessed primarily by Cronbach's alpha, was reported in Table 1 for most of the scales used in this study, based on information from earlier research. There was, however, no information about internal consistency for the Short Acculturation Scale. Also, the Table indicates that Cronbach's alpha reliability was assessed for the Framingham Safety Survey, but the value was not reported.

c. Three subscales of the Family Assessment Device had alphas of less than .70: Affective responsiveness (.69), Affective involvement (.64), and Behavior control (.52). Also, for the scale Media Quotient, three subscales had alphas less than .70: Media effects (.63), Media knowledge (.25), and Alternative activities (.66).

d. Test–retest reliability coefficients were reported for several scales, including the Schoolager's Coping Strategies Inventory (interval not specified), the Media Quotient (interval not specified), Health Self-Determinism Index-Children (2-week interval), and the Injury Behavior Checklist (1-month interval). The article also cited "moderate stability" for the Child's Health Self-Concept Scale, but a precise reliability coefficient was not stated, nor was the interval between testings indicated. For every scale and subscale for which test–retest reliability was reported, the values exceeded .70.

e. Validity information:
   • Self-Perception Profile: No information about validity of any type was reported in the article.
   • Child's Health Self-Concept Scale: Table 1 indicates that this scale had evidence of content validity, but actual CVI values were not presented. (Moreover, content validity in itself is relatively weak evidence of the scale's validity.)
   • Acculturation Scale: Construct validity information was reported. The article presented correlations between scale

scores and variables hypothesized to be correlated with acculturation, such as length of residents in the United States and age on arrival in the United States.

- Injury Behavior Checklist (IBC): Table 1 did not specify validity information for this scale. However, the text indicates that IBC scores are predictive of subsequent injuries, which could be construed as construct validity or criterion-related validity.

f. Kennedy and Chen presented reliability assessments from other researchers for most of their instruments, but there is no information in the report about the reliability of the scales in the study sample. That does not mean that the researchers did not compute reliability estimates—space constraints might have made it difficult to include comprehensive psychometric information. (One option, however, would have been to add another column to Table 1, and to present values of alpha from the study itself there.)

g. Table 1 noted that "specificity was adequate" for the Injury Behavior Checklist. It would have been useful if an actual value had been given, rather than just saying it was "adequate;" *adequacy* is open to different interpretations.

■ Chapter 15

EXERCISE C: QUESTIONS OF FACT (APPENDIX J)

a. The Nursing Teamwork Survey (NTS) was based on Eduardo Salas' theory of teamwork, called the "Big Five" framework of teamwork. Salas, who is not a nurse researcher, nevertheless participated in the development and testing of the NTS. Salas' framework was depicted in a conceptual map, Figure 1.

b. The authors acknowledged that "many survey tools have been developed to measure teamwork in general." The authors

presented a rationale for developing a new instrument specific to measuring teamwork among nurses in acute care settings.

c. The items were "generated on theoretical grounds, informed by the Salas teamwork model." In addition, qualitative data from focus group interviews with 170 nurses and nursing assistive personnel were a source of inspiration for item development.

d. A total of 74 items were originally developed and subjected to preliminary review. The scale subjected to psychometric testing comprised 45 items, and the final scale included 33 items.

e. The NTS was a summated rating scale, with five response options that indicated *frequency of occurrence* of certain phenomena. The response options were: 1 = rarely, 2 = 25% of the time, 3 = 50% of the time, 4 = 75% of the time, and 5 = always.

f. Higher scores on the scale represent a greater degree of teamwork—that is, that teamwork-related behaviors occur with greater regularity.

g. There was no information about a readability assessment. This scale was not, however, developed for a general population. The intended population for this scale is acute care nurses. All but 12.5% of the development sample had a Bachelor's degree or higher. Readability was unlikely to be an important concern.

h. The article did not state that the instrument was formally pretested, but that does not necessarily mean that pretesting did not occur—especially in light of the fact that the authors noted that there were 10 different versions of the instrument. No mention was made of cognitive questioning.

i. It appears that the researchers undertook several rounds of content validation, and that there were multiple expert panels. The panels included staff nurses, nurse managers, and experts in teamwork. Although specific information about the size of the panels and number of rounds of content validation was not provided, it appears likely that the researchers were extremely thorough in their content validation efforts. The multiple rounds led to considerable item refinements and item deletions. Information about I-CVIs was not provided, but the scale CVI was reported as 91.2. The paper did not report whether the method of calculating the CVI was the "universal agreement" or "averaging" method. We suspect, however, that the averaging method was used because if the UA method had been used, the S-CVI would be 91.1 (rather than 91.2) if 41 of 45 items were universally endorsed by the experts as relevant.

j. A total of 1,802 respondents from acute care units in a large academic healthcare center and a community hospital returned a questionnaire. After eliminating some cases due to extensive missing data and sample ineligibility, data from 1,758 people were analyzed. Respondents were RNs, LPNs, nursing assistive personnel, and unit secretaries. Sample members were predominantly female (90.8), well-educated, and had an average of nearly 10 years of experience. Most were employed more than 30 hours per week.

k. Yes, internal consistency of the scale, as revised on the basis of preliminary analyses, was assessed. The coefficient alpha for the overall scale (33 items) was .94. Alpha coefficients for the five subscales ranged from .74 (Team Leadership, a 4-item subscale) to .85 (Trust, a 7-item subscale).

l. The test–retest reliability of the scale was assessed, using a subsample of 49 nurses, who were readministered the scale 2 weeks after the initial administration. For the overall scale, the test–retest reliability coefficient was .92, with subscale reliabilities ranging from .77 to .87.

m. Yes, an EFA was undertaken with a randomly selected 50% subsample of respondents. Principal component analysis with Varimax (orthogonal) rotation was used. The EFA yielded 5 interpretable factors, which is also the number of components to Salas' framework. There was not, however, a one-to-one correspondence between the empirically derived factors and Salas' model. Yet the researchers concluded that the results suggest a "relatively strong fit." The first factor (Trust), with 7 items, had an eigenvalue of 11.85 and explained 35.9% of the variance. The second factor (Team Orientation), with 9 items, had an eigenvalue of 2.26 and explained 6.9% of the variance. Next, the factor called Backup (6 items) had an eigenvalue of 1.22 (percent of variance = 3.7%), followed by the factor called Shared Mental model, with an eigenvalue of 1.15 percent of variance = 3.5%). The factor with the lowest eigenvalue (1.04) was Team leadership (3.2% of the variance). The researchers indicated that they used a cutoff value of .40 for item loadings, and that 12 items that did not meet this criterion were dropped from the scale.

n. Yes, the article indicates that the researchers looked at the inter-item correlation matrix and identified "correlation coefficients less than .30." Presumably, those with lower coefficients were considered candidates for removal. The range of inter-item correlations was not stated.

o. Yes, a CFA was performed. The measurement model suggested by the EFA was tested with the other randomly selected half of the respondents. According to the authors, "The CFA yielded a 33-item five-factor structure that fit the data from the NTS very well··· the five-factor structure suggested by the earlier EFA was confirmed and resulted in a good model fit."

p. The authors undertook several validation activities. Concurrent validity was assessed by testing the relationship between teamwork scores and nurses' stated satisfaction with teamwork on their units. As hypothesized, the NTS had a strong correlation with satisfaction responses. Contrast validity using a known-groups approach was assessed by comparing NTS scores for nurses on inpatient teams with those of nurses on survival flight teams. Those in survival flight teams, as hypothesized, had low scores. Convergent validity was assessed by examining correlations between NTS scores and scores on another teamwork scale. The correlation of .76 provided support for convergent validity.

■ Chapter 16

EXERCISE B.1

a. Interval b. Ordinal c. Ratio d. Ratio
e. Nominal f. Ratio g. Interval h. Nominal
i. Interval j. Ratio

EXERCISE B.2

Unimodal, fairly symmetrical

EXERCISE B.3

Mean = 81.8; median = 83; mode = 84

EXERCISE B.4

a. 45 b. 3 c. 27.8% d. 2.2% e. 66.7%

EXERCISE B.7

Absolute Risk, exposed group (AR_E) = .60; Absolute Risk, nonexposed group (AR_{NE}) = .90; Absolute Risk Reduction (ARR) = .30; Relative Risk (RR) = .667; Relative Risk Reduction (RRR) = .333; Odds Ratio (OR) = .167; Number Needed to Treat (NNT) = 3.33

EXERCISE C.1: QUESTIONS OF FACT (APPENDIX F)

a. Yes, Jurgens and colleagues presented descriptive statistics about the demographic and clinical characteristics of their study participants in Table 2. The text

briefly commented on a few characteristics (e.g., "Functional capacity was low, with 82% of the participants classified as class 3 or 4 . . .").

b. Referring to Table 2:
   • Nominal-level: Gender, race/ethnicity, marital status, and presence versus absence of comorbid conditions (coronary artery disease, hypertension, diabetes)
   • Ordinal-level: As operationalized in this paper, education, household income, Charlson comorbidity category, and functional performance class were measured on an ordinal scale.
   • Interval-level: None
   • Ratio-level: None. Household income *could* have been measured on a ratio scale, but ordinal scales such as the one used are often preferable in encouraging people to answer.
   • The typical study participant was a white (non-Hispanic) married male with at least 12 years of education.
   • 44.2% of the sample had a household income less than $25,000 in the prior year.

c. Referring to Table 3:
   • This table presented percentages and medians
   • Presumably, the researchers used the median rather than the mean because the distribution was severely skewed.
   • The symptom that was experienced by the most study participants was dyspnea (88%).
   • The symptom that had the longest duration was weight gain (9 days).

d. Referring to Table 4:
   • This table presented means and standard deviations for six variables.
   • All the variables were measured on the interval scale; the scale are all composite measures of self-report items on the participants' physical, cognitive, and emotional response to symptoms.
   • The mean score of participants on the scale measuring seriousness of symptoms was 2.92.

EXERCISE C.2: QUESTIONS OF FACT (APPENDIX H)

a. Yes, McGillion and his colleagues presented descriptive statistics about the baseline characteristics of their sample members. Table 1 presented the sample's demographic characteristics, separately for participants in the treatment and control groups. Table 2 presented descriptive information on selected clinical characteristics at baseline for the two groups. The text highlighted key characteristics. For example, the text stated that "The majority of the sample was male, married or cohabitating, and Caucasian."

b. Referring to Tables 1 and 2:
- Nominal-level: Most characteristics were nominal-level. Examples include marital status, gender, employment status, race, presence vs. absence of various comorbid conditions, and use vs. nonuse of various medications.
- Ordinal-level: Canadian Cardiovascular Society Functional Class (three ordinal classes)
- Interval-level: None
- Ratio-level: Age; number of years living with angina, and number of revascularizations.

c. Referring to Tables 1 and 2:
- The descriptive statistical indexes presented in this table include percentages, means, and standard deviations.
- The mean age of subjects in the treatment group was 67 years.
- Seven subjects (11%) in the control group had thyroid problems as a comorbidity.
- There was more variability in the control group than in the treatment group with regard to length of time they had lived with angina ($SD = 8$ vs. 6).
- The two groups were most different in terms of incidence of diabetes: 27% of those in the treatment group, compared to 14% of those in the control group, had this comorbid condition.

■ Chapter 17

EXERCISE B.3

a. Chi-square test   b. *t*-test for independent groups   c. Pearson's *r*   d. ANOVA

EXERCISE B.4

a. 893   b. $-.134$ c. Yes, it is significant at $p < .001$; in SPSS, any probability value less than .001 (e.g., .0003 or .00009) is shown as .000.   d. $p < .001$ e. Number of doctor visits, SF-12 (physical health)   f. The correlation between the two scales (.168) is small. It indicates that there is a modest tendency for people who are in better physical health to be in better mental health. The modest correlation is highly significant because of the large sample size.

EXERCISE B.6

a. 344 in total, 172 per group   b. 194

EXERCISE C.1: QUESTIONS OF FACT (APPENDIX D)

a. In Table 2, the researchers reported the results of *t*-tests and Fisher's exact tests. In this study, which had a small sample size ($N = 58$), Fisher's exact tests were used in lieu of chi-square tests because some of the cell sizes would have had small numbers.

b. The independent variable in the analyses presented in Table 2 was group (treatment versus control). The dependent variables were the various subject characteristics such as age, gender, and so on.

c. The purpose of the tests presented in Table 2 was to assess the baseline comparability of the two groups—that is, to assess possible selection biases.

d. • Age: The null hypothesis is that the two groups were comparable with respect to age; *t*-test; the null hypothesis was retained, *p* = .1415
   • Race: The null hypothesis is that the racial composition was comparable in the two groups; Fisher's exact test; the null hypothesis was rejected, *p* = .0116
   • BMI: The null hypothesis is that the two groups had comparable BMIs; *t*-test; the null hypothesis was retained, *p* = .2262
   • Physical activity: The null hypothesis is that the two groups had comparable levels of baseline activity at baseline; *t*-test; the null hypothesis was retained, *p* = .7747

e. The mean age of participants in the treatment group (*M* = 48.2) was not significantly different from the mean age of those in the control group (*p* = 14).

f. The percentage of participants with incomes less than $20,000 was 9.1% in the treatment group and 90.9% in the control group. This difference was statistically significant at *p* = .0176.

g. Overall, two tests that compared group differences in baseline characteristics were significant—the tests for race and income.

h. The report stated that the researchers did a power analysis to arrive at an estimate of how many subjects would be needed in a full study, although details of the power analysis were not provided. The researchers then opted, because this was just a pilot study, to recruit a sample of 20% of what would be needed.

EXERCISE C.2: QUESTIONS OF FACT (APPENDIX H)

a. • Group differences for two of the characteristics (age and years of living with angina) would presumably have been tested using a *t*-test. Although Table 2 presents information about mean number of revascularizations, the very limited

variability (*SD* = 1) suggests that a *t*-test was probably not appropriate—perhaps a Mann-Whitney *U* test was used. Group differences for all other characteristics were probably tested using chi-square tests.
   • No, probability levels for these tests were not shown in the tables.
   • The article stated that all tests comparing the groups on baseline characteristics were nonsignificant. In other words, there was no evidence of selection bias, and randomization apparently did a good job in equalizing the two groups prior to any intervention.

b. Results from analyses of variance (*F*-tests) are presented in Tables 3 and 4. The researchers could also have used *t*-tests, given that there are only two groups, but *F* and *t* are mathematically related, and *F*-tests can always be used to compare means, but *t*-tests can only be used when there are only two groups.

c. In Tables 3 and 4, the independent variable was treatment group status. The dependent variables were change scores on the various outcomes—that is, the difference between a person's score at time 2 compared to time 1 (baseline).

d. Yes, the article stated that a power analysis was done, and that a moderate effect size was assumed. The researchers also took clinical significance, and not just statistical significance, into consideration in their power analysis. Their analysis indicated a need of 52 subjects per group, for alpha = .05 and power = .80. They recruited a larger number to allow for losses to follow-up.

■ Chapter 18

EXERCISE B.2

a. Logistic regression (or discriminant analysis)   b. ANCOVA   c. MANOVA   d. Multiple regression   e. Mixed design RM-ANOVA

EXERCISE C.1: QUESTIONS OF FACT (APPENDICES A, D, AND H)

a. The Kennedy and Chen study in Appendix A used stepwise multiple regression to examine factors that could predict the children's risk-taking and safety behaviors. The dependent variables were scores on scales of safety and risk-taking behavior 6 months after baseline. Baseline characteristics were the predictors. Table 3 lists only the predictors that were "stepped" into the equation and were significant. The significant predictors included problem solving (coping), affective involvement, media use, and television viewing time for predicting safety behaviors. The significant predictors of risk-taking scores were race, gender, affective response, and media consistency.

b. The McGillion and colleagues' article (Appendix H) stated that an ANCOVA was used, but ANCOVA results were not presented in tables. The researchers opted to use change scores as the outcome variables in their primary analyses, but did a sensitivity test by using ANCOVA to test whether the results would be different. In the ANCOVA, baseline outcome variables would have been the covariates, and group status (treatment versus control) was the independent variable.

c. MANOVA was used in the McGillion and colleagues' study (Appendix H). The studies in Appendices A and D used mixed modeling analyses, which were not described in the textbook.

d. None of the studies reported confidence intervals.

e. Yes, the Whittemore and colleague's study in Appendix D presented effect size estimates for the effect of the intervention on various outcomes in Table 4.

EXERCISE C.2: QUESTIONS OF FACT (APPENDIX F)

a. Jurgens and colleagues used hierarchical regression to enter variables into the multiple regression equation.

b. The researchers entered predictors in three steps. Age and gender were entered in the first step. Next, symptom distress was added. Finally, in the third step anxiety and perceived seriousness were added.

c. Referring to Table 5:
   • The dependent variable in the multiple regression analysis was duration of dyspnea.
   • Three predictors were significantly associated with the duration of dyspnea: gender, symptom distress, and anxiety. Age narrowly missed being significant ($p = .053$).
   • While controlling other predictors, symptom distress was most strongly predictive of the dyspnea duration ($p = .003$).
   • The value of R^2 was .29.
   • The table does not provide all elements of the regression equation for predicting new values of the dependent variable from raw scores—the value of the constant (a) is not shown. However, the full standardized equation is shown via the beta weights, because in a standardized equation the constant is zero.
   • The overall regression equation most likely is statistically significant, given that three predictors were significant. However, neither the table nor the text stated the value and significance of the overall F test.

d. Yes, the authors did assess the risk of multicollinearity for their regression analysis. They concluded that although intercorrelations among some of the predictors were fairly high (e.g., $r = .635$ between anxiety and perceived seriousness), tolerance limits were not problematic. The lowest tolerance was .527.

■ Chapter 19

EXERCISE C.1: QUESTIONS OF FACT (APPENDIX A)

a. There was no explicit information about how any missing data were handled, but the article did note that there was no subject loss (attrition) in this study. It is possible that there *were* no missing data.

b. The report did not state that tests were performed to assess the degree to which the data met assumptions for parametric tests. Given journal space constraints, this is not unusual and does not mean that the researchers failed to make such assessments.

c. The researchers stated that they compared subjects in the experimental and control groups in terms of baseline characteristics, primarily using *t* tests. Specific results of these analyses are not shown, but the article stated that "the groups were balanced in distribution by gender and ethnicity." It also stated the following: "Mean scores for the major child model variables did not differ significantly between the children in the two groups at baseline." Thus, there does not seem to have been any selection bias threats in this study.

d. There was no attrition in this study, so there was no need for an analysis of attrition bias.

e. The article did not explicitly state that the analysis was by intention-to-treat (ITT), but ITT analysis was in fact made possible because there was no loss of subjects over the 6-month study period.

f. No, the Discussion section did not discuss any methodological issues, nor did it comment on the quality of the evidence that the study provided.

g. Yes, in discussing and interpreting the findings, the researchers did link the study findings to other research.

h. The authors noted some possible limitations of the intervention, but not of the study design or methods. For example, they speculated that a reason for the absence of intervention effects on risk-taking behavior might be that the intervention "did not attend to the social identity and perceptions of other peers in the group." They also considered the possibility that with a sample of relatively low risk-takers, floor effects suppressed any benefits of the intervention.

EXERCISE C.2: QUESTIONS OF FACT (APPENDIX D)

a. The report stated that "mean substitution was employed for missing data of individual items on instruments (up to 15%). If more than 15% of items were missing (rare), the subscale or scale was coded as missing data." The researchers did not state how many scale scores were coded as missing.

b. The report did not specifically mention transformations. However, a note at the bottom of 2, 3, and 4 indicated that certain variables had been log transformed, presumably because the data were severely skewed. The transformation would have made the distribution more normal, which is an assumption underlying many parametric statistical tests.

c. Figure 1 shows that 58 people were randomized to the treatment or control group, but only 51 people completed the 6-month follow-up assessment, a rate of attrition of 12%. Six people in the treatment group withdrew from the treatment itself, and another person withdrew from the study. The researchers did do an analysis of attrition bias. Those who did not complete the study, compared to those who did, were significantly younger, had higher BMIs, and lower LDL.

d. The report stated that the effects of the intervention "was tested using an intent-to-treat repeated–measures mixed modeling procedure." Mixed modeling analyses do account for missing data within a repeated measures framework, so the authors' claim for having used intention-to-treat appears justified.

e. Yes, the discussion section considered findings within the context of results from earlier research. For example, in discussing the trend among those in the treatment group toward improvements in exercise behavior, they cited prior research that has found that increasing exercise has been the primary behavior associated with reduced risk of type 2 diabetes.

f. The purpose of a pilot study is to gain insights that can be applied to a larger endeavor and, commendably, the Discussion section of this paper did describe some "lessons learned" about how to improve the intervention. For example, the researchers noted the need to increase the intensity of the intervention and to encourage family participation at sessions.

■ Chapter 20

EXERCISE B.1

a. Grounded theory   b. Ethnography
c. Discourse analysis   d. Phenomenology

EXERCISE C.1: QUESTIONS OF FACT (APPENDIX E)

a. Beck's study was phenomenological. It did not have an ideological perspective.
b. This article noted that the method used includes elements of both descriptive and interpretive phenomenology, but the primary focus was descriptive.
c. The central phenomenon under study was mothers' experiences of caring for a child with an obstetric brachial plexus injury (OBPI).
d. No, this study was not longitudinal. Data were collected at a single point in time.
e. Beck noted that her inquiry was guided by the work of the phenomenologist Colaizzi. The article stated that bracketing itself was not used, but that Colaaizi urged phenomenologists to start their research by "investigating their own presuppositions about the investigated phenomenon to identify their beliefs, attitudes, and hypotheses regarding the phenomenon. It is personal, phenomenological reflection." Later in the article, Beck stated that she had kept a reflective journal throughout the inquiry.

f. Yes, the research question is completely congruent with a qualitative approach—specifically with phenomenological methods.

EXERCISE C.2: QUESTIONS OF FACT (APPENDIX G)

a. Rasmussen and colleagues' research was a grounded theory study.
b. The researchers cited Charmaz in the section on sampling procedures, but they cited two of Glaser's writings in the section on data analysis, so it is probably safe to conclude that the study was primarily Glaserian. However, a bit more elaboration would have been helpful.
c. The central phenomenon studied in this inquiry was the self-management of young women with type 1 diabetes during turning points and transitions in their lives.
d. No, the study was not longitudinal. Rasmussen and her colleagues did not follow the young women through periods of transition to observe how these transitions were negotiated and processed. Rather, the young women were asked to give retrospective accounts of their experiences.
e. This study was conducted in Victoria, Australia. Women were recruited through an advertisement in Diabetes Australia and on a support group website. The report did not state where data were collected, however. It seems likely that the interviews were conducted in the young women's homes, but it is possible they were conducted elsewhere, such as in a healthcare facility or at the researchers' university offices.
f. Yes, in the data analysis subsection, the researchers stated that "Constant comparative analysis method was used throughout the study." No further elaboration was provided.
g. Yes, Rasmussen and colleagues identified the basic social problem as *being in the grip of blood glucose levels.* The basic social process was called "creating stability."

h. Rasmussen and colleagues used a well-suited methodological approach, grounded theory, to get a rich, holistic understanding of the problems that young women with type 1 diabetes faced during life transitions and the processes used to successfully manage those transitions. Given the researchers' aims, no other qualitative approach would have been as suitable. Other qualitative traditions would not have discovered the major concern of "being in the grip" of blood glucose levels, nor the basic social process (creating stability) that described the young women's manner of addressing it.

i. The methods used in this study were congruent with a grounded theory approach. The researchers conducted lengthy conversational interviews with 20 young women, supplemented by conversations with relatives and health professionals. During the interviews, the researchers made observations of the women and recorded "nonverbal communication." They also analyzed relevant documents and newspapers—although details about these data sources were not provided.

j. No, this study did not have an ideological perspective. Even though all of the study participants were female, gender was not a key construct in helping the researchers interpret the data.

■ Chapter 21

EXERCISE C.1: QUESTIONS OF FACT (APPENDIX B)

a. Specific eligibility criteria were not stated in this report. All of the study participants were nurses who worked "in a level IV NICU in a freestanding children's hospital in the Northeastern United States."

b. The article stated that study information was provided to the nurses through staff meetings, the hospital's intranet, and individual encounters in the NICU. The article did not discuss specific recruitment procedures.

c. The article implies that maximum variation was used in sampling nurses: informants "were selected for maximal variety of infant feeding and NICU experiences." There is a further statement that nurses were "purposively selected to provide a wide-angle view of breastfeeding promotion."

d. The sample included 114 nurses who were general informants, out of 250 nurses employed in the NICU. For this general sample, 18 key informants were chosen who were followed more intensively and interviewed in-depth.

e. The article did not mention data saturation.

f. The article described background characteristics of the nurses in the sample. For example, of the 114 general informants, 96 were white and all but one were female. Among the 18 key informants, the mean age was 33, with a range between 22 and 51 years of age. There was also diversity in terms of education (from diploma to a master's degree) and level of expertise, from novice to clinical expert.

EXERCISE C.2: QUESTIONS OF FACT (APPENDIX G)

a. Specific eligibility criteria were not stated in this report. We can infer, however, that to be eligible, prospective participants had to be (a) female; (b) have a diagnosis of type 1 diabetes; (c) be an adult, for example, over 18 years of age; and (d) be able to speak and understand English. The title of the article indicates that the focus was on "young women," but the article did not stipulate an upper age limit for eligibility—only that the oldest person was 36 years old.

b. Participants were recruited through advertisements in a diabetes-focused newsletter (Diabetes Australia) and through announcements on the websites of local diabetes support groups.

c. The article stated that "both purposeful and theoretical sampling procedures were used." As described, however, the primary sampling approach appears to be sampling by convenience. Participants were women who volunteered in response to the recruitment advertisements. It does not appear that the researchers purposively selected particular types of young women, nor sought to maximize variation, select typical cases, and so on. In other words, the only "purposive" aspect of the sampling plan, it appears, is that the researchers deliberately selected young women with diabetes—but their participants were a convenience sample of those who met these criteria. Later in the study, however, the researchers expanded their sample to address theoretical concerns. For example, their theoretical needs led them to interview young women who had given birth, and they also interviewed family members of young women with diabetes and health professionals who worked with diabetes patients.

d. The main sample consisted of 20 women with type 1 diabetes.

e. The report did not mention saturation. (This does not mean that it did not occur.)

f. There is no mention of sampling confirming or disconfirming cases.

g. Characteristics of the 20 women were briefly described. The young women were, on average, 28 years old and had lived with diabetes for an average of 17 years. More than half the women had no family history of type 1 diabetes, but one-fourth had immediate family members with diabetes. It appears that all participants were white women of European descent. The marital status, educational background, and employment status of the women were not described. Even though the researchers stated that they had theoretically sampled women who had given birth, no information about childbearing histories of the 20 women was provided.

■ Chapter 22

EXERCISE C.1: QUESTIONS OF FACT (APPENDIX B)

a. Yes, the study involved in-depth unstructured interviews with the 18 key informants in this study, who were nurses working in the NICU. In addition to formal interviews, the key informants were informally interviewed several times over the course of the study.

b. The article did not describe the interviews in detail. The formal interviews involved "open-ended questions," which presumably means that a semi-structured format was used—that is, the interviewer asked a set of predetermined questions. It seems likely that for the informal interviews, an unstructured format was used—that is, questioning was probably more ad hoc, and was triggered by an event or activity that the researcher had observed.

c. No, examples of the questions asked in the interviews were not provided.

d. The article stated that the formal interviews lasted 1 hour.

e. The interviews were tape-recorded and subsequently transcribed verbatim.

f. Yes, participant observation was an important source of data in this study. There were a total of 128 observation sessions that lasted between 1 and 2 hours. The observations focused on "the nurses' behaviors during interactions with babies, families, nurses, and other healthcare professionals throughout everyday NICU activities." Examples included infant feedings, shift reports, and nurse-led breastfeeding support groups.

g. The article stated that "all observational and informal interview data were documented immediately after each session," presumably onto a computer file or in a handwritten set of notes.

h. The researcher gathered additional data through documents, such as breastfeeding standards of care, teaching plans, and written policies and procedures.

i. Cricco-Lizza herself collected the study data. The article stated that "the investigator introduced herself as a nurse researcher" and that her role "evolved from observation to informal interviews over time."

EXERCISE C.2: QUESTIONS OF FACT (APPENDIX E)

a. Yes, Beck collected all of her data via self-report. The phenomenon captured was the mothers' experiences of raising a child with an obstetric brachial plexus injury (OBPI).
b. Data were collected by personal interview (12 mothers) or by Internet interview (11 mothers) by means of a totally unstructured interview format.
c. Yes, the overarching question was stated as follows: "Please describe for me in as much detail as you can your experiences caring for your child with a BPI. Include all of your thoughts and feelings that you wish to share about these experiences."
d. No, there was no information about how long the in-person interviews took.
e. Responses to the Internet interviews were sent in an email to Beck by attachment. The in-person interviews were tape-recorded and then transcribed.
f. No, this study did not collect any observational data.
g. Not applicable.
h. Beck collected the data for this study.

■ Chapter 23

EXERCISE B.3

a. A grounded theory analysis would not yield themes—a phenomenological study involves a thematic analysis.
b. Texts from poetry are used by interpretive phenomenologists, not by ethnographers (unless the poetry is a product of the culture under study, which it is not in this case).

c. Phenomenological studies do not focus on domains, ethnographies do.
d. Grounded theory studies do not yield taxonomies, ethnographies do.
e. A paradigm case is a strategy in a hermeneutic analysis, not in an ethnographic one.

EXERCISE C.1: QUESTIONS OF FACT (APPENDIX E)

a. The report did not specifically mention that Beck used computer software to organize and manage her data. However, Beck (co-author of this book) does not use computer software in her analyses, but rather uses a file card system. She put each significant statement on a file card and then sorted the file cards into the themes.
b. Beck did not mention calculating any quasi-statistics, and did not do so.
c. Beck reported that she used Colaizzi's phenomenologic approach.
d. The report stated that Beck maintained a reflective journal and in-depth field notes.
e. Beck discussed the analytic process in terms of the steps outlined by Colaizzi, and she presented a figure depicting those steps. Colaizzi's process involves identifying *significant statements,* which are the units of analysis. Classification involved organizing the formulated meanings of the significant statements into clusters of themes.
f. Beck's analysis revealed six themes: In an instant: Dreams shattered; The arm: No escaping the reality; Tormented: Agonizing worries and questions; Therapy and surgeries: Consuming mothers' lives; Anger: Simmering pot inside; and So much to bear: Enduring heartbreak.
g. Yes, Beck provided rich supportive evidence for her themes, in the form of direct quotes from the women's narratives. The report also provided a timeline (Table 2) that provided a typical day in the life of one mother caring for a child with an obstetric brachial plexus injury.

EXERCISE C.2: QUESTIONS OF FACT (APPENDIX G)

a. Yes, the formal interviews with 20 young women were audiotaped, and then subsequently transcribed for analysis by the first author of the report (Rasmussen). The report did not indicate how many pages of transcription resulted, but it did say that interviews were between 30 and 140 minutes long. This likely resulted in a total of several hundred pages in the dataset that had to be read and re-read, coded, and analyzed.

b. Yes, the report indicated that "constant comparative analysis was used throughout the study."

c. The report provided no information about whether manual methods were used to organize and index the data, or whether computer software was used.

d. Rasmussen and her colleagues did not use quasi-statistics, but it is important to note that they did engage in (as do most qualitative researchers) a kind of qualitative "accounting." Here are two examples: "*All of the women* described personal interactions and social support as important factors that influenced how they stabilized their lives with diabetes" and "*Some of the women* explained how, when they were young, they met other children at diabetes camps, which they felt contributed to their having a sense of belonging."

e. The report did not explicitly state which grounded theory analytic method was adopted, but it did cite two of Glaser's writings (and none of Strauss and Corbin's writings) in the data analysis section, and so we assume they used a Glaserian approach.

f. Yes, the report indicated that Rasmussen (the first author) wrote memos throughout the study "to guide her in identifying links between categories, compare and identify differences in the data, develop new questions, and test assumptions."

g. The authors did not, unfortunately, say very much about the coding process. They

indicated that they began with open coding as they read the data line by line.

h. They noted that "Theoretical coding was applied simultaneously and involved connecting the developing categories through open coding with emerging relationships between categories and their properties." The authors did not, however, provide any specific examples of their theoretical codes.

i. The report indicated that the analysis revealed a basic social process that encompassed three subcategories: (a) the impact of being susceptible to fluctuating BGLs, (b) the responses of other people to the women's diabetes, and (c) the impact of the women's diabetes on other people's lives. Each of these subcategories had further subcategories. For example, *Impact of being susceptible to fluctuating BGLs* itself had three subcategories: Fearing complications, Fluctuating BGLs and entering the workforce, and Fluctuating BGLs during pregnancy and in transition to motherhood.

j. In this study, the core category was the basic social process, being in the grip of blood glucose levels. The core category "accounted for the greatest variation in the data, was related to all of the other categories in the data, and accurately described the problem the women experienced during transitional periods."

k. This report did not include a figure depicting the grounded theory and relationships among the categories.

■ Chapter 24

EXERCISE C.1: QUESTIONS OF FACT (APPENDIX E)

a. Yes, Beck had a subsection of the Methods section that was explicitly labeled "Quality Enhancement Strategies."

b. It could be said that Beck used method triangulation or data source triangulation.

She collected data from mothers over both the Internet and in person; therefore, she was able to "validate" what she learned from one source with data from a different source. Even though the question she asked in the two modalities was the same, by gathering self-report data in two different formats, she was able to rule out any "irrelevancies" associated with a single approach. Also, Beck observed mothers during the in-person interviews and maintained field notes, which provided another source of data.

c. Methods to enhance credibility:
  - The report stated that both prolonged engagement and persistent observation were used: "For over 21/2 years, the researcher was involved in UBPN (the United Brachial Plexus Network), getting to know its board of directors and mothers and their families." Beck spent time at two of the organization's biennial camps, and both observed and interacted with members.
  - With regard to member checks, Beck stated that "Two mothers who participated in the study reviewed the findings, and both agreed that the results captured their experiences."
  - There does not appear to have been a search for disconfirming evidence in Beck's study.
  - Beck's credibility as a researcher on maternal–child dynamics is extremely high—she has a worldwide reputation on issues relating to such issues as postpartum depression and birth trauma.
  - Beck described several other steps she took to enhance the credibility of her findings, including taking comprehensive field notes and maintaining a reflexive journal. The in-person interviews were audiotaped and transcribed, and each transcript was double checked for accuracy. Beck also described in some detail how she strived "to be totally

present to the participants" as they described their experiences and attended to their gestures and nuances of speech.

d. Methods used to enhance the following aspects of the study:
  - Dependability: Beck maintained careful documentation of her decision trail, which contributed to the dependability of her study. Member checking also enhances dependability.
  - Transferability: Beck's rich description of her study sample and their experiences contributes to transferability.
  - Authenticity: Many of the steps Beck took to enhance credibility also contributed to her study's authenticity (e.g., maintaining a reflexive journal, prolonged engagement, persistent observation, and verbatim transcription of audiotaped interviews).
  - Explicitness: Beck addressed the criterion of explicitness through careful documentation of decisions, thick and vivid description of the mothers' experiences, and explicit description of her quality enhancement efforts.

EXERCISE C.2: QUESTIONS OF FACT (APPENDIX G)

a. Yes, a specific section of the report was labeled "Rigor and Credibility." It was a subsection of the "Design and Methods" section of the report.

b. The researchers used method triangulation: their main data source, formal interviews with 20 young women, was supplemented with "informal interviews, relevant documents, newspapers," and observations of behaviors during the interviews, as recorded in field notes. The report did not mention that investigator triangulation was used, but—given that there were multiple authors—some level of investigator triangulation likely occurred.

c. Strategies used that were mentioned in the report:
- Prolonged engagement: The report specifically indicated that there was "lengthy contact with the women," and noted that this was designed as a method of achieving prolonged engagement. However, it is not clear what the authors meant by "lengthy contact." Each participant was interviewed only once and the interviews only lasted 30 to 140 minutes. The fact that data were collected over a period of 1 1/2 years does not in itself speak to "prolonged engagement"—it may reflect only the pace of recruitment into the sample.
- Peer review: The report indicated that the theory was "validated by peer review throughout the research process." They cited as an example that the abstract of the study was peer reviewed for conference presentations. This does not strike us as a good manner for peers to validate the credibility of the analysis and interpretation because the reviewers would have no access to the actual data or categorization process. Perhaps other forms of peer review were undertaken, but not described, that offered further opportunities for validation.
- Member checks: Member checking was not mentioned.
- Search for disconfirming evidence: If this strategy was used, it was not explicitly mentioned.
- Researcher credibility: The credentials of the researchers were not fully spelled out—we know only that they are doctorally prepared faculty at Deakin University in Australia. In fact, they are on the nursing faculty, although this was not mentioned. There was also no mention of the personal relevance of diabetes to any of them—that is, whether they or any family member has type 1 diabetes. The report did indicate, however, that the lead author had previously undertaken research on the topic of diabetes.

d. Methods used to address quality criteria:
- Dependability: Method triangulation enhances the reliability of the data and interpretation, but it does not appear that Rasmussen and her colleagues used formal approaches to enhancing dependability, such as would be achieved with an inquiry audit.
- Confirmability: An inquiry audit is a key approach to enhancing confirmability, and these do not appear to have been used. Investigator triangulation may have been used but was not discussed. Peer review and debriefing, if done more formally than what was described in the report, would also have contributed to confirmability.
- Transferability: The report provided a good description of the young women who participated in the study, and offered many good verbatim quotes, but perhaps a bit more about the context of their lives would have been helpful—especially, about the specific kinds of transitions with which they were faced and how many of the participants faced them.
- Authenticity: The report used rich verbatim quotes (made possible because the researchers had audiotaped and transcribed the interviews), and these strategies contribute to authenticity. As noted earlier, it is difficult to assess the extent to which prolonged engagement (another strategy for enhancing authenticity) was actually achieved.
- Explicitness: This criterion is primarily about auditability, and it is difficult to assess whether the researchers took steps to carefully document decisions. The report did indicate, however, that the researcher produced memos throughout the study and these would have had information about key decisions. The researchers are to be commended for having a section of their report devoted to quality-enhancement issues, although a bit more information would have been helpful.

■ Chapter 25

EXERCISE C.2: QUESTIONS OF FACT (APPENDIX F)

a. Yes, this was a mixed methods study. The purpose of the quantitative strand was to describe the duration of heart failure symptoms and to identify factors that influenced symptom duration prior to help seeking. The purpose of the qualitative strand was to enrich the description of the patient's symptoms, their responses to the symptoms, and their help-seeking behavior.

b. The quantitative strand had priority in the study design.

c. The design was concurrent—data for both strands were collected at the same time.

d. The design used in this study could be described as an embedded design. Qualitative data were used primarily in a supportive capacity.

e. Using the Creswell-Plano design types, the study design would be QUAN(qual). The researchers used a similar notation: QUAN/qual.

f. Jurgens and colleagues used identical sampling to obtain both qualitative and quantitative data from the same study participants.

g. No, quantitative data were not qualitized, and qualitative data were not quantitized.

h. The report stated that a matrix was created in the analysis of the qualitative data, and that "the final step in the data analysis was integration of the qualitative and quantitative data." It is not clear what this means, but it could mean that a meta-matrix method was used.

■ Chapter 26

EXERCISE C.1: QUESTIONS OF FACT (APPENDIX A)

a. Yes, Kennedy and Chen's intervention involved a 4-week program and would be considered complex. There was complexity on several dimensions, including number of sessions (four), activities in the sessions (knowledge acquisition, supportive practice, problem solving), number of groups targeted (children and parents), and complexity of the outcomes (safety and risk-taking behaviors).

b. Yes, the researchers used a multidisciplinary model called Cox's Interaction Model of Client Health Behavior. The article included a figure depicting the model graphically.

c. Yes, in the literature review section, the authors cited much of their earlier research, which contributed to the development of the intervention.

d. It does not appear that there was a pilot test of this intervention. There is no information in the article about how the researchers assessed the project's feasibility.

e. This study does not appear to have had any qualitative component. The article mentioned a process evaluation, but a review of the article they cited (by Kennedy & Floriani, 2008) does not suggest that any qualitative data were collected.

EXERCISE C.2: QUESTIONS OF FACT (APPENDIX D)

a. Yes, the Lifestyle Change Program is a complex intervention that involved multiple components (education, behavioral support, motivational interviewing) and multiple sessions. The behaviors required of the interventionists and the behavioral outcomes for the participants (diet and exercise) were complex. The program was delivered over a 6-month period.

b. The report stated that the intervention protocol was "based on behavioral science theories," but the theoretical background was not elaborated.

c. The researchers for this study have undertaken extensive research on diabetes and diabetes prevention. In this particular instance, most of the development work was done by other researchers, who had launched a "large clinical trial in the United States with an ethnically diverse sample of adults." Nevertheless, in the first phase of this particular study, Whittemore and colleagues used "an interpretive and participatory method with the purpose of modifying the intervention protocol" for use by nurse practitioners in primary care.

d. The present study was a pilot study and could, in fact, be conceptualized as a "pilot" for a Phase IV (effectiveness) study within the original Medical Research Council framework (Figure 26.1 of the textbook). The efficacy of the Diabetes Prevention Program (DPP) had previously been demonstrated, and the Whittemore and colleagues' study was a pilot to assess the feasibility of translating DPP into primary care settings.

e. Yes, this study was described as a mixed methods study. The quantitative component addressed several questions relating to the reach and efficacy of the program. Qualitative data were gathered during Phase I of the project and contributed to the modification and adaptation of the DPP protocol. Qualitative data were also gathered to better understand implementation processes during the course of the project.

f. The quantitative strand had priority in this study.

g. The design is probably best described as sequential, with qualitative work having contributed to the modification of the intervention protocol that was tested primarily (but not exclusively) through quantitative methods.

h. The design could perhaps best be diagrammed as follows: qual → QUAN (qual)—that is, an embedded design following a preliminary qualitative phase.

■ Chapter 27

EXERCISE C.1: QUESTIONS OF FACT (APPENDIX K)

a. As stated in the abstract, the objective of this meta-analytic study was to "determine the effectiveness of the intervention (interventions to promote mammography screening) among asymptomatic ethnic minority women." (The purpose was stated more ambiguously in the introduction: "The objective . . . was to describe mammography intervention approaches used for ethnic minority women in the United States." We would disagree that a description of intervention approaches was the purpose of this research—one would not need to do a meta-analysis for such a purpose.)

b. Four electronic databases were searched—CINAHL, Medline, PsychoInfo, and Web of Science. There does not appear to have been a special effort to identify relevant "grey literature," but the article noted that the investigators did some hand searching.

c. Only English language studies were retrieved. The sampling criteria also excluded studies with less than 40% minority women, studies that did not use an experimental or quasi-experimental design, studies not done in the United States, and studies published before September, 2000.

d. A total of 749 citations were originally obtained, and 142 full-text articles were reviewed. Of these, 23 studies met all criteria for inclusion in the meta-analysis.

e. No, studies were included only if the intervention was designed to promote mammography screening.

f. Each primary study was given a quality assessment score. The section "Study Coding" indicated that four study elements were appraised on a dichotomous scale (quality element present or not present). The highest possible score was 4 (all quality elements present), and the lowest was 0. Quality criteria were summarized in Table 1. Studies with scores of 3 or 4 were considered to be *high quality*, and those with 1 to 2 were considered *low quality*. The Results section indicated that 14 of the 23 studies were in the low-quality category. Two coders independently coded the studies and all discrepancies were resolved. Inter-rater agreement (kappa) was adequate, .86.

g. The researchers did not state an intention to remove low-quality studies. Quality was one of several factors examined for effects on heterogeneity.

h. The standardized mean difference (d) was used as the effect size measure. Effect sizes were weighted by the inverse of the estimated study variance.

i. A fixed effects model was used, and a random effects model was used when tests for heterogeneity suggested this would be appropriate. Forest plots were not presented, but the researchers used a formal test of heterogeneity of effects involving a Q statistic that was not described in the textbook.

j. Across all 23 studies, data from a total of 22,849 women were included in the meta-analysis.

k. The pooled effect size was .078 (95% CI = .043 to .113), indicating a modest positive effect of screening promotion interventions on mammography screening in minority women.

l. Yes, the researchers did a number of subgroup analyses to assess whether effects varied in relation to characteristics of the studies or the interventions. Seven characteristics were the basis for subgroup formation: type of intervention (e.g., individual, mass media), theory-based or not, individually tailored or not, use of various cultural strategies, type of setting, targeted ethnic groups, and high versus low study quality. Thus, subgroup variation included methodologic characteristics, subject traits, and intervention attributes.

m. Regarding information in Table 1:
  • Nineteen of the 23 studies involved individually directed interventions.
  • Among the intervention types, the ones that were described as "access enhancing" had the largest effect size, d = .155. Social networking interventions actually had a negative effect size (d = −.023),

but this was not statistically significant. Of the different types of interventions, only two (access enhancing and individually directed) had *significant* effects, as shown by having the lower limit of the 95% CI be greater than .00.
  • The interventions in healthcare settings had a larger effect size than those in community settings (d = .113 versus .067, respectively).
  • Intervention effects were significantly positive only for African American women.
  • No, the quality of the study did not play a major role in the size of the intervention effect. The effect size for *high-quality* studies (d = .099) was not much greater than that for *low quality* studies (d = .061). For both subgroups, effects were statistically significant.

n. It does not appear that a meta-regression was performed.

o. Yes, the researchers described several types of sensitivity analysis. They used an approach called "leave one out," which involved re-estimating effects when influential studies (e.g., those with a large sample size or an extreme effect size) were removed. They also studied the effect of restricting the sample to ones with high- (or low-) quality ratings.

p. Yes, the authors addressed publication bias. They constructed funnel plots and also used the fail-safe N approach. The authors concluded that publication bias was unlikely to have affected their conclusions.

EXERCISE C.2: QUESTIONS OF FACT (APPENDIX L)

a. Xu stated that the purpose of his metasynthesis was to provide insight into the experiences of Asian nurses who practice nursing in Western countries. The central phenomenon was the "collectively lived experiences" of these Asian nurses, who were defined as nurses whose home countries are in Asia.

b. Xu used a wide variety of approaches in searching for and identifying relevant studies. In consultation with a health sciences librarian (an excellent strategy), he searched CINAHL, Medline, PsychINFO, Sociological Abstract, and ERIC (a database for education literature). He also explicitly searched for unpublished literature through Proquest Dissertations and Theses. Search terms included *Asian nurses, foreign nurses, foreign-born nurses, internally educated nurses, internationally recruited nurses, immigrant nurses,* and the names of specific Asian countries such as Korea and Taiwan. In addition to electronic searchers, Xu used traditional "ancestry" type searches (i.e., retrieving studies cited in other relevant studies) and he also hand-searched journals that had a history of publishing research on the topic of interest. Commendably, Xu also made efforts to interact with the original researchers when, in several instances, he had questions about whether the primary study findings were applicable equally to Asian nurses as to other foreign-born nurses. One study was omitted because he did not get a response.

c. Xu explicitly stated that type of qualitative study had no bearing on his decision to use the study in the metasynthesis. In fact, he used data from mixed methods studies, as well as data from purely qualitative studies—although his metasynthesis ignored quantitative findings because they were not relevant to his inquiry. His metasynthesis included grounded theory studies, an ethnography, phenomenological studies, and qualitative descriptive studies.

d. The final sample for the metasynthesis was 14 studies. These studies were very nicely summarized (in terms of sample size, sample, characteristics, country, research tradition, and disciplinary orientation) in Tables 1 and 2.

e. The report did not indicate whether studies were appraised for quality. It is unlikely that any studies were excluded because of poor quality. Xu provided excellent information about his sampling decisions, and it seems quite likely that had there been exclusions, he would have mentioned this.

f. The data in the primary studies were obtained through interviews, focus-group interviews, open-ended questions in written questionnaires, and (in the case of one ethnographic study) observation.

g. Xu used Noblit and Hare's approach to doing a metasynthesis. He provided an excellent description of the seven phases of the approach. Xu stated a "detailed table of metaphors, themes and concepts from the 14 studies was constructed and translated into each other" and he shared this table in the report (Table 3).

h. No, a meta-summary is a strategy developed by Sandelowski and colleagues, and Xu did not follow this approach.

i. In all of the 14 studies combined, there were a total of 587 Asian nurses who served as study participants—a substantial number for a metasynthesis.

j. Xu identified four overarching themes: Communication as a daunting challenge; Differences in nursing practice; Marginalization, discrimination, and exploitation; and Cultural differences.

k. Xu included some powerful quotes from primary studies in support of his thematic integration. Many were small snippets of quotes, but a few were more extensive—for example, the quote from the nurse who had difficulty because of her short stature.

l. Xu's paper concluded with an excellent discussion section that provided a summary and a series of implications for knowledge development and future research, for nursing practice, and for public policy.

▪ Chapter 28

EXERCISE C: QUESTIONS OF FACT (APPENDICES A–L)

a. All of the articles in Appendices A through L were published in journals that have an impact factor rating. The article by McGillion and colleagues (Appendix H) was published in the *Journal of Pain & Symptom Management*. This journal is not listed in Table 28.2 because it is not a nursing journal, even though nurses do publish in this multidisciplinary journal. It is listed in the Science edition of *Journal Citation Reports*, in two subject categories: (1) Health Care Sciences and Services, and (2) Medicine, General and Internal. The impact factor of this journal in 2009 was 2.423.

b. With the exception of one article (Cricco-Lizza's article in Appendix B, published in *MCN, American Journal of Maternal/Child Nursing*), all were published in journals with an impact factor greater than 1.00 in 2009.

c. With some minor variations (especially in the introduction and method sections), all of the articles followed a traditional IMRAD format (although "Results" were reported in a section called "Findings" in several). The article that deviated the most was the article by Yackel and colleagues (Appendix C), which is not surprising given that this paper summarized an EBP project rather than primary research.

d. The majority of articles had multiple authors, with the exception of the papers by Cricco-Lizza (Appendix B), Beck (Appendix E), and Xu (Appendix L). In none of the multiple-authored papers were the authors listed alphabetically.

e. None of the reports used first-person narratives. The authors used third-person narrative to describe their own actions ("The researcher referred to her field notes . . ."), or used the passive voice ("Ten interviews were conducted . . .").

▪ Chapter 29

EXERCISE C.1: APPENDIX M

a. No, this program announcement (PA) funded projects through the R01 and R21 mechanisms, as described in the section "Mechanisms of Support."

b. For R01 applications, this PA expired July 30, 2006 (unless it was reissued).

c. Nine other institutes within NIH, besides NINR, participated in this PA.

d. Yes, the PA specifically indicated that research on behavior-related interventions was being sought.

e. Yes, the PA specifically mentioned an interest in studies that explored "basic mechanisms of the conscious perception of pain and the affective responses to pain."

EXERCISE C.2: QUESTIONS OF FACT (APPENDIX M)

a. Total direct costs = $175,000; Total requested funds: $259,000

b. May 1, 2006 to April 30, 2008

c. Five people were listed as key personnel. The PI (McDonald) was proposed at a 20% level for 2 academic years, and at a 50% level in the summers.

d. Yes, the Specific Aims section started on page 14, and the Research Design and Methods section ended on page 28, for a total of 15 pages. (For this PA, the four major sections of the grant application were restricted to 15 pages.)

e. McDonald presented her hypothesis in the Specific Aims section, which is consistent with guidelines.

f. McDonald described her own prior research on pain communication in the "Preliminary Studies" section. She mentioned nine prior studies.

g. McDonald's "Research Design and Methods" section had the following subsections: Design, Sample, Procedure, Video Clip Experimental Manipulation, Measures, Content Analysis, Summary of the Methods, Analysis, Hypothesis, and Summary of the Analyses.

h. McDonald proposed a double blind random assignment (experimental) design.

i. McDonald proposed a total sample of 300 participants, and based this estimate on a power analysis.

j. Blinding was proposed for study participants, the graduate assistant administering the "treatment," and the people doing the content analysis of participants' responses.

k. Yes, it was proposed that participants be compensated with a $20 money order, and a publication about pain management.

l. Yes, multivariate analysis of covariance was proposed.

EXERCISE 3: APPENDIX M

a. R21, an Exploratory/Developmental Research Grant Award

b. Nursing Science: Adults and Older Adults (NSAA)

c. The score was 167, on a scale that ranged from 100 (most meritorious) to 500.

d. The study section had human subjects concerns. Two reviewers requested a data and safety monitoring plan, and another had concerns about future use of the project audiotapes.

Answers to Crossword Puzzles

```
 E V I D E N C E - B A S E D .
 M . . . . . . . . . . . E B M
 P A R A D I G M . . . N A T .
 I . E . E . . H . . . E . E .
 R . P O S I T I V I S M . R X
 I . L . C . . E . M . M . P .
 C . I . R . N C N R . T R I A L
 A . C . I . . . A . H . N . A .
 L . A P P L . Q . R . . I . N .
 . . T . T . U . C L U B S . M .
 C L I N I C . A . H . . . M . T
 . . O . O . L . Y . U . . . I .
 . . N I N R . I . . T . F . O .
 A . . . . . T R A D I T I O N .
 H I S T O R Y . . . . L . E .
 R . . . . . . . . . . I . L .
 Q . . G E N E R A L I Z . D E D
```

Chapter 1

```
 A . D . . . B . C . . . . .
 G U I D E L I N E . T R I P .
 R . F . B . M . S . . I . R .
 E . F . P . P O T E N T I A L
 E . U . L . . . . . . I . C .
 . . S Y S T E M A T I C . T .
 . . I . . M O . . O . A . I . K
 . F O R E . D . P . L . C . N
 H . N O . . E . I . . E . . O
 I . . G . S . L . C . . . . W
 E X P E R T I S E . P . . . L
 R . . R . E . . I . . P . . E
 A R R S . T . B A C K G R N D
 R . . . L . M . O . . O . . G
 C O S T B E N E F I T . B . E
 H . . C . R . T . . . . . . .
 Y . R R R . B A R R I E R S .
```

Chapter 2

Chapter 3

Chapter 5

Chapter 4

Chapter 6

Chapter 7

Chapter 9

Chapter 8

Chapter 10

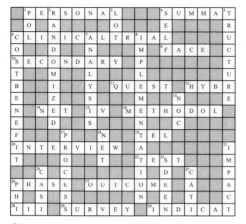

Chapter 11

Chapter 13

Chapter 12

Chapter 14

Chapter 15

Chapter 17

Chapter 16

Chapter 18

Chapter 19

Chapter 21

Chapter 20

Chapter 22

Chapter 23

```
W . . . . . M E M B E R . . A
O . T H E M E S . . A . . X
R E D . . E . M . S U B I
D O M A I N . L E V E L I . A
. P . . M T . C I R C L E
C O L A I Z Z . E A . O
. A . . R . P A T T E R N
F I T . G I O R G . H A E
A E . P . E O X . . P
M . B E N N E R O . D A T A
I M C . N T . N . R
L E O . F L O W . H A
I M M E R S I O N . I M . O D
E O B . O L I L I
S . I K T C O D I N G
V A N M A N E N R S M
A A S D A T A
S C H E M E E I
S E T . . . U T R E C H T
```

Chapter 25

```
T R I A N G U L A T I O N . . D
E N . P N . O . O
D A T A . P R A G M A T I S M . I
D E . C E L . A . N
L A G . O R Y . M T R A N S F
I R N . S A I . A E
E A . C O N V E R T O . N R
. T U O S R N . T
P R I O R I T Y . I . . E
L O R E . M I X I N G . M
U N E S . D . B B
S N . M E . D R I V E
I N S T R U M E N T . I A D
E T . P A S S D
M S E Q U E N T I A L G E
E T C A R R O W D
T H E O R E T I C A N A
A D L O M U L T I
```

Chapter 24

```
A U D I T C R E D I B I L I T Y
R N P I
T R I A N G U L A T I O N M
H I E D E P E N D
E X P L I C I T G G I
O H R A S
T R A N S F E R A B I L I T Y C
Y C T I A O
I K Y V U N
N D E C I S I O N T E T F
V A R H I
E T C O N G R U E N C E N M
S P A C E R U S N M
T L E B T R V I
I N T E R N A L A V I V I D R
G A T G C
A I N Q U I R Y O
T V O B S E R V A T N
```

Chapter 26

```
S T A K E H O L D E I Q
G W M O N E Y U
S E T T I N G B T P A
N E R E T E N T I O N
P I T F A L L S D R L F
S M E D E V E L O P M E
D S A F E E T A
E X P E R T S D N V S
S L O M T N A I
C H A L L E N G E D I S T A L B
R N I S D O E I I
I N N I N O N D L
P R E F E R E N C E S I
T D A B E L I E F T
I R E V I E W T R Y
V Y A
E F F E C T I V E N E S S M R C
P L E X
```

Chapter 27

```
F A I L   F R E Q U E N C Y
O         X     F         P
R A N D O M   T   F O R M A L
E   O   R E G R   E   E   O
S   B   T   A   S C A L E   T
T O L E R A N C E   T   I
  I   S   T   N   P
E   T   U   S U B G R O U P
N   S U M   L   R O
C H I   M O D E L   E L I
O   A   X   Y   N
D I F F E R E N C E   Q   T
E   I   Y   L   U E
  X   P U B L I C A I N
S E N S I T   D   N L S
  D I   E   E I I
    Z   T T
H E T E R O G E N E I T Y   Y
```

Chapter 29

```
O   G   S P E C I F I C
I N D I R E C T       C O
  E   A   U   S   S   N
  N   D I R E C T   T
G R A N T   Y   G   A R
  S   S   R F A
  P M   E G O V T   C
A R E A   C       T
  I N   T M
T W O S   P I L O T
R   R H   O   D   S F
A   I I   N   U   U
I   T O P I C   L L A M S
N   Y       A   M
I     O V E R H E A D
N R S A       R
G     P R I M A R Y
```

Chapter 28

```
C O N S O R T   D   P A P E R
O       T I T L E   R   E
R E V I E W   S   E   E
R     A N S F E R   S
E   A   E   E   E
S   U T H E M E S   N   D
P O S T E R   I   T   I
O   H I   N   I M P A C T
N   O R A L A   A T   O
D   R L   T   N I   R
I J N S S   I   U O
N   H   N O N   S N
G F I R S T N   C   Q
  P   A   I M R A D U
C   O B   I   E
A C K N O W L E D G P O W E R
L   S E   T   Y
L E T T E R S   P A S S I V E
```